Progress in Anterior Eye Segment
Research and Practice

Volume in Honour of
Prof. John E. Harris, Ph.D., M.D.

Documenta Ophthalmologica Proceedings Series volume 18

Editor H.E. Henkes

Dr. W. Junk bv Publishers The Hague-Boston-London 1979

Progress in Anterior Eye Segment
Research and Practice

Volume in Honour of
Prof. John E. Harris, Ph.D., M.D.

Edited by O. Hockwin & W.B. Rathbun

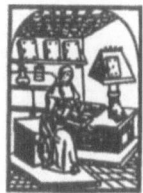

Dr. W. Junk bv Publishers The Hague-Boston-London 1979

ISBN-13:978-90-6193-158-4   e-ISBN-13:978-94-009-9609-0
DOI: 10.1007/978-94-009-9609-0

CONTENTS

FOREWORD OF THE EDITORS

On December 27, 1978, John Edward Harris, Ph.D., M.D., Professor and Head of the Department of Ophthalmology, University of Minnesota, will celebrate his 65th birthday, and will retire.

The laudations offered by his closest friends and colleagues preface the present issue, and explain why we decided on dedicating this book as a token of respect together with our heartfelt congratulations.

The Editors want to express their thanks to the invited authors for readily submitting their latest results in order to honour one of their most distinguished colleagues.

We feel sure that it is in accordance with Professor Harris' intentions to present in 'Progress in Anterior Eye Segment Research and Practice' a selection of current concepts in our field of science which will be of equal importance to ophthalmologists and research workers.

We are greatly indebted to Professor Henkes who kindly placed Volume 18 of Documenta Ophtalmologica Proceedings Series at our disposal. Dr. Junk Publishers have done their utmost to further publication and to attend to our detailed requests.

Appreciation is expressed to Mrs. Marlis Hagin and Mrs. Wiebke Naefe, Bonn, and to Mrs. Pearl Bergad, Miss Shirley Hanson, Mrs. Shirley Sethna, and Miss Patricia Williams, Minneapolis, for preparatory work on this book.

Otto Hockwin, Bonn
William B. Rathbun, Minneapolis

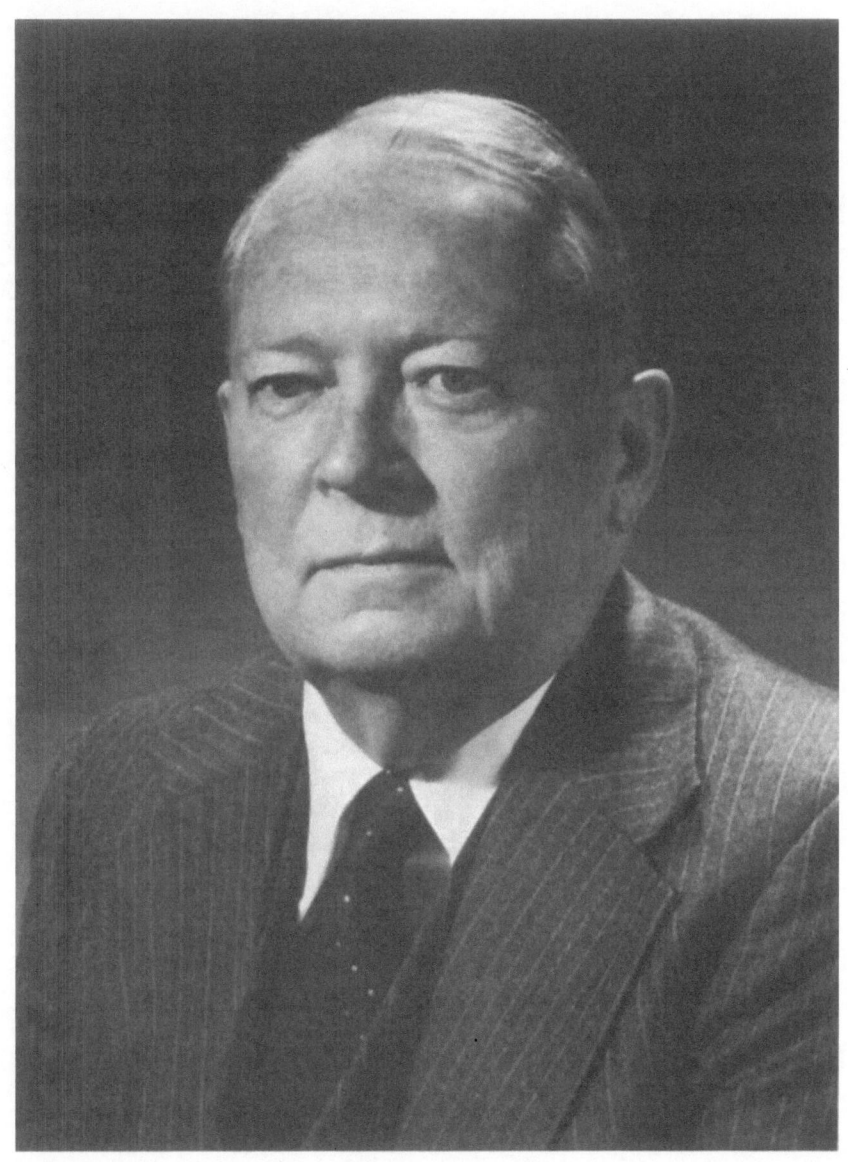

John E. Harris

Docum. Ophthal. Proc. Series, Vol. 18

JOHN E. HARRIS – I. THE SCIENTIST

John E. Harris has been a much admired colleague and friend for over thirty years. His affable manner and warm personality have endeared him to all his associates.

John Edward Harris was born December 27, 1913 in Toledo, Ohio. That year disastrous floods took the lives of more than seven hundred people when the Ohio and Indiana rivers went on a rampage. However, John and his family survived and he spent his first twenty-two years there, attending Libbey High School and the University of Toledo. He graduated in 1935 with a B.S. degree in Chemistry.

From 1936 to 1940 John attended the State University of Iowa earning a M.S. degree in 1938 and a Ph.D. in biochemistry in 1940. In 1938 he also gained a valuable and charming asset when he married Bessie Hatherly who was a graduate student at the time.

Upon receiving his Ph.D. he was given an appointment as Research Associate at the State University of Iowa for 1940-1941. At that time he became interested in problems relating to the red blood cell, a field in which he would shortly make a major scientific contribution. This was a period when it was generally thought that the high concentration of potassium and low content of sodium in red blood cells, like most other living cells that are bathed by fluids in which the relative concentrations are reversed, were maintained by impermeability of the cell membranes to these cations. This belief was seriously weakened in the early 1940's by the discovery that the red blood cell was, in fact, permeable to radioactive isotopes of sodium and potassium.

Dr. Harris was the first to demonstrate that extrusion of sodium and accumulation of potassium in red blood cells against their electro-chemical gradients depended upon active transport mechanisms or pumps which were fueled by anaerobic metabolism of the cell, thus explaining how concentration gradients could exist even though cell membranes are permeable to both ions.

The demonstration of the existence of such cation pumps had far reaching significance in physiology generally and, as Dr. Harris was soon to show, in several structures of the eye in particular.

In 1939, for his exhibit on Biochemical Aspects of Blood Preservation, he was awarded a Gold Medal by the American Medical Association.

Dr. Harris left Iowa in 1941 to accept a National Research Fellowship for a year's study with Dr. M.H. Jacobs in the Department of Physiology at the University of Pennsylvania. World War II then intervened and John spent the years 1942 to 1946 as an aviation physiologist in the U.S. Army Air Corps, attaining the rank of Major.

Along with Harris' great interest in biochemistry, he also had a lifelong desire to go to medical school. Dr. Kenneth C. Swan, a friend from the State University of Iowa, had become head of the Department of Ophthalmology at the University of Oregon Medical School. He appointed John as a Research Associate for the period 1946-1950. During this time John fulfilled his ambition of attending medical school, earning his degree in 1950. That year a report of his studies on the significance of changes in potassium and sodium in the lens was voted the best paper at the national meeting of the Association for Research in Ophthalmology.

Dr. Harris pioneered in physiologic studies involving cation transport and hydration of the ocular lens by demonstrating that excessive sodium aquired by lenses chilled to 0°C was extruded and potassium levels were restored toward normal when lenses were reheated to body temperature. This technique, now generally referred to as the temperature reversal cation shift, was employed by Harris extensively to study the metabolic requirements of the lens. His extensive investigations on the lens showed, among other things, that most of the energy needs were met normally by glycolysis, for which the substrate is almost exclusively glucose.

In 1955 Dr. Harris showed that corneas whose cation composition and water content had been altered by refrigeration were capable of reversing these changes when incubated at 37°C. He concluded that the normal dehydrated state of the cornea involved active transport mechanisms and he was the first to suggest that the endothelium played a dominant role in elimination of fluid from the cornea. His contributions in this field of research were recognized in 1957 when he was given the first Jonas S. Friedenwald Award. His acceptance lecture was appropriately entitled, 'The Physiologic Control of Corneal Hydration'. Dr. Harris' views on the importance of the endothelium in preventing corneal swelling have now been amply confirmed by others.

John Harris' research in basic ophthalmology has by no means been confined to studies on the effect of temperature on cation fluxes in ocular tissues. He has published a number of papers on aqueous humor formation. His work emphasized the importance of osmotic fluxes to the volume flow of aqueous resulting from active secretion of such ions as ascorbic acid and bicarbonate. While it now appears that neither of these substances constitute the primary moving force for bulk flow of aqueous in eyes of primates, it having since become more probable that secretion of sodium plays a dominant role, the ideas were, nevertheless, justified on the basis of information available at the time.

More recent studies by Harris and co-workers have centered around the important subject of the mechanism of cataract formation. They have studied rats in which experimental cataracts were induced by oral administration of triparanol. An important aspect of this research is that triparanol-induced cataracts are reversible, thus permitting experimental studies of the repair mechanisms. The eventual solution of the cause and possible therapy for human cataracts may well be accelerated by knowledge gained from studies of this additional model of experimental cataract formation and reversal.

John Harris has been a pioneer in bringing the basic sciences and teaching of ophthalmology together. He has been helpful in stimulating interest and providing training in basic ophthalmic research to residents and medical students.

During a period that spans more than thirty years the present writer has enjoyed many stimulating discourses on ophthalmic research with John Harris. John has the capacity to listen to another point of view and to engage in a kindly and intelligent analysis of both sides of a question. May there be many more such discussions in the years ahead.

V. Everett Kinsey, Ph.D.
Institute of Biological Sciences
Oakland University

JOHN E. HARRIS – II. THE CLINICIAN

John E. Harris was born in Toledo, Ohio on December 27, 1913 and received his early education there. In 1936 he enrolled in the Graduate School of the State University of Iowa. It was here that John Harris and William Hart, as graduate students, and Kenneth C. Swan, as a resident in Ophthalmology, worked in adjacent laboratories in an isolated corner of the University Hospital in Iowa City. A lasting friendship was established, along with an interest in ophthalmic research. Later, all three were to become Professors and Chairmen of Ophthalmology Departments in American medical schools. John Harris received his Ph.D. in Biochemistry, then carried out research at the State University of Iowa and University of Pennsylvania. This was followed by four years in the Army. In 1946 he joined the Department of Ophthalmology at the University of Oregon Medical School, where Dr. Kenneth Swan had become Chairman. Dr. Harris continued his investigative work as a Research Associate while completing requirements for the degree in medicine, which he received in 1950. Although he devoted considerable time to research, John Harris had the outstanding scholastic record of his medical school class and was elected to the honorary medical society, Alpha Omega Alpha, in his third year.

Dr. Harris served an internship at the Walter Reed Army Hospital in Washington, D.C. and then returned to the University of Oregon Medical School as an Assistant Professor (1951-1955) to continue investigative work, to teach the basic sciences related to ophthalmology, and to complete clinical training in ophthalmology. In 1952 he became the first member of the faculty of the University of Oregon Medical School to be selected as a Markle Scholar in Medicine. He was instrumental in the organization of the John E. Weeks Memorial Laboratory in Ophthalmology and advanced to the rank of Associate Professor (1955-1958). Fundamental research which he conducted in his laboratory formed the basis for the first Jonas Friedenwald Memorial Award, which Dr. Harris received in June of 1957.

In 1959 John E. Harris became the first full-time Professor and Chairman of the Department of Ophthalmology at the University of Minnesota. Under his leadership the Department of Ophthalmology has become an outstanding example of an academically oriented clinical department. Its programs of teaching, research, patient and community services are balanced and the department has actively participated in institutional affairs and contributed to the programs of the national and regional scientific societies.

Under Dr. Harris' leadership, educational programs have been established at all levels; undergraduate, graduate, and continuing education. Research laboratories with excellent facilities, equipment and staff have been developed. The clinical services of the department are diversified and combine clinical research with patient service. The department serves as a consultation center for physicians of the region. Community services include the establishment of the regional eye bank which provides donor tissue to physicians over a large area. Dr. Harris and his staff have participated in the Prevention of Blindness activities of the Minnesota Society and he is a member of the Board of the National Society for the Prevention of Blindness. At the national level, the department has been well represented, participating in the NIH sponsored study of diabetic retinopathy, and the staff have been regular contributors to scientific programs. Dr. Harris has served as Trustee and Chairman of the Association for Research in Vision and Opthalmology and has held numerous committee appointments.

In addition to developing a strong department of opthalmology, John Harris has contributed to the advancement of ophthalmology in other ways. His nearly 100 publications testify to his continued research efforts but he also has supported the cause of research by serving for two decades on various committees of the National Institutes of Health. Few individuals in any field of biomedical research have served as long or in as many capacities.

John Harris met Bessie Hatherly at the University of Toledo. They were married in 1938 and moved to the State University of Iowa where both continued their studies as graduate students; John Harris in biochemistry and Mrs. Harris in the social sciences.

Mrs. Harris has continued her interest in social problems and has been active in community service in Minnesota. In the minds of their friends, John and Bessie Harris are inseparable. Somehow, they have found a formula for integrating demanding professional responsibilities with an active family and social life with their three sons and their families.

Kenneth C. Swan, M.D.
Chairman, Department of Ophthalmology
University of Oregon Medical School

Docum. Ophthal. Proc. Series, Vol. 18

JOHN E. HARRIS – III. NATIONAL SCOPE

Dr. John E. Harris is among the very few individuals in ophthalmology who have managed to combine successfully a career in clinical medicine with one in basic research, excelling in both fields, and making valuable contributions to each. This combination of skills has made him very much in demand by those involved in national biomedical research policymaking, in particular for the past nine years, by the National Eye Institute (NEI) which has sought his advice and counsel on numerous occasions. He was a member from 1969 to 1971 of the very first National Advisory Eye Council and has just completed a second term on this distinguished body. Before NEI.s formation, the Vision Research Training Committee, the Sensory Disorders Study Section, and the National Advisory Council to the then National Institute of Neurological Diseases and Blindness (NINDB) also benefitted from Dr. Harris' participation. He also successfully chaired a committee for determining National Manpower Needs in the field of Ophthalmology. The first International Symposium was organized and hosted by Dr. Harris in Minneapolis under the sponsorship of NINDB.

Dr. Harris' great interest in diabetic retinopathy and his early advocacy of a controlled clinical trial to evaluate new treatments for this disease were reflected in his leadership as a member of the NINDB Council in initiating plans for the nationwide Diabetic Retinopathy Study which came to fruition under the sponsorship of the National Eye Institute. Dr. Harris is a principal investigator in this study at the University of Minnesota, one of the first clinical centers to join in this landmark trial of photocoagulation.

Dr. Harris has had no less of an impact on vision science as a result of his basic studies on the physiology of the eye, particularly the lens. He was the first to demonstrate active transport of cations across membranes against a concentration gradient in this tissue, a concept that is now fundamental in cell physiology. Using the technique he developed in early research on blood cells, Dr. Harris later demonstrated the role of active transport of cations in maintaining the electrolyte content, and therefore the hydration, of the cornea and lens. This work lead to his receipt in 1957 of the first Freidenwald Award, the highest research award of the then Association for Research in Ophthalmology.

Continuing to pursue his foremost research interest, Dr. Harris' recent studies of the reversible triparanol cataract implicated a disturbance in lens permeability as the cause of water accumulation and swelling of the lens which leads to this type of lens opacity. This is both a major contribution to our understanding of lens physiology and the etiology of cataract, and a further example of Dr. Harris' brilliance as an investigator.

It is a pleasure to join with all of Dr. Harris' many colleagues and friends in congratulating him on his many achievements and in expressing particular appreciation for his contributions to the programs of the NEI and the National Institutes of Health.

Carl Kupfer, M.D.
Director
National Eye Institute

Docum. Ophthal. Proc. Series, Vol. 18

JOHN E. HARRIS – IV. DEPARTMENTAL CHAIRMAN AND FRIEND

My introduction to John Harris and research was in the Weeks Laboratory at the University of Oregon Medical School in 1955. His desk was located in the laboratory and he would periodically disappear to see patients but would return, whistling, to let us know of his approach. Later he moved to an office with a view of Mt. Hood and the lab was never quite the same. His crew was an assortment of graduate and medical students, student's wives, and others. The hospitality of the Harris' was well known and enjoyed. Dr. Harris was a master at barbecuing and Mrs. Harris provided delicious accompaniments without stealing his 'show'. I early found he had an utter disregard for time. (This eventually resulted in him receiving a gift of a watch without hands). It was not unusual to work until two or three in the morning or all weekend. However, our lab was in a core of basic science labs and people were always there too. Researchers just worked all hours in those days.

When Dr. Harris told me he was going to the University of Minnesota as Head of the Department I thought, 'He won't like it; he's a scientist – not an administrator'. How wrong I was. He simply turned some of his energy towards administration and teaching without giving up his interest in research and patients. From this point on, a list of his accomplishments may sound like a history of the department, and well it might, because in my mind they are almost synonymous.

Dr. Harris was the first full time Head, in fact, the first full time faculty member in the Department of Ophthalmology. When he arrived at the University of Minnesota Hospitals, eye clinics were held only in the mornings. Three residents were based at the University and they were taught by a part-time volunteer staff. Clinic personnel included a nurse, an aide, and a volunteer secretary when clinic was in session. There was an eye pathology laboratory with a histology technician who is still in the department and a secretary.

The clinic area was small and one of his first priorities was enlarging and redesigning the space in order to eliminate examination of several patients in the same room. The clinic area has increased several – fold in the intervening years but not in proportion to the numbers of patients seen so that once again the practice of examining several patients in one room has resumed.

9

The Ophthalmology Outpatient Clinic has more patient visits than any other clinic at the University of Minnesota Hospitals. Patients frequently have long waits but their complaints are few because they appreciate the care they receive. In the interest of providing better eye care and resident training, he has added to the clinical staff and it now includes specialists in anterior segment (his chief interest), retina, pediatric ophthalmology, neuro-opthalmology, and opthalmic pathology. There are usually nine residents based at the University Hospitals. Ancillary clinic staff includes opthalmic technicians, an orthoptist, photographers, nurses, aides, and secretaries. In the fall of 1978 the clinic is scheduled to move into a new, large, well-equipped space. This will include an area designated as the Minnesota Lions Children's Eye Clinic. Under the sponsorship of the Lions the Minnesota Eye Bank was established in 1961, which allowed Dr. Harris to start a corneal transplant program. The Lions have also supported research in organ culture storage of corneas and keratoplasty is now done on a regularly scheduled basis.

When Dr. Harris arrived at the University of Minnesota he was sole lecturer to the medical students in ophthalmology. Now, students also spend time in the clinic or laboratory during their medical school career. Many have been accepted into eye residency programs. Initially the residency training was fractionated with residents being appointed and trained at several hospitals, meeting jointly only for lectures. It is now an integrated residency with 18-20 residents rotating through the affiliated hospitals. Residents who have trained under Dr. Harris number over 100. Some have taken further training and have remained in academic ophthalmology. Several now practice in Minnesota but others have moved great distances. Many people who never met John Harris are indirectly benefiting from his knowledge and dedication. He is a great example of a caring physician.

Temporary laboratory space was provided by the Departments of Physiology and Biochemistry until the ophthalmology research laboratories were completed. Present laboratory personnel include two Ph.D's., numerous technicians and varying numbers of residents and medical students. Dr. Harris has been instrumental in obtaining both federal and private funds to support research and training. He has had one or more NIH grants funded continuously since 1951. In the new Ophthalmology area, clinical faculty offices are strategically located between the laboratory and the clinic. Out of necessity Dr. Harris's own time in research diminished but he always encouraged and supported those engaged in it. However, in 1977 he took a single quarter leave and returned to the laboratory bench — this time with Professor Otto Hockwin at the Klinisches Institut für experimentelle Ophthalmologie der Universität Bonn, Bonn, Germany.

He has been active in many organizations at the University, local, state, and national level. Many of these have required travel, and on several occasions I stayed with their sons while Mrs. Harris accompanied him. There were also many Saturday nights when, after working all day, Dr. Harris would say, 'Come home and have hamburgers with us'. A close friendship with the family evolved. This contribution is a tribute to Dr. Harris but I would also like to pay tribute to his wife who encouraged and supported him in his endeavours even though his dedication to his profession often impinged on their family life. Harris was a social worker and he often used her as a sounding board when a patient's personal problems concerned him. Although none of the sons pursued medicine, all are working in service fields. All have lovely wives and children whom the Harris' enjoy.

Recreation time has been limited but perhaps his enjoyment of it has been heightened because of its rarity. He is a warm affable man who enjoys people. He can read a book, watch football on TV, and take part in a conversation simultaneously. He is an avid Minnesota Gopher Football fan. He enjoys the Harris cabin on the lake. He likes to golf and play bridge.

It has been a great honour to work for and enjoy the friendship of John Harris these many years.

Louise Gruber, M.S.
Department of Ophthalmology
University of Minnesota

JOHN E. HARRIS – V. PUBLICATIONS

DeGowin, Elmer L., Harris, John E. & Plass, E.D. Changes in human blood preserved for transfusion. *Proc. Soc. exp. Biol. Med.* 40: *126-128* (1939).

DeGowin, Elmer L., Harris, John E. & Plass, E.D. Studies on preserved human blood. I. Various factors influencing hemolysis. *J. Am. med. Ass.* 114: *850-855* (1940).

DeGowin, Elmer L., Harris, John E. & Plass, E.D. Studies on preserved human blood. II. Diffusion of potassium from the erythrocytes during storage. *J. Am. med. Ass.* 114: *855-857* (1940).

DeGowin, Elmer L., Hardin, Robert C. & Harris, John E. Studies on preserved human blood. III. Toxicity of blood with high plasma potassium transfused into human beings. *J. Am. med. Ass.* 114: *858-859* (1940).

Harris, John E. modified silver cobaltinitrite method for potassium determination. *J. biol. Chem.* 136: *619-627* (1940).

Harris, John E. The influence of the metabolism of human erythrocytes on their potassium content. *J. biol. Chem.* 141: *579-595* (1941).

DeGowin, Elmer L., Harris, John E. & Bell, Joy. Rates of hemolysis in human blood stored in dextrose solutions and in other mixtures. *Proc. Soc. exp. Biol. Med.* 49: *481-484* (1942).

DeGowin, Elmer L., Harris, John E., Bell, Joy & Hardin, Robert C. Osmotic changes in erythrocytes of human blood during storage. *Proc. Soc. exp. Biol. Med.* 49: *484-488* (1942).

Harris, John E. & Gehrsitz, Leta B.: The movement of monosaccharides into and out of the aqueous humor. *Am. J. Ophthal.* 32: *167-176* (1949).

Harris, John E. & Gehrsitz, Leta B. The aqueous: plasma steady-state ratios: their variations and significance. *Am. J. Ophthal.* 34: *113-120* (1951).

Harris, John E. & Gehrsitz, Leta B. Significance of changes in potassium and sodium content of the lens: a mechanism for lenticular intumescence. *Am. J. Ophthal.* 34: *131-138* (1951).

Harris, John E. The aqueous humor problem. *Eye Digest* 1: *17-22* (1952).

Harris, John E., Gehrsitz, Leta B. & Nordquist, Loretta. The in vitro reversal of the lenticular cation shift induced by cold or calcium deficiency. *Am. J. Ophthal.* 36: *39-49* (1953).

Harris, John E. Annual Review – Pharmacology and Toxicology. *A.M.A. Archs. Ophthal.* 50: *192-247* (1953).

Harris, John E., Hauschildt, James D. & Nordquist, Loretta T. Lens metabolism as studied with the reversible cation shift. I. The role of glucose. *Am. J. Ophthal.* 38: *141-147* (1954).

Harris, John E., Hauschildt, James D. & Nordquist, Loretta T. Lens metabolism as studied with the reversible cation shift. II. The effect of oxygen and glutamic acid. *Am J. Ophthal.* 38: *148-152* (1954).

Harris, John E. Annual Review – Pharmacology and Toxicology. *A.M.A Archs. Ophthal.* 52: *275-327* (1954).

Harris, John E. & Nordquist, Loretta T. Factors affecting the cation and water balance of the lens. *Acta XVII Conc. Ophthal.* 1: *1002-1012* (1954).

Harris, John E., Gehrsitz, Leta B. & Heinrichs, Daniel J. The effect of dibenamine and certain of its congeners on aqueous humor dynamics. *Acta XVII Conc. Ophthal.* 3: *1589-1597* (1954).

Hauschildt, James D., Harris, John E. & Nordquist, Loretta T. Changes in the phosphate fractions of the lens under various conditions which influence cation transport. *Am. J. Ophthal.* 39: *155-160* (1955).

Harris, John E., Hauschildt, James D. & Nordquist, Loretta T. Transport of glucose across the lens surfaces. *Am. J. Ophthal.* 39: *161-169* (1955).

Harris, John E. Annual Review – Pharmacology and Toxicology. *A.M.A. Archs. Ophthal.* 54: *262-299* (1955).

Harris, John E. & Nordquist, Loretta T. The hydration of the cornea: I. The transport of water from the cornea. *Am. J. Ophthal.* 42: *100-110* (1955).

Harris, John E., Gehrsitz, Leta & Gruber, Louise. The hydration of the cornea: II. The effect of the intraocular pressure. *Am. J. Ophthal.* 42: *325-329* (1956).

Harris, John E. & Gruber, Louise. The hydration of the cornea: III. The influence of the epithelium. *Am. J. Ophthal.* 42: *330-336* (1956).

Heinrichs, Daniel J. & Harris, John E. Lens metabolism with the reversible cation shift: IV. The ability of various metabolites to replace glucose. *Am. J. Ophthal.* 42: *358-362* (1956).

Heinrichs, Daniel J. & Harris, John E. Lens metabolism as studied with the reversible cation shift: III. The effect of lens age (size). *A.M.A. Archs. Ophthal.* 57: *207-213* (1957).

Harris, John E., Carlson, A. Eugene, Gruber, Louise & Hoskinson, Gertrude. The aqueous: serum sodium and potassium steady-state ratios in the rabbit, and the influence of Diamox and Dibenamine thereon. *Am. J. Ophthal.* 44: *409-418* (1957).

Harris, John E. Remarks on acceptance of Friedenwald memorial plaque. *Am. J. Ophthal.* 44: *258-260* (1957).

Harris, John E. The physiologic control of corneal hydration: the first Jonas S. Friedenwald Memorial Lecture. *Am. J. Ophthal.* 44: *262-280* (1957).

Giles, Kenneth M. & Harris, John E. Radioelectrophoretic patterns of aqueous and plasma: after intravenous injection of I^{131} – labelled insulin into rabbits. *Am. J. Ophthal.* 46: *196-203* (1958).

Harris, J.E. Active transport across the lens surface. *Acta XVIII Conc. Ophthal.* 1: *735-743* (1958).

Harris, John E., Rowell, Peter P. & Beaudreau, Olive. The adaptation of Virac, a new iodophore, to clinical use. *A.M.A. Archs. Ophthal.* 60: *206-214* (1958).

Harris, John E., Gruber, Louise & Hoskinson, Gertrude. The effect of methylene blue and certain other dyes on cation transport and hydration of the rabbit lens. *Am. J. Ophthal.* 47: *387-395* (1959).

Talman, Ellen L. & Harris, John E. Ocular changes induced by polysaccharides: II. Detection of hyaluronic acid sulfate after injection into ocular tissues. *Am. J. Ophthal.* 47: *428-436* (1959).

Giles, Kenneth M. & Harris, John E. The accumulation of C^{14} from uniformly labeled glucose by the normal and diabetic rabbit lens. *Am. J. Ophthal.* 48: *508-516* (1959).

Tanner, K.N. & Harris, John E. The effect of artificial osmotic loads on the intraocular pressure. *Am. J. Ophthal.* 48: *487-499* (1959).

Harris, John E., Gruber, Louise, Talman, Ellen, & Hoskinson, Gertrude. The influence of oxygen on the photodynamic action of methylene blue on cation transport in the rabbit lens. *Am. J. Ophthal.* 48: *528-534* (1959).

Talman, Ellen L. & Harris, John E. Ocular changes induced by polysaccharides: III. Paper chromatographic fractionation of a biologically active hyaluronic acid sulfate preparation. *Am. J. Ophthal.* 48: *560-572* (1959).

Lewis, Richard P., Talman, Ellen L. & Harris, John E. The effect of oxygen tension on glucose uptake by the isolated rabbit lens. *Am. J. Ophthal.* 50: *974-984* (1960).

Harris, John E. Transport of fluid from the cornea, in The transparency of the cornea (eds. Duke-Elder, Sir Stewart & Perkins, E.S.), Blackwell Scientific Publications, Oxford, 1960, pp. *73-86.*

Harris, John E. Factors influencing corneal hydration. *Invest. Ophthal.* 1: *151-157* (1962).

Harris, John E. & Gruber, Louise, The electrolyte and water balance of the lens. *Expl. Eye Res.* 1: *372-384* (1962).

Harris, John E. Contributions of biochemistry to clinical ophthalmology. *Am. J. Ophthal.* 57: *731-737* (1964).

Kanter, Yale C. & Harris, John E. Retinoblastoma occurring in one of a pair of identical twins. *Archs. Ophthal.* 72: *783-787* (1964).

Carter, Charles B. & Harris, John E. Use of high energy light in the treatment of ocular disease. *Med. Bull. Univ. Minn.* 35: *186-188* (1964).

Harris, John E. Cardiovascular renal agents as they impinge on ophthalmic practice. *Invest. Ophthal.* 3: *481-488* (1964).

Harris John E. Corneal wound healing, in The cornea world congress (eds. King, John Harry Jr. & McTigue, John W.) Butterworths, Washington D.C., 1965, pp. *73-79.*

Clausen, Donald, F. & Harris, John E. Experiments in intraocular hydrodynamics: I. Inflow rate − pressure relationships in the intact eyes of living and dead cats. *Expl. Eye Res.* 4: *67-70* (1965).

Harris, John E. Editor and Chairman of organizing committee, Symposium on the lens, C.V. Mosby, St. Louis, 1965.

Harris, John E. & Becker, Bernard, Cation transport of the lens. *Invest. Ophthal.* 4: *709-722* (1965).

Clausen, Donald F. & Harris, John E. Experiments in intraocular hydrodynamics: II. The effect of dichlorphenamide on dextrose − induced ocular hypertension. *Expl. Eye Res.* 4: *71-75* (1965).

Clausen, Donald F, Cockrell, Carl V. & Harris, John E. Experiments in intraocular hydrodynamics: III. Some effects of experimentally induced changes in aqueous salt concentration. *Expl. Eye Res.* 4: *76-82* (1965).

Householder, James, R., Clausen, Donald F. & Harris, John E. Experiments in intraocular hydrodynamics: IV. The IOP sensitivity of the anterior chamber appearance time of intra-arterially injected fluorescein. *Expl. Eye Res.* 4: *83-86* (1965).

McClanahan, William S., Harris, John E., Knobloch, William H., Tredici, Louis M. & Udasco, Rolando L. Ocular manifestations of chronic phenothiazine derivative administration. *Archs. Ophthal.* 75: *319-325* (1966).

Householder, James R. & Harris, John E. Anesthetic drugs in ophthalmology, in Ocular therapy: complications and management (ed. Leopold, Irving H.) C.V. Mosby, St. Louis, 1966, pp. *88-121.*

Harris, John E. The temperature-reversible cation shift of the lens. *Trans. Am. Ophthal. Soc.* 64: *675-699* (1966).

Harris, John E. Current thoughts on the maintenance of corneal hydration in vivo. *Archs. Ophthal.* 78: *126-132* (1967).

Harris, John E. Problems in drug penetration, in Ocular therapy III (ed. Leopold, Irving H.) C.V. Mosby, St. Louis, 1968, pp. *96-105.*

Harris, John E., Letson, Robert D. & Buckley, Joseph J. The use of CI-581, a new parenteral anesthetic, in ophthalmic practice. *Trans. Am. Ophthal. Soc.* 66: *206-213* (1968).

Harris, John E. & Gruber, Louise. The reversal of triparanol induced cataracts in the rat. *Doc. Ophthal.* 26: *324-333* (1969).

Harris, John E., Letson, Robert D. & Buckley, Joseph J. Sedation of children in ophthalmic office practice, in Symposium on ocular therapy, Vol. IV (ed. Leopold, Irving H.) C.V. Mosby, St. Louis, 1969, pp. *127-135.*

Harris, J.E. The natural history of diabetic retinopathy, in Modern problems in ophthalmology, Vol 9, Karger, Basel, 1971, pp. *101-103.*

Harris, John E. Management and complications of systemic corticosteroid therapy, in Symposium on ocular therapy, Vol. V (ed. Leopold, Irving H.) C.V. Mosby, St. Louis, 1972, pp. *70-76.*

Harris, John E. & Rathbun, William B. Ocular tissues, in Transplantation (eds. Najarian, John S. & Simmons, Richard L.) Lea and Febiger, Philadelphia, 1972, pp. *613-626.*

Harris, John E. & Gruber, Louise. Reversal of triparanol-induced cataracts in the rat: II. The exchange of ^{22}Na, ^{42}K, and ^{86}Rb in cataractous and clearing lenses. *Invest. Ophthal.* 11: *608-616* (1972).

Harris, John E. Prophylaxis of ophthalmia neonatorum, in Symposium on ocular therapy, Vol VI (ed. Leopold, Irving H.) C.V. Mosby, St. Louis, 1973, pp. *39-43.*

Harris, John E. & Byrnes, Patrick. Reversal of induced hydration of human corneas stored in a moist chamber at refrigeration temperatures for various periods of time, in Corneal Preservation (eds. Capella, Joseph A., Edelhauser, Henry F. & Van Horn, Diane L.), Charles C. Thomas, Springfield, 1973, pp. *81-95.*

Summerlin, William T., Miller, George E., Harris, John E. & Good, Robert A. The organ-cultured cornea: an in vitro study. *Invest. Ophthal.* 12: *176-180* (1973).

Harris, John E. & Gruber, Louise. The reversal of triparanol-induced cataracts in the rat: III. Amino acid content and uptake of ^{14}C α-AIB in cataractous and clearing lenses. *Invest. Ophthal.* 12: *385-388* (1973).

Rathbun, William B., Harris, John E., Vagstad, Gary & Gruber, Louise. The reversal of triparanol-induced cataract in the rat: IV. Reduced sulfhydryl groups in soluble protein and glutathione. *Invest. Ophthal.* 12: *388-390* (1973).

Boone, W. Benton, Doughman, Donald J. and Harris, John E. Ophthalmia neonatorum: value of prophylactic treatment. *Minn. Med.* 56: *940-943* (1973).

Doughman, Donald J., Van Horn, Diane, Harris, John E., Miller, George E., Lindstrom, Richard, Summerlin, William & Good, Robert A. Endothelium of the human organ cultured cornea: An electron microscopic study. *Trans. Am. Ophthal. Soc.* 71: *304-328* (1973).

Doughman, Donald J., Van Horn, Diane L., Harris, John E., Miller, George E., Lindstrom, Richard, & Good, Robert A. The ultrastructure of human organ – cultured cornea: I. Endothelium *Archs. Ophthal.* 92: *516-523* (1974).

Harris, John E. Use of cellulose gums in ophthalmology, in Symposium on ocular therapy, Vol. VII (ed. Leopold, Irving H.) C.V. Mosby, St. Louis, 1974, pp. *62-67.*

Mizuno, G., Ellison, E., Chipault, J.R. & Harris, J.E. Lipids of the triparanol cataract in the rat. *Ophthal. Res.* 6: *206-215* (1974).

Van Horn, Diane, Doughman, Donald J., Harris, John E., Miller, George E., Lindstrom, Richard & Good, Robert A. Ultrastructure of human organ cultured cornea: II. Stroma and epithelium. *Archs. Ophthal.* 93: *275-277* (1975).

Warshawsky, Robert S., Hill, Charlotte W., Doughman,Donald, J. & Harris, John E. Acrodermatitis enteropathica: corneal involvement with histochemical and electronmicrographic studies. *Archs. Ophthal.* 93: *194-197* (1975).

Doughman, Donald J., Harris, John E. & Schmitt, Mary Kay. Penetrating keratoplasty using 37°C organ cultured cornea. *Trans. Am. Acad. Ophthal. and Oto-lar.* 81: *778-793* (1976).

Priluck, Ira A., Doughman, Donald J. & Harris, John E. Tissue adhesives, in Symposium on ocular therapy, Vol IX (eds. Leopold, Irving H. & Burns, Robert P.) Wiley & Sons, New York, 1976, pp. *137-153.*

Lindstrom, Richard L, Doughman, Donald J., Van Horn, Diane L., Dancil, Diane & Harris, John E. A metabolic and electronmicroscopic study of human organ-cultured cornea. *Am. J. Ophthal.* 82: *72-82* (1976).

Doughman, Donald J., Miller, George E., Mindrup, Elizabeth A. & Harris, John E. The fate of experimental organ cultured corneal xenografts. *Transplantation* 22: *132-137* (1976).

Rathbun, W.B., Hough, Margiolina, Gruber, Louise & Harris, J.E. The reversal of triparanol-induced cataract in the rat. V. Activity levels of ATPase and three enzymes of glutathione metabolism. *Interdiscpl. Topics Geront.* 12: *000-000* (1978).

Bours, J., Gruber, L., Hockwin, O. & Harris, J. The crystallins of the rat lens with triparanol induced cataracts, also related to aging. *Interdiscpl. Topics Geront.* 12: *000-000* (1978).

Schlüter, G., Hockwin, O., Harris, J.E. & Gruber, L. The reversal of triparanol-induced cataract in the rat. VI. ultrastructural changes. *Doc. Ophthal. Proc. Ser.* 9: *000-000* (1978).

Doughman, Donald J., Harris, John E., Lindstrom, Richard L. & Schmitt, Mary Kay. Corneal preservation using 37°C. organ culture incubation. *Contact Intraocular lens med. J.* In Press.

Compiled by William B. Rathbun, Ph.D. & Pearl L. Bergad, M.S.

SENILE CATARACTOGENESIS AND LENS LIPID

J. STEVENS ANDREWS

(Nashville, U.S.A.)

Senile cataracts are those cataracts which develop in elderly individuals (generally over sixty years old). These cataracts have no apparent causative agent and the distribution of the opacified region is principally either cortical or nuclear.

The cortical cataract is characterized by areas of enlarged fiber cells with occasional liquid-filled areas between the cells. These discontinuities in refractive index result in light-scattering and the observed opacities. On the other hand, a nuclear cataract has been explained as the result of conversion of soluble protein to an insoluble form and/or accumulation of pigment. Both the increase in index of refraction due to protein insolubility and the accumulation of pigment are responsible for the loss in visual acuity (Maraini & Mangill, 1973).

A large number of agents and some diseases have been associated with cataract formation in humans. Application of these agents to or induction of appropriate diseases in laboratory animals has been attempted in order to develop an animal model for cataractogenesis. The goal in any model system is to be able to apply knowledge obtained from the animal model to the prevention of the ultimate clinical outcome in humans. Since it is difficult, if not impossible, to find a precise animal model for a geriatric condition such as senile cataract, the assumption is made that all forms of cortical cataractogenesis may have a common underlying mechanism. Therefore, causitive agents may be used and the general observation applied to obtain an understanding of the process. For the biochemist, the most successful and popular model system for the study of cataractogenesis is the feeding of high levels of galactose (30 to 50%) to weanling rodents. Within two weeks a cortical cataract develops due to the accumulation of dulcitol (a metabolic product of galactose) within the cortical fiber cell (Kinoshita, 1965). This cataract is an excellent model for the galactosemic infant who is unable to metabolize the galactose from ingested lactose due to a genetic defect. It is also a good model for diabetic cataract where sorbitol accumulates (Dvornik et al., 1973; Pirie, 1965). On the other hand, with one exception, (Barber, 1968)

* Preparation of this review was supported in part by PHS Grant ROI-EY01852, and an Unrestricted Grant from Research to Prevent Blindness, Inc.

an osmotic agent has not been invoked as the cause of senile cortical cataract. However, due to a generally common histological appearance for all cortical cataracts, it may be possible to glean an underlying mechanism for cortical cataractogenesis if the correct common denominator can be ascertained. Since cortical opacity depends on swelling of the lens fiber cell due to water uptake, it seems that fiber cell membrane integrity may be the common denominator (Kinostia, 165; Dvornik et al., 1973; Pirie, 1965; Barber, 1968; Sanders, et al., 1974; Machiko et al., 1975). Although membrane integrity may play a role in nuclear opacification an equally likely common denominator for this type of cataract may be the rate at which soluble fiber cell proteins become insoluble (Spector et al., 1974; Jedziniak et al., 1972).

Most cell or plasma membrane research has been conducted on erythrocytes or bacteria. Theoretical studies have been conducted with liposomes (lipid vesicles in aqueous solutions) which seem to possess some of the physical characteristics of membranes. Plasma membranes, however, are a mixture of both lipid and protein whose structure is uncertain. On the basis of both liposome and erythrocyte membrane permeability studies, it has been established that a relationship exists between the lipid composition of a membrane and its permeability to ions. The more condensed a membrane, in terms of the lipid present, the less its ion permeability (Van Deenen, et al., 1972). This property has been observed in both liposome and cell membrane studies. In the latter case, modification of the lipid composition has been accomplished by simple exchange or by the use of mutants unable to synthesize certain fatty acids which then incorporate fatty acids from the medium into their membranes. These studies have established that an increase in the cholesterol content of a membrane reduces the surface area (condensation) and confers a greater degree of ionic impermeability on the membrane (Van Deenen et al., 1972).

Every membrane appears to have incorporated in its structure some protein of low polarity which forms a complex with the membrane lipid. This complex is referred to as proteolipid and has the unusual property of being soluble in organic solvents. This protein seems to be a structural unit of cell membranes and its hydrophobic binding properties appear to contribute to membrane structural integrity.

Lens fiber cell membranes account for the bulk of the lipid present in mammalian lens. Although lipid metabolism in the lens is low, (Hammar, 1965) a number of investigators have analyzed the lipid content, (primarily phospholipid) (Feldman & Feldman, 1965; Broekhuyse & Veerkamp, 1968; Broekhuyse, 1969, Anderson et al., 1969) with the view that the results of such analyses would shed light on changes in membrane lipid composition and thus on fiber cell membrane composition. By analyzing normal human lenses from different age groups, data would be acquired on normal membrane composition as it changed with age. Comparison of the lipid composition from the cataractous lenses from comparable age groups would furnish information on changes which might be related to loss of membrane integrity. The results of such analyses have demonstrated no differences in total phospholipid between normal and cataractous lenses of the same age

20

(Broekhuyse, 1969). On the other hand, where the amount of proteolipid or the lipid complexed to proteolipid was investigated, significant differences between normal and cataractous lenses were found (Feldman & Feldman, 1965; Broekhuyse, 1969). The decrease in the amount of the proteolipid complex in cataractous lenses was interpreted as a sign of membrane disintegration.

More recently investigation of the relationship between ageing and the lipid composition of lens anatomical fractions has brought to light certain changes within the phospholipids of the fiber cell membrane. In this investigation, the lens was fractionated into epithelium, cortex and nucleus at different ages and the phospholipids analyzed. From the results it was concluded that as the lens aged the sphingomyelin content in the cortex and nucleus increased principally at the expense of phosphatidyl choline and phosphatidyl ethanolamine (Broekhuyse, 1973; Broekhuyse et al., 1974). Recently it was observed that there was an increase in ceramide (acyl sphingosine) in cataractous lenses as opposed to normal lenses of the same age (Tao & Cotlier, 1975). The relationship between sphingomyelin and phosphatidyl choline in lens fiber cells may be direct since there is evidence that the latter is a choline donor for sphingomyelin synthesis in membranes (Diringer et al., 1972).

In summary, cataractogenesis appears to be associated with a defect in a specific sphingomyelin subspecies synthesis which possibly results in membrane instability and probably with changes in ion permeability which could result in cortical fiber cell swelling and membrane breakdown.

However, this simplified view must be broadened to include two other areas. One is deficient membrane protein synthesis (Broekhuyse, 1969) and the other is cholesterol incorporation. Lens fiber cell membranes are isolated in a pure form only with difficulty (Bloemendal, et al., 1972; Broekhuyse & Kuhlman, 1974; Alcala' et al., 1975; Broekhuyse et al., 1976) and at present direct investigation of their synthesis is just beginning (Vermorken, et al., 1977). On the other hand, the primary defect leading to a breakdown in sphingomyelin synthesis could result from insufficient production of membrane protein. However, it is unlikely that much progress in this area will be made until the methodology for membrane protein isolation improves.

The other lens cell membrane constituent which needs investigation is cholesterol. Early analyses of cholesterol content in human lens were variable between laboratories, presumably due to differences in techniques and ages of the lenses (Feldman, 1967). Unfortunately, this problem persists today — perhaps for some of the same reasons. For instance, there are two major lipid-extracting solutions and two methods of subsequent purification. Both extraction methods use some combination of chloroform and methanol. The major difference arises in the purification step which can be either an aqueous wash (Folch et al., 1957; Bligh & Dyer, 1959) or a sephedex G-25 column procedure (Siakotos & Rouser, 1965). Ganglioside loss into the aqueous wash occurs and requires subsequent purification from this fraction. Gangliosides, as a class, are eluted in a separate but contaminated fraction from the column. This fraction can be assayed directly for gangliosides by thin-layer chromotography.

In the human lens lipid field, further confusion has been added by Feldman who advocated saturating the chloroform methanol (2:1) extracting mixture with water in order to break down the proteolipid complex as the solvents were removed (Feldman & Feldman, 1965). In our laboratory use of these methods, including freezing and thawing the extracts on single fresh stored or lyophylized lens yielded consistently lower amounts of lipid after sephadex purification than when the paired lens was extracted with anhydrous chloroform-methanol (2:1). These results were assayed by bulk weight of the sephadex-purified lipid fraction and by a visual examination of the same fraction after either one or two dimensional thin-layer chromotography.

Because of variations in methods of reporting lens cholesterol, it is difficult to make direct comparisons between the results obtained by different laboratories. Feldman & Feldman (1965) used both dry weight and per lens as a basis for calculating cholesterol concentration. Obara, et al. (1976) reported their results using both these methods as well as per mg of protein. The only common basis for all data in both reports is weight of cholesterol per lens. Another difference between these reports, particularly with results reported on a per lens basis, is that Feldman extracted whole lenses while Obara, et al. used decapsulated lenses. However, without histological estimation of the number of epithelial cells adhering to the stripped capsule the assumption that all epithelial cells are removed from the lens is unjustified (Vermorken et al., 1977). Estimation of the average dry weight from the data in the Obara, et al. (1976) publication vary from 52 to 60 mg per lens. Feldman reported an average dry weight of 65-66 mg per whole lens in agreement with data obtained in our laboratory. A summary of these data, together with unpublished data from our laboratory, is presented in Table 1. (The data attributed to Obara, et al. (1976) represent an average of all data appearing in Table 1 of their publication.)

Table I. Cholesterol Concentrations In Human Normal And Cataractous Lenses.

Parameter	Age-matched Normal Lenses	Cataractous Lens
Av. dry weight (mg)*	65	66
Av. nutral lipid (μg/lens)*	1690	1114
Av. dry weight (mg)**	55.8	55.1
Av. cholesterol (μg/lens)**	994	1054
Av. dry weight (mg)***	65	–
Av. cholesterol (μg/lens)***	1120	–

*   Feldman & Feldman, 1965.
**   Obara et al., 1976.
*** Andrews & Campbell, unpublished results.

The normal lens cholesterol concentration estimated by Obara and ourselves are in substantial agreement but the neutral lipid fraction reported by Feldman appears to be substantially higher. However, it was calculated by adding the unbound and proteolipid-bound neutral lipid fractions together and thus represents both cholesterol and glyceride. Since Feldman has never reported proteolipid-bound cholesterol, the glyceride correction for this fraction is unknown. Approximating the glyceride concentration from the unbound neutral lipid fraction reduces the total human lens cholesterol concentration to 1311 μg/lens. This figure is much closer to the other figures appearing in Table 1, although the grounds for such a correction are questionable. Further confusion is added to Feldman's published results by his inclusion of a normal human lens cholesterol value of 775 μg/lens in a later publication (Feldman, 1967) without specifying whether this value represented total or unbound lens cholesterol. It seems probable that this value represents unbound cholesterol since it is of the correct magnitude and a pool of 200 cataractous lenses yielded a higher figure of 966 μg/lens.

Obara, et al. (1976) state that their figures for normal human lens cholesterol concentration are in agreement with Feldman because no difference in cholesterol content were found between normal and cataractous lenses. However, as can be seen from Table 1, this does not mean that the concentration of cholesterol in the normal human lens is the same in both publications. Indeed, in the final analysis, Feldman has never published a figure specifically representing the total concentration of cholesterol in either the normal or cataractous human lens, J.F.R. Kuck, Jr. (1970) quotes Feldman as saying 0.3% of the wet weight of a normal human lens is cholesterol. For a 250 mg lens, 0.3% represents only 750 μg of cholesterol/lens. Broekhuyse (1973), on the other hand, has published a concentration figure of 1350 μg cholesterol/normal lens from individuals between 60 and 70 years of age (Broekhuyse, 1973). Thus, it appears by consensus that the amount of cholesterol present in normal human lenses 50-70 years of age is 1100 to 1350 μg.

Obara, et al. (1976) found, however, that fractionation of cataractous lens with chaotropic agents significantly increased the apparent total cholesterol content of these lenses (Obara, 1976). Subjecting normal lenses of the same age to this process resulted in a slight, but not significant, increase in the amount of cholesterol/lens over the pooled and individually extracted normal lenses. These results suggest that proteolipid breakdown in the cataractous lens is releasing more cholesterol for assay than in the normal lens. However, all attempts in our laboratory to duplicate Feldman's published results (Feldman & Feldman, 1965) have been unsuccessful. Adding water to the extracting solution reduced the total yield of extractable lipid (wt.) as well as cholesterol. Application of the sephadex-purified extract to a silicic acid column resulted in weight yields in excess of 100% due to silicate contamination of the fractions — even after extensive washing of the column. These results do not negate the presence of proteolipid but merely demonstrate that the extraction procedures are probably complete. Broekhuyse (Broekhuyse, 1969) has observed that a less polar solvent will extract more cholesterol from a cataractous lens than from an age-matched normal lens with the implication that the total amount of cholesterol present is the same in both types of lens. Thus, the observation by Obara, et al. (1976) of increased cholesterol in chaotropic agent-treated cataractous lenses remains puzzling and, as yet, unconfirmed. One possible explanation for this observation is that certain types of cataracts are more efficient at non-specifically adsorbing aqueous lipoprotein cholesterol than others. On the other hand, human aqueous cholesterol levels are lower than in either rabbit or beef aqueous (Andrews & Campbell, unpublished results). However, this observation may be due to the elapsed time after death before these eyes come to the laboratory. Still, the long term course of cataract development coupled with the continuous exposure to a significant but low level of cholesterol in the aqueous might lead to increased deposition of exogenous cholesterol in certain of these lenses.

The significance of aqueous humor lipoprotein as a source of lens cell membrane cholesterol has never been adequately investigated. The assumption that the capsule prevents the uptake of lipoprotein cholesterol presupposes that the size of the aqueous lipoproteins are the same as those in the serum. Immunological examination of the human aqueous for serum lipoprotein has demonstrated the presence of low levels of the smallest lipoprotein — the high-density serum lipoprotein (Schmut & Zirm, 1974). Preliminary investigation in our laboratory suggests the presence of two different lipoproteins in rabbit aqueous. If aqueous humor contains a unique lipoprotein then this complex may be able to penetrate the capsule and make a significant contribution to lens cell membrane cholesterol in a manner analagous to low-density serum lipoprotein (Brown & Goldstein, 1976).

Finally, there is the question of the total lipid content of human lens compared to animal lenses. Aside from Feldman's work (Feldman & Feldman, 1965), there is little information available on this question. In our laboratory we have confirmed that approximately 4% of the normal dried human lens (60 to 70 years in age) is lipid. This figure is in contrast to rabbit and beef lenses where the amount of lipid present is approximately 0.5% of the dry weight (Andrews & Campbell, unpublished results). It seems possible that this difference represents a greater number of cells in the human lens due to the substantially longer life span of *Homo sapiens*. The only supporting evidence for this hypothesis, however, is the percentage replacement of glycerophosphatides by sphingomyelin in human lens as compared to animal lens phosphatide composition (Broekhuyse, 1969). According to this hypothesis, a much higher percentage of total lens lipid weight should be present in the nucleus of the human lens than in the nucleus of animal lenses.

In summary, there appears to be little difference in total lipid composition (neutral lipid vs phospholipid) between human normal and cataractous lenses. However, when individual molecular classes are examined, e.g. ceramide and possibly cholesterol, differences between the normal and diseased state may exist. Although it may seem that the primary defect resides in the proteolipid protein because of its greater extractability in the cataractous lens, its retention by the membrane may depend on either or both hydrophyllic or hydrophobic interactions. At present, there is still the possibility that the proteolipid complex is incompletely extracted from normal lenses. Perhaps what is needed in this area of investigation is a different approach, i.e. isolation of cell membranes followed by lipid extraction of the different membrane density classes. This might allow the differentation of epithelial intracellular membranes, lens fiber cell membranes and perhaps even tight junctions. The membrane defect may be localized in this last area and the significant differences are thus 'swamped out' by a preponderance of other membraneous structures.

REFERENCES

Alcala', J., Lieska, N. & Maisel, H. Protein composition of bovine lens cortical fiber cell membranes. *Expl. Eye Res.* 21: *581-595* (1975).

Anderson, R.E., Maude, M.B. & Feldman, G.L. Lipids of ocular tissues. I. The phospholipids of mature rabbit and bovine lens. *Biochim. biophys. Acta* 187: *345-353* (1969).

Andrews, J.S. & Campbell, C. Unpublished results.

Barber, G.W. Free amino acids in senile cataractous lenses: possible osmotic etiology. *Invest. Ophthal.* 7: *564-583* (1968).

Bligh E.G. & Dyer, W.J. A rapid method of total lipid extraction and purification. *Can. J. Biochim. Physiol.* 37: *911-917* (1959).

Bloemendal, H., Zweers, A., Vermorken, F., Dunia, I. & Benedetti, E.L. The plasma membranes of eye lens fibers, Biochemical and structural characterization, *Cell Diff.* 1: *91-106* (1972).

Broekhuyse, R.M. Phospholipids in tissues of the eye. III. Composition and metabolism of phospholipids in human lens in relation to age and cataract formation. *Biochim. biophys. Acta* 187: *354-365* (1969).

Broekhuyse, R.M. Membrane lipids and proteins in ageing lens and cataract in 'The human lens in relation to cataract', *Ciba Fn. Sympo.*, Associated Scientific Publishers, Amsterdam and New York, 19: *135-149* (1973).

Broekhuyse, R.M. & Kuhlman, E.D. Lens membranes. I. Composition of urea trated plasma membranes from calf lens. *Expl. Eye Res.* 19: *297-302* (1974).

Broekhuyse, R.M., Kuhlman, E.D. & Stols, A.L.H. Lens Membranes II. Isolation and characterization of the main intrinsic polypeptide (MIP) of bovine lens fibre membranes. *Expl. Eye Res.*, 23: *365-371* (1976).

Broekhuyse, R.M., Roelfzema, H., Breimer, M.E. & Karlson, K.A. Lipids in tissues of the eye. X. Molecular species of sphingomyelin from different parts of the calf lens in relation to differentiation and ageing. *Expl. Eye Res.* 19: *477-484* (1974).

Broekhuyse, R.M. & Veerkamp, J.H. Phospholipids in the tissues of the eye. II. Composition and incorporation of ^{32}Pi of phospholipids of normal rat and calf lens. *Biochim. biophys. Acta* 152: *316-324* (1968).

Brown, M.S. & Goldstein, J.L. Receptor – mediated control of cholesterol metabolism. *Science* 191: *150-154* (1976).

Diringer, H., Marggraf, W.D., Koch, M.A. & Anderer, F.A. Evidence for a new biosynthetic pathway of sphingomyelin in SV 40 transformed mouse cells. *Biochim. biophys. Res. Commun.* 47: *1345-1352* (1972).

Dvornik, D., Simard-Duquesne, H., Krami, M., Seslanj, K., Gabbay, K.H., Kinoshita, J.H., Varma, S.D. & Merola, L.D. Polyol accumulation in galactosemic and diabetic rats: Control by an aldose reductase inhibitor. *Science* 182: *1146-1148* (1973).

Feldman, G.L.: Human Ocular Lipids: their analysis and distribution. *Survey of Ophthal.*, 12: *207-243* (1967).

Feldman, G.L. & Feldman, L.S. New concepts of human lenticular lipids and their possible role in cataracts. *Invest. Ophthal.* 4: *162-166* (1965).

Folch, J., Lees, M. & Sloane-Stanley, G.H. A simple method for the isolation and purification of total lipids from animal tissues. *J. biol. Chem.*, 226: *497-509* (1957).

Hammar, H. The formation of amino acids in vitro from glucose-U-[14] C in the eye lens of rats and the influence of sodium fluoride and alloxan diabetes. *Acta Ophthal.* 43: *543-556* (1965).

Jedziniak, J.A., Kinoshita, J.H., Yates, E.M., Hocker, L.O. & Benedek, G.B. Calcium-induced aggregations of bovine lens alpha crystallins. *Invest. Ophthal.* 11: *905-915* (1972).

Kinoshita, J.H. Cataracts in galactosemia. *Invest. Ophthal.* 4: *786-799* (1965).

Kuck, J.F.R. Jr. In 'Biochemistry of the eye,' (ed. Graymore, C.) Academic Press, London, New York, 1970, p. *215.*

Machiko, S., Kuwabara, T., Kinoshita, J.H. & Fukui, H. Swelling of lens fibres. *Expl. Eye Res.* 21: *381-394* (1975).

Maraini, G. & Mangili, R. Differences in proteins and in the water balance of the lens in nuclear and cortical types of senile cataract. *Ciba Fn. Sympo.* (new series) in The Human Lens in Relation to Cataract, Associated Scientific Publishers, Amsterdam & New York, 19: *79-97* (1973).

Obara, Y., Cotlier, E., Lindberg, R. & Horn, J. Cholesterol, cholesterol ester and sphingomyelin complexed to protein of normal human lens and senile cataracts, Doc. Ophthal. Proceedings Series, 8: *193-203* (1976).

Pirie, A. Epidemiological and biochemical studies of cataracts and diabetes. *Invest. Ophtal.* 4: *629-637* (1965).

Sanders, D., Cotlier, E., Wyhinny, G. & Millman, L. Cataracts induced by surface active agents. *Expl. Eye Res.* 19: *35-42* (1974).

Schmut, O. & Zirm, M. Immunological determination of aqueous humor lipoproteins. Albrecht v. Graefesi. *Arch. klin. exp. Ophthal.*, 191: *19-23* (1974).

Siakotos, A.N. & Rouser, G. Analytical separation of nonlipid, water-soluble substances and gangliosides from other lipids by dextran gel column chromatography. J. *Am. Oil Chem. Soc.* 42: *913-919* (1965).

Spector, A., Li, S. & Seligman, J. Age-dependent changes in the molecular size of human lens proteins and their relationship to light scatter. *Invest. Ophthal.*13: *795-798* (1974).

Tao, R.V.P. & Cotlier, E. Ceramides of human normal and cataractous lens. *Biochim. biophys. Acta* 409: *329-341* (1975).

VanDeenen, L.L.M., DeGier, J. and Demel, R.A. Relations between lipid composition and permeability of membranes, in 'Current Trends in the Biochemistry of Lipids' (ed. Ganguly, J. + Smellie, R.M.S.) *Biochem. Soc. Symp.* 35: *377-382* (1972).

Vermorken, A.J.M., Hilderink, J.M.H.C., Dunia, I., Benedetti, E.L., & Bloemendal, H. Changes in membrane protein pattern in relation to lens cell differentiation. FEBS Lett. 83: *301-306* (1977).

Author's address:
Department of Ophthalmology
Vanderbilt University School of Medicine
Nashville, Tennessee 37232 USA

FREE AMINO ACIDS AND OTHER SOLUTES IN THE LENS DURING FORMATION AND REVERSAL OF TRIPARANOL CATARACTS*

G. WINSTON BARBER AND KATHRYN GOODWIN

(Philadelphia, U.S.A.)

ABSTRACT

Triparanol, 0.075% in a pelleted diet, was fed to 100 weanling rats. Slight but definite inhibition of net synthesis of protein was discernible by 4 weeks, and at 6 weeks the total of proteogenic amino acid levels, per lens, was 33% greater than in control lenses. Nuclear opacities began to appear after 8 weeks, and all except 5 of the 82 remaining rats had bilateral cataracts by 10 weeks. With progression of nuclear opacification, which was classifiable into 4 stages, sodium and water increased markedly and calcium and magnesium increased moderately. Protein, amino acids, and free phosphate decreased steadily. Potassium, labile phosphate, ascorbate, glutathione and lactate were decreased in the earliest cataracts, but did not decrease further with increased opacification. Twenty rats with bilateral cataracts were transferred to the control diet at 60 days, and during the ensuing 10 months, most opacities disappeared completely, with return toward normal of hydration and all solutes except ascorbate.

INTRODUCTION

Experimental triparanol-induced cataracts in rats were reported by Von Sallmann et al. (1963) and by Kirby (1967), although both reported high mortality among their animals. Other investigators were unable to produce cataracts by feeding triparanol to rats (Feldman, 1967). In contrast, Harris & Gruber (1969, 1972; 1973) have produced cataracts consistently using a pelleted diet containing 0.05-0.075 percent of triparanol, and mortality has not been mentioned as a problem.

But more importantly, Harris & Gruber (1969) reported that triparanol cataract in rats is unusual in that it is completely reversible after removing triparanol from the diet, whereas nuclear cataracts induced in rats by other agents are reversible only in the sense that subsequent overgrowth of normal lens fibers can produce a lens with a clear cortex and a nuclear opacity of reduced size (Fournier & Patterson, 1970; Barber, 1973).

John Harris and his coworkers have reported that loss of glutathione (Rathbun et al., 1973) and potassium (Harris & Gruber, 1972) from triparanol cataracts is slight compared to losses observed in other types of nuclear cataract in rats. They also concluded that the free amino acids, excluding taurine, of control, cataractous, and cleared lenses were essentially the same

* This work was supported by U.S. Public Health Service Grant No. EY-00225.

when examined 6-8 months after restoration of a normal diet (Harris & Gruber, 1973). No study was made, however, of free amino acids in precataractous lenses or during cataract formation.

The objectives of the work reported here were: (1) to determine lens levels of free amino acids, including taurine, before and during development of nuclear cataracts; (2) to determine, in the same lenses, levels of sodium, potassium, calcium, magnesium, free and labile phosphate, glutathione, ascorbate, lactate, and total protein, with the hope that correlation of such data might shed additional light on the mechanism of cataractogenesis; and (3) to confirm the unique reversibility of triparanol cataract in the rat.

METHODS

Because none could be obtained from the Merrell Company, triparanol was synthesized according to their patent (Allen et al., 1959). A pelleted diet of 0.075% triparanol in Purina rat chow was prepared by General Biochemicals. This was fed ad lib to 100 weanling (35 ± 5 gm), female, Sprague-Dawley strain rats obtained from Taconic Farms, Germantown, N.Y. Control rats were fed Purina rat chow and water was constantly available.

Rats were killed with nembutal at biweekly intervals preceding nuclear opacification and at daily intervals after opacification began. Lenses were removed and examined under magnification. By analogy to galactose cataracts (Sippel, 1966; Cotlier, 1962), nuclear opacities were graded as stage 4A, 4B, or 4C, corresponding to diameters of approximately 1/4, 1/2, and 3/4 of the lens diameter, or as stage 5 if completely opaque. At 60 days, 20 rats with nuclear cataracts were switched to the control diet and were observed for 25-36 more weeks.

Each lens was homogenized in 0.2 ml of water, and during the reversal period only, an aliquot was removed for chloride determination. Protein was precipitated by adding an equal volume of 10% trichloroacetic acid (TCA). Aliquots of the supernatant were used to determine glutathione and free amino acids by amino acid analyzer. Sodium and potassium were determined by flame photometry, and ascorbate (Deutsch & Weeks, 1965) and calcium and magnesium (Diehl, 1964) were measured by fluorimetry. Phosphate (Eibl & Lands, 1969) and lactate (Hullin & Noble, 1953) were measured colorimetrically. Labile phosphate was determined as the additional amount released by incubating equal volumes of TCA supernatant and 6 N HCl for 18 hours at 20°C. Protein in the TCA precipitate was determined by a biuret procedure (Reinhold, 1953) and lens water was estimated as the difference between wet weight and total protein.

RESULTS

There was no spontaneous mortality among our rats, and nuclear opacities appeared in all except 5 of the 82 animals kept as long as 10 weeks. These 5 were killed at 70 days and were considered to represent the latest precataractous stage, although they might have been resistant animals. Nuclear opacities appeared simultaneously in both lenses of every rat, so it was not possible to obtain any with unilateral cataracts. Opacification began in the center of the lens and enlarged slowly, so that 4-10 days were required for complete opacification. Most stage 4A and 4B cataracts were collected on the day of first appearance, and stage 4C cataracts were collected from the 2nd through 4th days.

In the rats returned to normal diet after feeding triparanol for 60 days, regression of cataract was slow. Both lenses of one rat cleared after 3 months, and the lenses of two more rats cleared within 6 months. By nine months, half of the remaining lenses had cleared and half still contained nuclear opacities. In 3 rats, clearing was unilateral.

Figure 1 presents the changes of total protein and total free amino acids, excluding taurine. This total is the sum of the individually determined amounts of those amino acids (proteogenic amino acids) which could be derived from hydrolysis of protein. The total is a convenient condensation

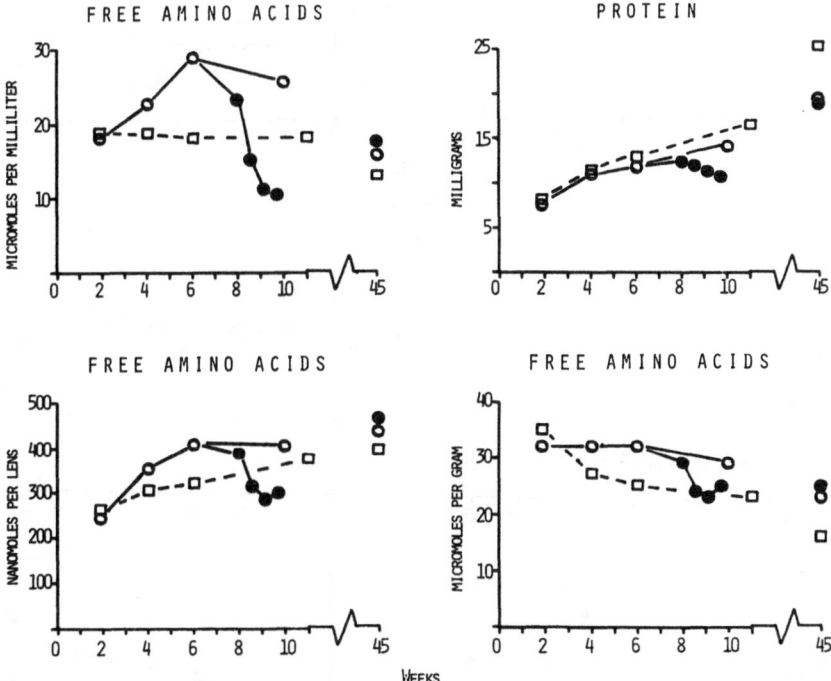

Fig. 1-6. Each symbol represents the mean for 6 or more lenses. Standard error bars are omitted because most would be within the diameters of the symbols. Squares represent control lenses, open circles represent clear, precataractous lenses of triparanol-fed rats, and filled circles represent the four stages of nuclear opacification, plotted arbitrarily at 56, 60, 64 and 70 days. There were 10, 16, 34 and 54 lenses, respectively, with stage 4A, 4B, 4C and 5 opacities. Data at 45 weeks are for rats switched to the control diet after feeding triparanol for 60 days.

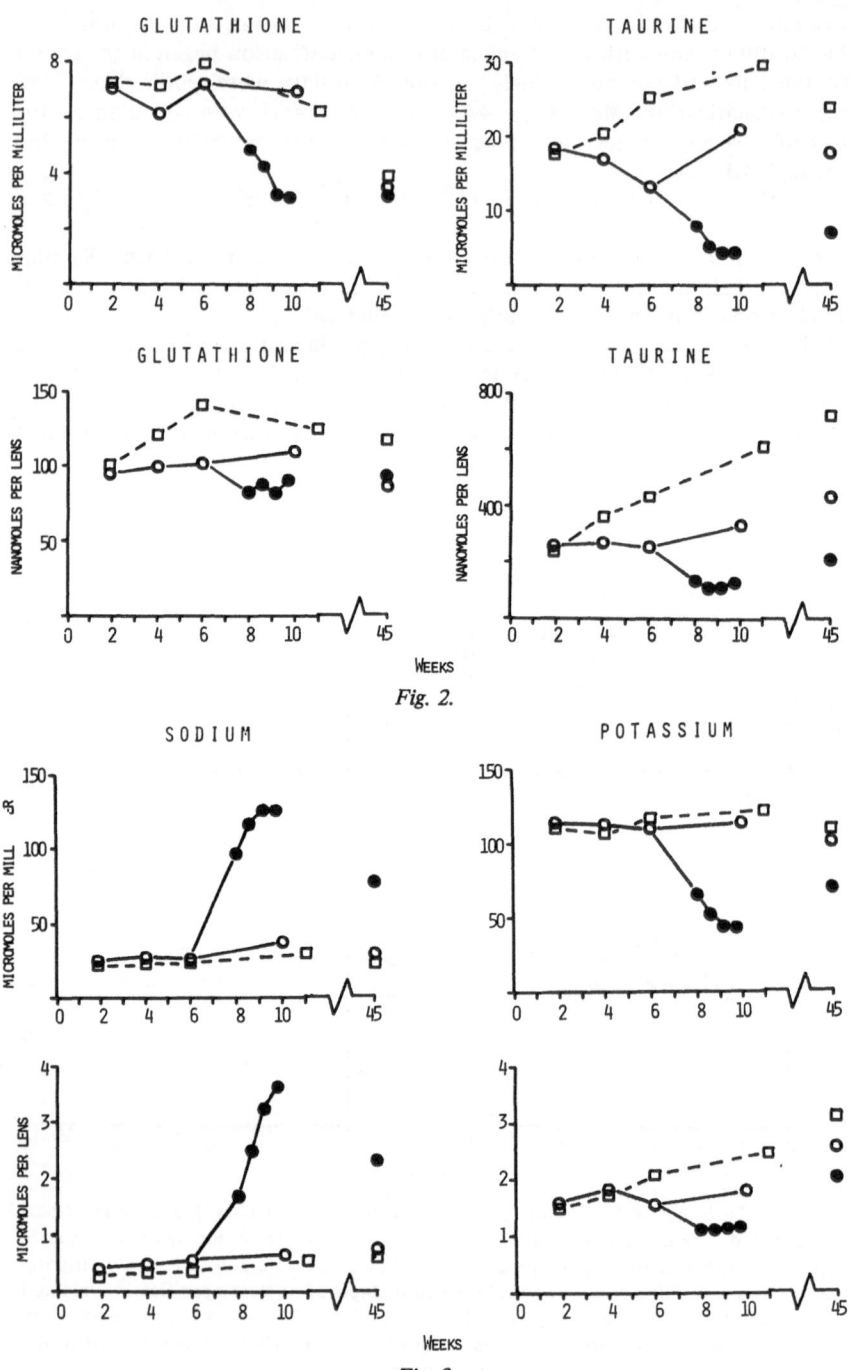

GLUTATHIONE

MICROMOLES PER MILLILITER

TAURINE

MICROMOLES PER MILLILITER

GLUTATHIONE

NANOMOLES PER LENS

TAURINE

NANOMOLES PER LENS

WEEKS

Fig. 2.

SODIUM

MICROMOLES PER MILL

POTASSIUM

MICROMOLES PER LENS

WEEKS

Fig. 3.

30

of a large amount of ... and ... which is not ... illustrated in the ... of the ... of the poor of this ... ...

To ... ... and ... ... water. The ... ... total of ... ... the ... in ... ... of ... in ... the ... ... lower.

During the ... ... there was ... ... of ... ... the ... ... The ... of ... ... there was not ... ... chart.

Changes of ... ... the ... ... shown in ... ... in ... ...

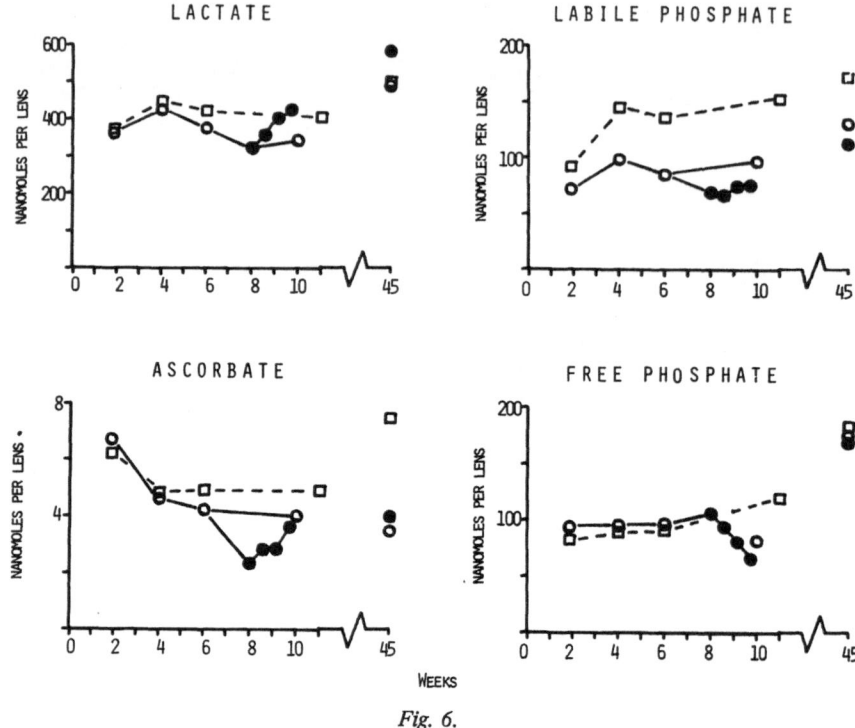

Fig. 6.

of a large amount of data and provides a qualitatively accurate illustration of the changes in levels of each of the constituents of the pool of free proteogenic amino acids.

In precataractous lenses of triparanol-fed rats, the levels of proteogenic amino acids increased compared to controls, whether expressed per lens or on the basis of wet weight or lens water. This increase was most evident at 6 weeks when the total of proteogenic amino acids, per lens, was 33% greater than the total in control lenses. This may have resulted from inhibited synthesis of lens protein, for the total protein of these precataractous lenses was less than in control lenses.

During the formation of nuclear opacities, there was actual loss of protein, probably by direct leakage from the lens, for there was no further accumulation of free amino acids. The loss of amino acids during opacification was not great, however, and generation by proteolysis could have been overshadowed by rapid efflux.

Changes of taurine, the principal amino acid of rat lenses, and of glutathione are shown in Figure 2, on both per lens and concentration bases. Both constituents remained relatively constant in precataractous lenses compared to increases in control lenses so that deficiencies were relative. With nuclear opacification, there was initial loss of about 35% glutathione and about 60% of taurine, but losses did not increase with increased opacification.

Figure 3 shows changes of lens sodium and potassium. Both were essentially normal in precataractous lenses, although potassium was slightly decreased, per lens, at 6 weeks. With nuclear opacification, the initial additional loss of potassium was not progressive, but there was steady increase of lens sodium. Figure 4 demonstrates that the influx of sodium during nuclear opacification, expressed as the total of sodium and potassium, was accompanied by increases of lens weight, lens water and percent water. Also shown is the loss of water from precataractous lenses at 6 weeks, which paralleled the loss of potassium so that potassium concentration was unchanged.

Lens calcium and magnesium increased progressively in cataractous lenses (Figure 5), but concentration changes were minimal and the calcium: magnesium ratio did not change much.

In precataractous lenses, levels of lactate, ascorbate and free phosphate differed insignificantly from levels in control lenses and losses during opacification were slight (Figure 6). Labile phosphate remained constant in precatar-

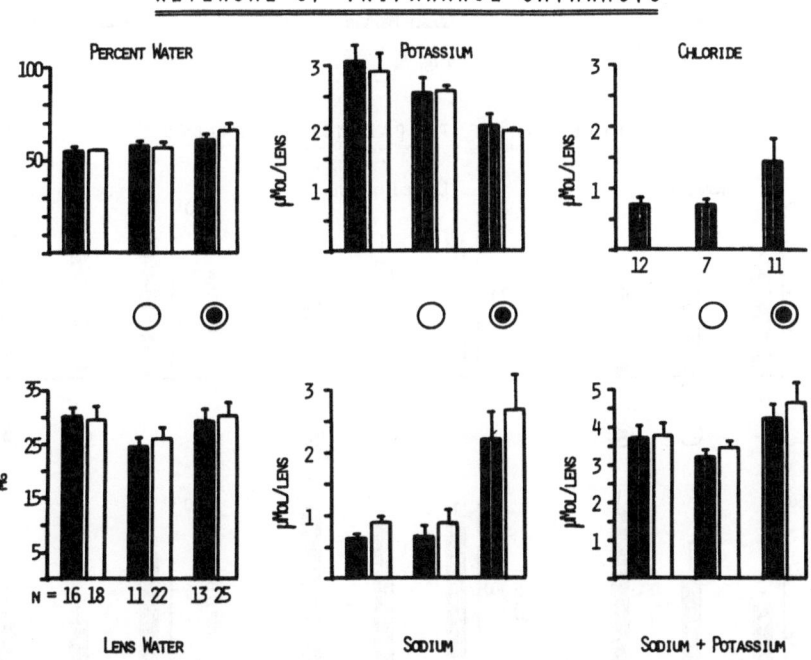

Fig. 7-9. Composition of reversing cataracts. Filled bars represent our data. Open bars are the data of Harris and coworkers. In each graph the first pair of bars represent control lenses, the second pair represent grossly clear reversed cataracts and the third pair represent persistent nuclear cataracts.

33

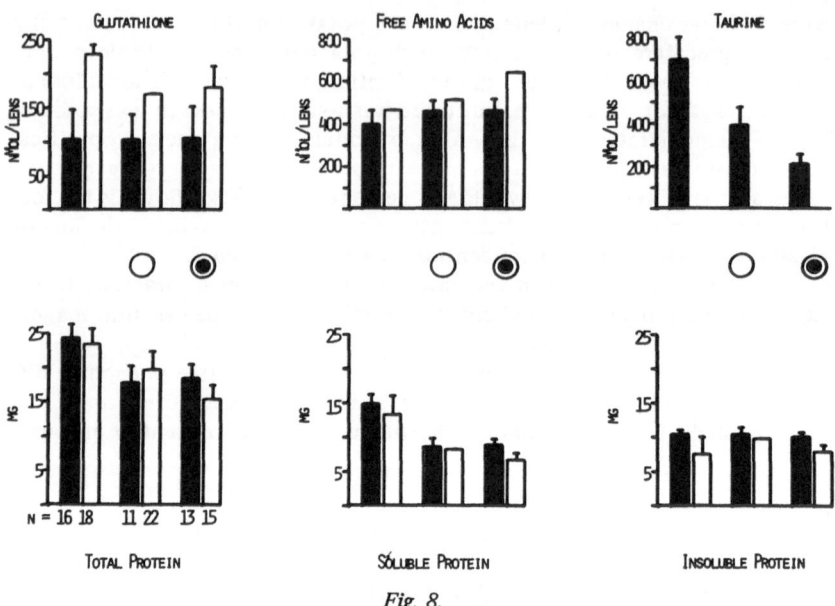

Fig. 8.

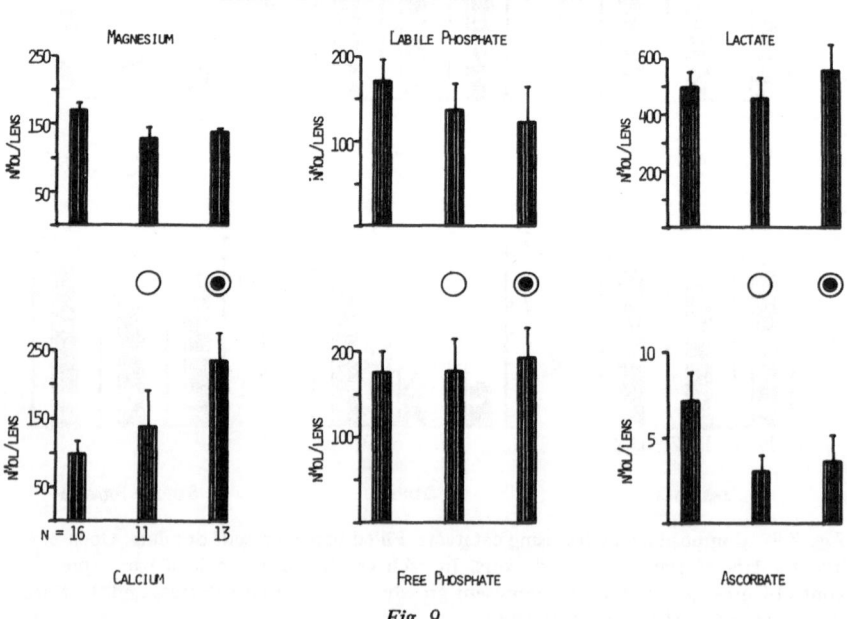

Fig. 9.

actous lenses, being deficient only in comparison to control lenses. There was little if any loss during opacification.

In Figures 7-9, our data (the filled bars) for reversing triparanol cataracts were compared with the data of Harris and coworkers (the open bars) for animals of comparable ages (Harris & Gruber, 1973; Rathbun et al., 1973). In each case rats were fed triparanol for about 60 days, followed by normal rat chow for 25-30 weeks. The principal differences between cleared and cataractous lenses were the levels of sodium, potassium and chloride (Figure 7), taurine (Figure 8) and calcium (Figure 9). Differences of water content were slight (Figure 7) and there were no important differences of soluble protein, insoluble protein or glutathione (Figure 8). Here the open bars are the data of Rathbun et al. (1973) for non-protein sulfhydryl, while the filled bars represent chromatographically determined glutathione.

DISCUSSION

Harris and his coworkers concluded that influx of sodium and water is the primary cause of nuclear opacification in lenses of triparanol-fed rats. Unlike other nuclear cataracts in rats, there was little loss of potassium or glutathione from opaque lenses. Reversal of triparanol cataracts was accompanied by loss of sodium and water and regain of potassium. These results are confirmed by our own, although we have found somewhat greater loss of potassium and glutathione during nuclear opacification. We also observed loss of both potassium and water from precataractous lenses after 6 weeks on the triparanol diet. This is reminiscent of the volume-regulating mechanism described by Patterson & Fournier (1976) but is puzzling because there was no antecedent swelling or obvious need for volume regulation. There was accumulation of proteogenic amino acids at six weeks, but the loss of taurine was greater. There was no accumulation of any other solute measured, but chloride was not determined in precataractous lenses

With the progression of nuclear opacification, there was steady accumulation of sodium and water and moderate accumulation of calcium and magnesium. Total protein and all proteogenic amino acids steadily decreased as opacification progressed, but the initial decreases of taurine and glutathione were not progressive. Losses of potassium and labile phosphate were also not progressive, and surprisingly, both lactate and ascorbate increased with increasing opacification. All these changes were small when compared to nuclear cataracts induced by feeding galactose to rats, and it seems possible that any increased permeability of cell membranes is more limited in triparanol cataract.

If protein synthesis is inhibited, one might expect proteogenic amino acids to accumulate, provided that amino acid transport and efflux are unchanged. This appeared to occur in precataractous lenses, starting after 4 weeks on the diet, with maximal accumulation of proteogenic amino acids, compared to control lenses, after 6 weeks. Since there was no accumulation of taurine, it seems unlikely that increased transport could have caused the selective accumulation of all proteogenic amino acids.

35

Since the accumulation of proteogenic amino acids in the precataractous stage of triparanol cataract was much less than we have observed in galactose cataracts (Barber, 1972), it seems probable that only the proteolytic component of normal protein turnover is active in triparanol cataract, without any additional autolysis ascribable to release of lysosomal proteases. This is speculative at present, but such a limitation could be a plausible explanation for the complete reversibility of triparanol cataracts.

As John Harris has reported, the propensity of triparanol cataracts to reverse after removal of the drug is truly unique, for nuclear opacities induced by other agents rarely disappear completely (Barber, 1973). Reversal of triparanol cataracts was slow, requiring 6 to 9 months recovery, but eventually most lenses became completely clear to gross inspection although slight cortical irregularities could often be seen under magnification. Cleared lenses were smaller and contained less protein than controls of the same age, and probably should be compared to younger controls.

Harris & Gruber (1972) suggested that active extrusion of sodium is only partially deficient in triparanol cataracts, so that Donnan swelling caused by sodium influx is limited. Specifically, they suggested that only one of two sodium pumps is inhibited, namely a ouabain-insensitive, non-electrogenic pump. Recently, histochemial assay of Na,K-ATPase in reversing triparanol cataracts revealed little difference between cleared lenses and persistent cataracts (Rathbun et al., 1978).

An alternative possibility is that membrane permeability is only slightly increased in triparanol cataracts so that relatively normal sodium transport limits Donnan swelling. The membrane enzyme, γ-glutamyltranspeptidase was relatively unaffected in clearing and cataractous lenses, and glutathione reductase activity in cataractous and normal lenses was the same (Rathbun et al., 1978). This may explain the small loss of glutathione from triparanol cataracts. Glutathione peroxidase activity was decreased about 35 percent in cataractous lenses, which might have permitted some oxidative damage to lens membranes.

Our own data are compatible with limitation of Donnan swelling for either of the reasons suggested, and such limitation could explain the reversibility of triparanol cataracts. Comparison with nuclear cataracts induced in rats by galactose, however, suggests that the hydration and swelling during formation of triparanol cataracts, and their reversal during clearing, are not sufficient to account completely for the changes of transparency. Recently, it has been suggested that altered lipid metabolism may also play a role in triparanol cataract formation.

Cataracts have been produced in rats by at least two other inhibitors of cholesterol synthesis, 20,25-diazacholesterol (Peter et al., 1973) and trans-1,4-bis(2-chlorobenzylaminomethyl)cyclohexane (AY 9944) (Sakuragawa et al., 1977). Accumulation of the cholesterol precursors, desmosterol and 7-dehydrocholesterol, has often been suggested as the cause of the manifold tissue effects of the inhibitors (Peter et al., 1973; Mizuno et al., 1974), but no direct evidence of toxicity of desmosterol or 7-dehydrocholesterol has been presented. By substituting for cholesterol in cell membranes, the intermediates conceivably could after membrane permeability, but there is direct evidence that deficiency of cholesterol can have marked effects on membrane permeability (Demel &DeKruyf, 1976) and on active transport of sodium (Giraud et al., 1976).

Sakuragawa et al. (1977) have reported that AY 9944 fed to rats caused decreased levels of sphingomyelinase in several tissues, including the lens, and resulted in the formation of electron-dense, lamellar inclusion bodies which were 'abundantly present in the epithelium and fibers of the lens', although cells were otherwise normal in appearance (Sakuragawa, 1976).

Sphingomyelinase deficiency may not be the explanation for the formation of these inclusion bodies, however, for quite similar formations can be induced by a large selection of amphiphilic drugs with widely varying pharmaceutical actions, and it has been suggested that these drugs bind strongly to phospholipids and inhibit their catabolism by altering the substrates rather than by inhibiting enzymes (Seydel & Wassermann, 1976).

Von Sallmann et al. (1963) described the presence of vesicular, sudanophilic deposits in lens fiber cells of triparanol-fed rats, with larger complexes of lipid between fibers. Membrane-limited, electron-dense inclusion bodies have been reported frequently in other tissues of animals fed triparanol, diazacholesterol, or AY 9944 (Yates et al., 1967; Chen & Yates, 1967; Dietert & Scallen, 1969). The inclusions have been considered to be autophagic vacuoles or engorged lysosomes. They are rich in phospholipid and a variety of lamellar, reticular and crystalline structures have been described. In triparanol-fed hamsters, inclusion bodies isolated from adrenal homogenates contained triparanol, desmosterol and sphingomyelins (Yates et al., 1967).

If such inclusion bodies are engorged lysosomes, their formation and probable distribution in the lens seems an improbable cause of selective nuclear opacification, but the presence of such inclusions may predispose lenses to opacification so that nuclear cataracts can appear as the result of moderate hydration and swelling which would otherwise be insufficient to cause opacification. In any event, it seems clear, as John Harris concluded, that accumulation of sodium and water play a major role in the formation of triparanol cataracts.

REFERENCES

Allen, R.E., Palopali, F.P., Schumann, E.L. & Van Campen, M.G. Amine derivatives of triphenylethanol. U.S. Patent 2, 914, 562 (1959)

Barber, G.W. Physiological chemistry of the eye. Annual review. *Arch. Ophthalmol.* 87: *72-106* (1972).

Barber, G.W. Physiological chemistry of the eye. Annual review. *Arch. Ophthalmol.* 89: *236-255* (1973).

Chen I. & Yates, R.D. An ultrastructural study of opaque cytoplasmic inclusions induced by triparanol treatment. *Am. J. Anat.* 121: *705-726* (1967).

Cotlier, E. Hypophysectomy effect on lens epithelium mitosis and galactose cataract development in rats. *Arch. Ophthalmol.* 67: *476-482* (1962).

Demel, R.A. & De Kruyf, B. The function of sterols in membranes. *Biochim. biophys. Acta* 457: *109-132* (1976).

Deutsch, M. & Weeks, C. Microfluorimetric assay for vitamin C. J. Ass. Off. Analyt. Chem. 48: *1248-1256* (1965).

Diehl, H. Calcein, calmagite and o,o'-dihydroxyazobenzene. Titrimetric, colorimetric and fluorimetric reagents for calcium and magnesium C.F. Smith Chemical Co., Columbus, Ohio, 1964.

Dietert, S.E. & Scallen, T.J. An ultrastructural and biochemical study of the effects of three inhibitors of cholesterol biosynthesis upon murine adrenal gland and testis. *J. Cell Biol.* 40: *44-60* (1969).

Eibl, H. & Lands, W. A new, sensitive determination of phosphate. *Analyt. Biochem.* 30: *51-57* (1969).

Feldman, G.L. Human ocular lipids: Their analysis and distribution. *Surv. Ophthal.* 12: *207-243* (1967).

Fournier, D.J. & Patterson, J.W. Lens regeneration after mature galactose cataract formation. *Proc. Soc. exp. Biol. Med.* 135: *377-379* (1970).

Giraud, F., Claret, M. & Garay, R. Interactions of cholesterol with the Na pump in red blood cells. *Nature* 264: *646-648* (1976).

Harris, J.E. & Gruber, L. The reversal of triparanol induced cataracts in the rat. *Doc. Ophthal.* 26: *324-333* (1969).

Harris, J.E. & Gruber, L. Reversal of triparanol-induced cataracts in the rat. II. Exchange of ^{22} Na, ^{42} K and ^{86} Rb in cataractous and clearing lenses. *Invest Ophthal.* 11: *608-615* (1972).

Harris, J.E. & Gruber, L. The reversal of triparanol-induced cataracts in the rat. III. Amino acid content and uptake of ^{14} C AIB in cataractous and clearing lenses. *Invest Ophthal.* 12: *385-388* (1973).

Hullin, R. & Noble, R. The determination of lactic acid in microgram quantities. *Biochem. J.* 55: *289-291* (1953).

Kirby, T.J. Cataracts produced by triparanol (Mer 29). *Trans. Am. Ophthal. Soc.* 65: *493-543* (1967).

Mizuno, G., Ellison, E., Chipault, J.R. & Harris, J.E. Lipids of the triparanol cataract in the rat. *Ophthal. Res.* 6: *206-215* (1974).

Patterson, J.W. & Fournier, D.J. The effect of tonicity on lens volume. *Invest. Ophthal.* 15: *866-869* (1976).

Peter, J.B., Andiman, R.M., Bowman, R.L. & Nagatomo, T. Myotonia induced by diazacholesterol: Increased (Na$^+$ + K$^+$) ATPase activity of erythrocyte ghosts and development of cataracts. *Expl. Neurol.* 41: *738-744* (1973).

Rathbun, W.B., Harris, J.E., Vagstad, G. & Gruber, L. The reversal of triparanol-induced cataract in the rat. IV. Reduced sulfhydryl groups in soluble protein and glutathione. *Invest. Ophthal.* 12: *388-390* (1973).

Rathbun, W.B., Hough, M., Gruber, L. & Harris, J.E. The reversal of triparanol-induced cataract in the rat. V. Activity levels of ATPase and three enzymes of glutathione metabolism. Interdiscpl. Topics Geront. In press (1978).

Reinhold, J. Total protein, albumin, and globulin. Stand. Meth. Clin Chem. 1: *88-97* (1953).

Sakuragawa, M. Niemann-Pick disease-like inclusions caused by a hypocholesterolemic agent. *Invest. Ophthal* . 15: *1022-1024* (1976).

Sakuragawa, N., Sakuragawa, M., Kuwabara, T., Pentchev. P., Barranger, J. & Brady, R. Niemann-Pick disease experimental model: Sphingomyelinase reduction induced by AY-9944. *Science* 196: *317-319* (1977).

Seydel, J.K. & Wassermann, O. NMR studies on the molecular basis of drug-induced phospholipidosis. II. Interaction between several amphiphilic drugs and phospholipids. *Biochem. Pharmac.* 25: *2357-2364* (1976).

Sippel, T.O. Changes in water, protein, and glutathione contents of the lens in the course of galactose cataract development in rats. *Invest. Ophthal.* 5: *568-575* (1966).

Von Sallmann, L., Grimes, P. & Collins, E. Triparanol induced cataract in rats *Arch. Ophthalmol.* 70: *522-530* (1963).

Yates, R.D., Arai, K. & Rappoport, D.A. Fine structure and chemical composition of opaque cytoplasmic bodies of triparanol treated Syrian hamsters. *Expl. Cell Res.* 47: *459-478* (1967).

Authors' address:
Wills Eye Hospital and Research Institute
1601 Spring Garden Street
Philadelphia, Pa. 19130 USA

Docum. Ophthal. Proc. Series, Vol. 18

CATION TRANSPORT IN THE LENS AND THE Na-K-ACTIVATED ATPase SYSTEM

S.L. BONTING & J.J.H.H.M. DE PONT

(Nijmegen, the Netherlands)

ABSTRACT

The evidence for the existence of an active cation transport in the lens and its relation to the epithelial Na-K activated ATPase system is reviewed. The properties and mechanism of the latter enzyme system are briefly described. Four aspects from our own work are treated in more detail: phospholipid requirement, the presence of an essential arginine group and of a vital sulfhydryl group in the ATP-binding center, and the identity of the phospho-enzymes formed by ATP and by inorganic phosphate.

CATION TRANSPORT

It is a pleasure to honor John E. Harris with this paper on a subject dear to his heart. Not only was he the first one to discover the active transport of sodium and potassium in the lens (Harris & Gehrsitz, 1951), he was one of the first to explain the cation gradients across a cell membrane as the result of an active transport system working against a passive diffusion by means of his reversible cation shift experiments (Harris, 1941). Applying these experiments to the lens he demonstrated that inhibition of lens metabolism in vitro by refrigeration or metabolic inhibitors causes Na to enter and K to leave the rabbit lens (Harris & Gehrsitz, 1951). He also showed that the cation shift due to refrigeration can be reversed upon incubation at 37°C (Harris et al., 1953), and that this requires the presence of glucose (Harris et al., 1954a), without an absolute requirement of oxygen (Harris et al., 1954b, 1959). From these experiments he concluded that a cation transport system keeps the potassium content of the rabbit lens high and the sodium content low, that this is located at or near the lens surface, that it requires (anaerobic) metabolic energy for its function, and that this system is essential for preventing swelling of the lens and thus for the preservation of lens clarity (Harris, 1958).

In subsequent years, Kinoshita and his associates (1961) confirmed most of these findings for cattle lens. In addition, they established a correlation between the high-energy phosphate level and the extent of the reversal of the cold-induced cation shift. This suggested that high energy phosphate bonds, derived from glycolysis, supply the energy required for cation transport in the lens. They also demonstrated that the cardiac glycoside ouabain is a potent inhibitor of this cation transport system. Becker (1962) studied the accumulation of ^{86}Rb by the rabbit lens, and found that rubidium ions compete with potassium ions for the active transport system. He confirmed that the system is inhibited by glycolytic inhibitors and by cardiac glycosides (digoxin and ouabain), but not by the absence of oxygen. These studies thus indicated that the cation transport system of the lens is sensitive to cardiac glycosides and is dependent on high-energy phosphate bonds, presumably adenosine triphosphate.

DISCOVERY OF Na-K ACTIVATED ATPase

In this same period Skou (1957, 1960) detected an ouabain-sensitive ATPase, activated by Na$^+$ plus K$^+$ions (Na-K ATPase) in crab nerve, which he postulated to be related to the cation transport system in the nerve membrane. Post et al. (1960) and Dunham & Glynn (1961) demonstrated its presence in the erythrocyte membrane and its close relationship to the cation transport system of the erythrocyte.

Our own studies showed the wide distribution of the enzyme in tissues of the cat, including the lens epithelium (Bonting et al., 1961), and its occurrence in all tissues known at that time to have a cardiac glycoside sensitive cation transport system (Bonting et al., 1962). We also demonstrated an equivalence of active cation flux values and Na-K ATPase activities over a 25,000 fold range in six tissues with an average ratio of nearly 3 equivalents cation transported per mole ATP hydrolyzed (Bonting & Caravaggio, 1963). In subsequent years a primary and rate-limiting role of the enzyme in various secretion systems could be shown: formation of aqueous humour, cerebrospinal fluid and pancreatic fluid, sodium transport in toad bladder, avian salt gland and elasmobranch rectal gland (review: Bonting, 1970).

Na-K ACTIVATED ATPase IN THE LENS

The similarity of various properties of the lens cation transport system and of the Na-K ATPase system, and our earlier detection of the enzyme in cat lens epithelium (Bonting et al., 1961) prompted us to study its possible role in the lens (Bonting et al., 1963; Bonting, 1965).

Its distribution in the lens of cat, calf and rabbit was found to be very consistent: only the epithelium has a significant and high activity (Table 1). This implies that active cation transport would only take place through the anterior face of the lens in these species, while passive diffusion can take place on both sides. This has been confirmed in the rabbit lens for ^{86}Rb uptake by Becker & Cotlier (1962) and for ^{42}K uptake by Kinsey & Reddy (1965). Recent histochemical studies corroborate the exclusive localization of the enzyme in the epithelial cells, where it appears to be mainly located in the lateral cell membranes (Palva & Palkama, 1976).

Various other properties of the epithelial Na-K ATPase system have been determined and compared with the related properties of the cation transport system (Table 2). The excellent agreement, both qualitatively and quantitatively, strongly indicate that the enzyme is identical with or very closely related to the cation transport system of the lens. Cation/ATP ratios close to 3 are found (Table 2, bottom three lines), in good agreement with those generally observed for the Na-K ATPase system (Bonting, 1970, p. 272, Table 5) and indicating a primary and rate-limiting role of the enzyme system in active cation transport of the lens.

MECHANISM OF Na-K ACTIVATED ATPase

The properties of the Na-K activated ATPase system from many tissues and species have been shown to be remarkably similar (Bonting, 1970,

Table 1. Distribution of Na-K activated ATPase activity in lens of cat, calf and rabbit.

Structure	Cat Activity	Cat % of total ATPase	Calf Activity	Calf % of total ATPase	Rabbit Activity	Rabbit % of total ATPase
Anterior capsule	.0	–	.1	–	.1	–
Epithelium + capsule	41.5*	73*	90.0*	66*	149.0*	72*
Cortex	.6	15	.6	16	1.8	18
Nucleus	.3	–	.1	–	.7	–
Posterior capsule	.3	–	.0	–	.0	–

Activities expressed in millimoles ATP per kg. wet wt. per hr hydrolyzed at 37° C.
* Significantly different from zero at the P = 0.05 level.
After Bonting et al. (1963)

Table 2. Properties of the cation transport and epithelial Na-K activated ATPase systems of the lens.

Property	Cation transport	Na-K ATPase
Location	epithelium	epithelium
Substrate	ATP	ATP
Cation requirements	Mg^{2+} (?), Na^+, K^+, Rb^+ competes with K^+	Mg^{2+}, Na^+, K^+; Rb^+ can replace K^+
pH optimum (rabbit)	7.5	7.3
Temperature coefficient, Q_{10} (rabbit)	2	2.4
Ouabain effects	inhibits	inhibits
pI_{50}, calf	7.0-7.4	7.10
pI_{50}, rabbit	6.0	5.95
Rates (μmole/lens/hr)		ratio:
Calf	2.6 (K^+), 3.1 (Na^+)	0.78 (ATP) 3.6
Rabbit	6.5 (K^+), 3.9 (Na^+)	1.56 (ATP) 3.3
	3.9 (Rb^+)	1.34 (ATP) 2.9

After Bonting et al. (1963)

p. 264-270). Thus it seems permissible to use evidence obtained for the enzyme isolated from other tissues instead of from lens epithelium, which is difficult to obtain in considerable quantities. We routinely use rabbit kidney outer medulla microsomes, which after sodium dodecyl sulfate extraction and zonal gradient centrifugation yield a highly pure ($>$ 90% on protein basis), active (ca. 2 mol ATP/g protein/hr) and stable enzyme preparation.

The enzyme has a molecular weight of 250,000, and consists of two subunits α and β. The α-subunit has a molecular weight of ca. 90,000, is phosphorylated by ATP in the presence of Mg^{2+} and Na^+ and by inorganic phosphate in the presence of Mg^{2+} (Schuurmans Stekhoven et al., 1976), and carries the ouabain binding site. The β-subunit is a sialoglycoprotein with a molecular weight of ca. 50,000, is not phosphorylated, and may function as a cation carrier with a specificity for Na^+ ions (review: Bonting & de Pont, 1977, pp. 153-161). The enzyme complex seems to consist of an $\alpha_2\beta$ trimer or an $\alpha_2\beta_2$ tetramer.

The reaction mechanism involves binding and phosphorylation, trans-phosphorylation or conformational change of the phosphorylated intermediate and dephosphorylation:

$$E_1 + ATP \rightleftharpoons E_1 \cdot ATP \underset{Na^+}{\overset{Mg^{2+}}{\rightleftharpoons}} E_1 \sim P + ADP \tag{1}$$

$$E_1 \sim P \rightleftharpoons E_2 \sim P \rightarrow E_2 - P \tag{2}$$

$$E_2 - P + H_2O \overset{K^+}{\rightarrow} E_2 + P_i \tag{3}$$

$$E_2 \rightleftharpoons E_1 \tag{4}$$

Phosphorylation requires Mg^{2+} and Na^+, and is not inhibited by low concentrations of ouabain. Reaction ③ requires K^+ and is very sensitive to ouabain; its rate can be measured as a K^+-stimulated phosphatase activity. The phosphoenzyme $E \sim P$ can be isolated by treating the enzyme with terminally ^{32}P-labelled ATP in the presence of Na^+ and Mg^{2+}, followed by precipitation with trichloroacetic acid. This also allows measurement of the rate of reaction ①. Proteolytic treatment of the phosphoenzyme yields a phosphorylated tripeptide, which appears to have the phosphate group bound to an aspartyl group. It is assumed that E_1 is a conformation of the enzyme with inwardly oriented cation binding sites with high affinity for Na^+ and low affinity for K^+, while E_2 would be a conformation with outwardly oriented cation binding sites with low affinity for Na^+ and high affinity for K^+. During reaction ③ exchange of Na^+ for K^+ would take place, while the reverse exchange would take place during reaction ④. Uncertain is whether during reaction ② the phosphate group shifts from the aspartyl group to another group, or merely a conformational change occurs.

PHOSPHOLIPID REQUIREMENT

Being a membrane-bound enzyme, the Na-K ATPase requires a phospholipid environment for its activity. Removal of the phospholipids from the enzyme preparation by treatment with detergents, phospholipases or organic solvents leads to its inactivation. Addition of various lipids to a partially delipidated preparation restores the activity, at least in part. Some investigators find that the negatively charged phosphatidylserine is the most effective of the reactivating lipids, and have suggested that this phospholipid is essential for the Na-K ATPase activity (Wheeler & Whittam, 1970).

Since delipidation is a rather drastic treatment, we have applied another approach: treatment of the enzyme preparation with phosphatidylserine decarboxylase converts phosphatidylserine (PS) quantitatively into its decarboxylation product, phosphatidylethanolamine (PE), without any other changes in the phospholipid pattern (de Pont et al., 1973). A purified Na-K ATPase preparation shows no significant loss in enzyme activity upon this treatment (Table 3). The same is true upon specific removal of the other negatively charged phospholipid phosphatidylinositol (PI) by PI-specific phospholipase, and for neutral phospholipid removal by phospholipase C, as well as for combinations of these treatments. Only combined treatment removing both PI and PS leads to a significant 40% loss in enzyme activity (de Pont et al., 1978). This indicates that there is no absolute requirement for any particular phospholipid, although in the absence of both negatively charged phospholipids PS and PI the activity is lowered somewhat.

ESSENTIAL ARGININE GROUP IN THE ATP-BINDING CENTER

Information about the active center of the enzyme can be obtained by studying the effects of chemical modification of particular residues in the enzyme complex. The purified enzyme preparation has been treated with the arginine reagent butanedione (de Pont et al., 1977). This leads to a reversible inactivation of the Na-K ATPase activity. The reaction shows second-order kinetics, indicating that modification of a single arginine residue (one out of 90 present per enzyme molecule!) results in complete inactivation.

ATP in micromolar concentrations strongly protects the enzyme against butanedione. It does so under non-phosphorylating conditions (absence of Mg^{2+}), indicating that binding of ATP protects the essential arginine group. This suggests that the arginine residue is involved in substrate binding, probably attracting the negative β-γ-phosphate groups to its positively charged guanidinium group. This is further confirmed by the fact that K^+ ions, which reduce ATP binding, also reduce inactivation by butanedione. Conversely, Na^+ ions make the arginine group more accessible to both ATP and butanedione, indicating two conformational states of the enzyme in the presence of either Na^+ or K^+.

The K^+ stimulated phosphatase activity and the phosphorylation by inorganic phosphate are much less sensitive to butanedione than the Na-K ATPase activity and the Na^+-Mg^{2+} stimulated phosphorylation by ATP. This suggests that the enzyme has two phosphorylation sites, one with high affinity for ATP (sensitive to butanedione) and one with low affinity for ATP

45

Table 3. Effect of treatment of the Na-K ATPase with various phospholipid converting enzymes on phospholipid composition and enzyme activities.

phospholipid	un-treated	PS-decarb.	PI-PL-ase	PL-ase C	PI-PL-ase +PL-ase C	PS-decarb. +PL-ase C	PI-PL-ase +PS-decarb.
				mol phospholipid/mol Na-K ATPase			
PC	95	104	100	5	7	8	104
PS	35	0	29	34	42	0.5	1.6
PI	15	14	0	18	0.5	18	0.5
PE	74	101	74	26	16	54	97
Sph	48	48	46	17	24	18	50
Total	267	267	249	100	90	99	253
				activity in percent of control activity			
Na-K ATPase	$\equiv$100	87±7 (7)	101±3 (11)	80±6 (7)	82±6 (3)	90±15 (7)	56±2 (4)
K-Phosphatase	$\equiv$100	–	99±4 (11)	90±8 (12)	85±6 (3)	75±16 (7)	64±8 (4)

Abbreviations: PC = phosphatidylcholine, PS = phosphatidylserine, PI = phosphatidylinositol, PE = phosphatidylethanolamine, Sph = sphingomyelin, PL-ase = phospholipase, PS-decarb. = phosphatidylserine decarboxylase.

After de Pont et al. (1978)

(less sensitive to butanedione). The Na-K ATPase reaction would require phosphorylation of both sites, the K^+-phosphatase reaction would require phosphorylation of the low affinity site only.

ROLE OF SULFHYDRYL GROUPS

Reaction of purified Na-K ATPase with the sulfhydryl reagent N-ethylmaleimide (NEM) inhibits the overall activity and the partial activities (phosphorylation by ATP and by inorganic phosphate, and the K^+ phosphatase activity) in parallel fashion (Schoot et al., 1977). The inhibition follows second order kinetics, indicating that NEM reacts with one site at the time. The parallel inhibition of all activities indicates that NEM does not primarily and exclusively inhibit the $E_1 \sim P \rightarrow E_2 - P$ transition (reaction 2), as had been suggested.

ATP and other nucleotides protect the enzyme under non-phosphorylating conditions, suggesting that the vital sulfhydryl group, modified by NEM, is involved in substrate binding. This group probably interacts with the adenine group of ATP.

The parallel inhibition of the overall activity and the partial reactions suggests that more is involved than only the ATP binding center. Therefore, a search for other reactive sulfhydryl groups was made with the sulfhydryl reagent dithiobis-nitrobenzoic acid (DTNB). A total of 36 reactive SH-groups per enzyme molecule have been demonstrated with DTNB in the presence of the detergent sodium dodecyl sulfate (SDS) (Schoot et al., 1978). Twelve of these groups react with both NEM and DTNB, including one that is vital for the enzyme activity. Another 14 SH-groups react with NEM only, including one that is vital. The remaining 10 SH-groups react with neither NEM nor DTNB in the absence of detergent. The 12 SH groups are located on the hydrophilic surface of the enzyme, the 14 in a more hydrophobic environment, and the remaining 10 in very inaccessible parts of the molecule which are only exposed upon denaturation with SDS. The vital SH-group in the hydrophilic region is probably located in the ATP-binding center, while the hydrophobic SH-group is not. All (or virtually all) reactive SH-groups appear to be present in the α-subunit.

IDENTITY OF THE TWO PHOSPHOENZYMES

We have mentioned that the Na-K ATPase system can be phosphorylated both by ATP and by inorganic phosphate. Phosphorylation in both cases takes place in the α-subunit (Schuurmans Stekhoven et al., 1976). The maximal amounts of phosphoenzyme formed by either substrate are equimolar.

One would expect the phosphoenzyme, resulting from phosphorylation by inorganic phosphate, to have a low energy phosphate bond, while the phosphate bond resulting from phosphorylation by ATP would be a high energy bond. It would then be quite likely that the phosphate group would be attached to different residues in the two phosphoenzymes.

In order to check this, we have prepared the two phosphoenzymes from

γ-^{32}P ATP and ^{32}P-phosphate respectively, subjected them to pronase treatment, and compared the resulting phosphopeptides (Schuurmans Stekhoven, Swarts, de Pont, Bonting, to be published). They show identical behaviour in electrophoresis (isoelectric point 3.8), binding to diethylaminoethyl cellulose, thin layer chromatography on cellulose and molecular sieve chromatography over Bio-Gel P-2. The latter procedure yields a molecular weight of 295, suggesting that they are dipeptides. We must, therefore, conclude that the two phosphoenzymes are chemically identical, and that their different energy content is due to conformational differences.

CONCLUDING REMARK

It will be clear from this brief survey that 37 years after Harris' characterization of the cation transport system we have acquired a great deal of relevant information, although much still has to be discovered about this fascinating system which plays a crucial role in the preservation of the clarity of the lens.

REFERENCES

Becker, B. Accumulation of rubidium 86 by the rabbit lens. *Invest. Ophthal.* 1: *502-506* (1962).

Becker, B. & Cotlier, E. Distribution of ^{86}Rb accumulated in the rabbit lens. *Invest. Ophthal.* 1: *642-645* (1962).

Bonting, S.L. Na-K activated ATPase and active cation transport in the lens. *Invest. Ophthal.* 4: *723-738* (1965).

Bonting, S.L. Na-K activated ATPase and cation transport, in Membrane and Ion Transport, ed. Bittar, E.E., vol. 1, pp. *257-363*; Wiley Interscience, London (1970).

Bonting, S.L. & Caravaggio, L.L. Studies on Na-K activated ATPase. V. Correlation of enzyme activity with cation flux in six tissues. *Arch. Biochem. Biophys.* 101: *37-46* (1963).

Bonting, S.L. & de Pont, J.J.H.H.M. Active transport. In: Mammalian Cell Membranes, (ed. G.A. Jamieson & D.M. Robinson) vol. 4, pp. *145-183* Butterworths, London (1977).

Bonting, S.L., Simon, K.A. & Hawkins, N.M. Studies on Na-K activated ATPase. I. Quantitative distribution in several tissues of the cat. *Arch. Biochem. Biophys.* 95: *416-423* (1961).

Bonting, S.L., Caravaggio, L.L. & Hawkins, N.M. Studies on Na-K activated ATPase. IV. Correlation with cation transport sensitive to cardiac glycosides. *Arch. Biochem. Biophys.* 98: *413-419* (1962).

Bonting, S.L., Caravaggio, L.L. & Hawkins, N.M. Studies on Na-K activated ATPase. VI. Its role in cation transport in the lens of cat, calf and rabbit. *Arch. Biochem. Biophys.* 101: *47-55* (1963).

de Pont, J.J.H.H.M., van Prooyen, A., Bonting, S.L. Studies on (Na$^+$ + K$^+$)-activated ATPase. XXXIV. Phosphatidylserine not essential for (Na$^+$-K$^+$)-ATPase activity. *Biochim. Biophys. Acta* 323: *487-494* (1973).

de Pont, J.J.H.H.M., Schoot, B.M., van Prooyen, A. & Bonting, S.L. Studies on Na-K activated ATPase. XL. An essential arginine residue in the ATP-binding center of Na-K ATPase. *Biochim. Biophys. Acta* 482: *213-227* (1977).

de Pont, J.J.H.H.M., van Prooyen, A. & Bonting, S.L. Studies on Na-K activated ATPase. XXXIX. Role of negatively charged phospholipids. *Biochim. Biophys. Acta*, (1978) in press.

Dunham, E.T. & Glynn, I.M. Adenosinetriphosphatase activity and active alkalimetal-ion mobility. *J. Physiol.* 156: *274-293* (1961).

Harris, J.E. The influence of the metabolism of human erythrocytes on their potassium content. *J. biol. Chem.* 141: *579-595* (1941).

Harris, J.E. Active transport across the lens surface. *Acta XVIII Conc. Ophthal.* 1: *735-743* (1958).

Harris, J.E. & Gehrsitz, L.B. Significance of changes in potassium and sodium content of the lens *Am. J. Ophthal.* 34: *131-138* (1951).

Harris, J.E., Gehrsitz, L.B. & Nordquist, L.T. In vitro reversal of the lenticular cation shift induced by cold or calcium deficiency. *Am. J. Ophthal.* 36: *39-50* (1953).

Harris, J.E. Gruber, L., Talman, E. & Hoskinson, G. Influence of oxygen on the photodynamic action of methylene blue on cation transport in rabbit lenses. *Am. J. Ophthal.* 48: *528-534* (1959).

Harris, J.E., Hauschildt, J.D. & Nordquist, L.T. Lens metabolism as studied with the reversible cation shift. I. The role of glucose. *Am. J. Ophthal.* 38: *141-147* (1954a).

Harris, J.E., Hauschildt, J.D. & Nordquist, L.T. Lens metabolism as studied with the reversible cation shift. II. The effect of oxygen and glutamic acid. *Am. J. Ophthal.* 38: *148-152* (1954b).

Kinoshita, J.H., Kern, H.L. & Merola, L.O. Factors affecting the cation transport of calf lens. *Biochim. Biophys.Acta* 47: *458-466* (1961).

Kinsey, V.E. & Reddy, D.V.N. Studies on the crystalline lens. XI. The relative role of the epithelium and capsule in transport. *Invest. Ophthal.* 4: *104-116* (1965).

Palva, M. & Palkama, A. Electronmicroscopical, histochemical and biochemical findings on the Na-K activated ATPase activity in the epithelium of the rat lens. *Expl. Eye Res.* 22: *229-236* (1976).

Post, R.L., Merritt, C.R., Kinsolving, C.R. & Albright, C.D. Membrane ATPase as a participant in the active transport of Na- and K in the human erythrocyte. *J. biol. Chem.* 235: *1796-1802* (1960).

Schoot, B.M., de Pont, J.J.H.H.M. & Bonting, S.L. Studies on Na-K activated ATPase. XLII. Evidence for two classes of sulfhydryl groups. *Biochim. biophys. Acta* 522: *602-613* (1978).

Schoot, B.M., Schoots, A.F.M., de Pont, J.J.H.H.M., Schuurmans Stekhoven, F.M.A.H. & Bonting, S.L. Studies on Na-K activated ATPase. XLI. Effects on N-ethylmaleimide on overall and partial reactions. *Biochim. biophys. Acta* 483: *181-192* (1977).

Schuurmans Stekhoven, F.M.A.H., van Heeswijk, M.P.E., de Pont, J.J.H.H.M. & Bonting, S.L. Studies on (Na$^+$ + K$^+$)-activated ATPase. XXXVIII. A 100 000 molecular weight protein as the low-energy phosphorylated intermediate of the enzyme. *Biochim. biophys. Acta* 422: *210-224* (1976).

Skou J.C. The influence of some cations on ATPase from peripheral nerve. *Biochim. biophys. Acta* 23: *394-401* (1957).

Skou, J.C. A Mg- and Na-activated ATPase, possible related to the active, linked transport of Na and K ions across the nerve membrane. *Biochim. Biophys. Acta* 42: *6-23* (1960).

Wheeler, K.P. & Whittam, R. The involvement of phosphatidylserine in adenosine triphosphatase activity of the sodium pump. *J. Physiol., Lond.*, 207: *303-328* (1970).

Authors' address:
Dept. of Biochemistry
University of Nijmegen
Nijmegen, the Netherlands

Docum. Ophthal. Proc. Series, Vol. 18

THE REVERSAL OF TRIPARANOL-INDUCED CATARACT IN THE RAT.

VII. THE CRYSTALLINS OF THE CORTEX AND NUCLEUS RELATED TO AGEING[1]

J. BOURS, LOUISE GRUBER, O. HOCKWIN & J.E. HARRIS

(Bonn-Venusberg F.R.G., Minneapolis U.S.A.)

ABSTRACT

Cataracts were induced in rat lenses by feeding of triparanol. In a number of animals a reversal of these cataracts occurred. Thin-layer isoelectric focusing was carried out to separate crystallins in pre-α-, α-, 12 β- and 8 γ-crystallin components. Compared to the normal lens, the cataractous lens cortex and nucleus show a decrease of γ-crystallins and a considerable increase of albuminoid. In the cataractous lens that cleared again an almost complete recovery of transparency was observed, accompanied by a diminishment of the albuminoid content and an augmentation of the content of all watersoluble crystallins. In the clearing cataractous lens there is a tendency to return to normal values of lens wet weight, and water-soluble and insoluble dry weight. The feeding of triparanol appears to cause an artificial ageing of the rat lens.

INTRODUCTION

In a previous paper Bours et al (1978) reported that most of the cataractous lenses which developed in rats fed triparanol, cleared after returning the rats to a normal diet. Some animals never developed cataracts. The composition of the water-soluble crystallins of the lenses aged from 98 to 781 days from the normal and the triparanol fed rats was examined by thin layer isoelectric focusing and separated into α-crystallin, 12 β-crystallin components and 8 γ-crystallin components. The cataractous lenses showed a loss of γ- and β-crystallin components compared to the normal. In lenses where the induced cataract cleared the damage was less pronounced, and the change was similar to that seen during the ageing process.

It is the aim of the present report to examine the crystallins by thin layer isoelectric focusing and the albuminoid by determination of the water − -insoluble dry weight from the lens cortex and nucleus during the cataractous and the clearing stages of the triparanol cataract in the rat.

1 Supported in part by the 'Deutsche Forschungsgemeinschaft' (Ho 249/8, Oh 32/1), and by the U.S. Public Health Service Grant EY 01200-03. This paper was included in this special issue without the prior knowledge of John E. Harris.

MATERIALS AND METHODS

Weanling female wistar rats (21-day-old) were fed a diet containing 0.075% triparanol for 67-73 days, according to Harris & Gruber (1969, 1972). For the purpose of this article lenses are divided into 3 groups: (1) controls; (2) cataractous and (3) cataractous with subsequent clearing. The wet weight of the lenses was determined, and the lenses were dissected to obtain the cortex and the nucleus. These parts were weighed and lyophilized to determine the dry weight and the water-content, homogenized and centrifuged at 38,000 g for 1 h. The sediments were washed 3 times to free them from the water-soluble crystallins, and the total amounts of water-soluble and insoluble dry weights were determined by weighing. The ratios of the water-soluble crystallins and the water-insoluble albuminoid were calculated from the dry weights of all samples. The water-soluble crystallins were separated by thin-layer isoelectric focusing at a voltage of 220-1,200 V during 90 min and at an amperage of 20-11 mA, and stained with Coomassie Brilliant Blue according to Bours (1977). The percentage of the various lens crystallins present in each sample which were separated by isoelectric focusing was calculated from the densitometric tracings. Patterns of crystallin composition with regard to age dependence were made from the percent values by calculation of the linear regression lines of the crystallins and their components.

RESULTS

Table 1 gives the protocol of the experiments: the age and number of animals, the number of days on triparanol, the onset of cataract and the onset of clearing.

Figure 1 gives: a) the wet weight, b) the dry weight, c) the water-soluble dry weight, d) the water-insoluble dry weight, e) the ratio and f) the percent of water as determined for three groups of protein samples:

1. The normal lens in dependence on age (CONTR)

The normal whole lens and the cortex showed an increase of the wet and dry weight (Fig. 1a, b), and in the nucleus the wet and dry weight showed a constant level. The water-soluble and -insoluble dry weight (Fig. 1c, d) decreased in the whole lens and in the nucleus. The percent of water (Fig. 1f) of the whole lens, the cortex and the nucleus demonstrated a gradual decrease in dependence on age.

2. The cataractous lens (CAT)

The cataractous lens had a lower wet and dry weight, and a lower water-soluble and -insoluble dry weight. This is due to the synthesis of a lower amount of water-soluble and water-insoluble crystallins. Also the ratio was lower in the cataractous lens (Fig. 1e), due to a lower water-soluble protein

Table 1. triparanol cataracts induced in rats of the same age (21-day-old)

Age (days)	Number of days on triparanol	Age at onset of cataract (days)	Age at onset of clearing (days)	Number of animals	Lens part	Refers to figure	Comments
123	–	–	–	2	C	2a; 5, 7, 9a, b	CONTR
					N	2b; 6, 8, 10a, b	
193	–	–	–	2	C	2e; 5, 7, 9a, b	CONTR
					N	2f; 6, 8, 10a, b	
227	–	–	–	2	C	3a; 5, 7, 9a, b	CONTR
					N	3b; 6, 8, 10a, b	
122	73	97	NC	2	C	2c; 5, 7, 9c, d	CAT
					N	2d; 6, 8, 10c, d	
192	70	78	NC	2	C	2g; 5, 7, 9c, d	CAT
					N	2h; 6, 8, 10c, d	
225	67	93	NC	1/2	C	3c; 5, 7, 9c, d	CAT
					N	3d; 6, 8, 10c, d	
194	70	88	158	2	C	2j; 5, 7, 9e, f	CAT & CLR
					N	2k; 6, 8, 10e, f	
225	67	87	195	1/2	C	3e; 5, 7, 9e, f	CAT & CLR
					N	3f; 6, 8, 10e, f	

Legend: C = lens cortex; N = lens nucleus; CAT = cataract; CAT & CLR = cataract and clearing; CONTR = control experiment; NC = no clearing; – = not of application.

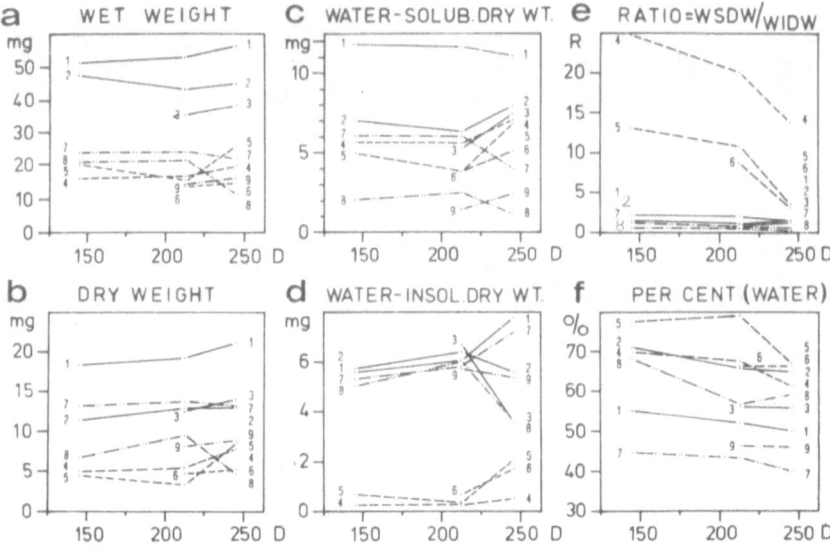

Fig. 1. *Determination of various parameters of normal and triparanol-induced cata-*
ractous lenses. 1, 4, 7 = control experiment (normal values); 2, 5, 8 = cataract; 3, 6, 9
= cataract and clearing.
●————● = whole lens; ●————● = cortex; ●—··——··—● = nucleus.

content. A marked swelling of the cataractous whole lens was noted due to
a higher water content than in the normal case. There was a decrease in
water-soluble protein in both the cortex and the nucleus, as well as a decrease in water-insoluble proteins in the nucleus; explaining why the ratios in
the cortex and nucleus were also lower. Both the nucleus and the cortex had
higher water content than found in the corresponding parts of the normal
lens.

3. *The cataractous lens that cleared again (CAT & CLR)*

In the clearing cataractous lens there was a tendency to attain normal values
again, which may be understood as an almost complete recovery of the
cleared lens. This tendency of return to normal values was observed in the
wet weight, the dry weight, the water-soluble and -insoluble dry weight and

Fig. 2. *Thin-layer isoelectric focusing patterns* of the crystallins of the rat lens with
triparanol-induced cataracts (c, d; g, h), with subsequent clearing (j, k) and of normal
lenses (control: a, b; e, f). C = lens cortex, N = lens nucleus, d = age in days. The
samples a-k contained 400 μg of protein. The scale shows the pH-values along the gel,
measured at 4° C. The Roman numerals I-IV and I-III denote the groups of β- and
γ-crystallin components. The numbers β_{1-12} and γ_{1-8} indicate the single crystallin
components isofocused.

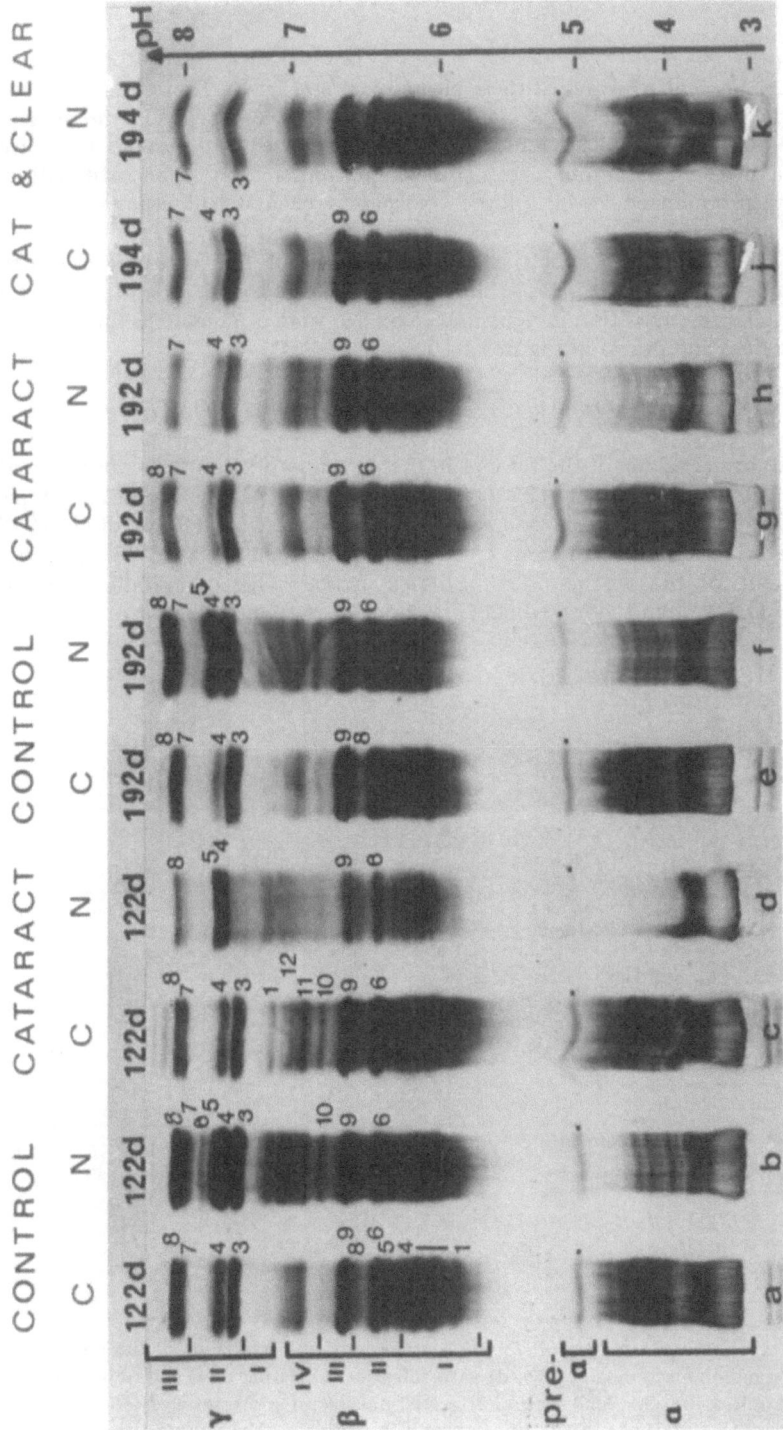

in the percent of water of these cleared lenses (Fig. 1). There was a decrease in the water-insoluble material in the whole lens, especially in the nucleus. The ratio in the whole lens and in the lens cortex and nucleus was lower than in the cataractous case. This can be understood as an artificial and more pronounced ageing of the transparent cleared lens compared to the normal lens.

The thin-layer isoelectric focusing patterns of the 3 groups of protein samples as mentioned above are given in Figure 2 and 3. The patterns of crystallin composition in dependence on age were calculated as linear regression lines and drawn in Figures 4-10.

The normal ageing, control experiments (CONTR)

The normal ageing of the rat lens in the present work concerns only 3 events in the growth curve: 122 days (Fig. 2a, b), 192 days (Fig. 2e, f) and 226 days (Fig. 3a, b), in contrast to the previous work (Bours et al., 1978) where the ageing of the lens covered the time span of 98- to 781 days. The percent of the water-soluble proteins increases for α-crystallins and decreases for β- and γ-crystallins (Fig. 4-6a) in the whole lens, the cortex and

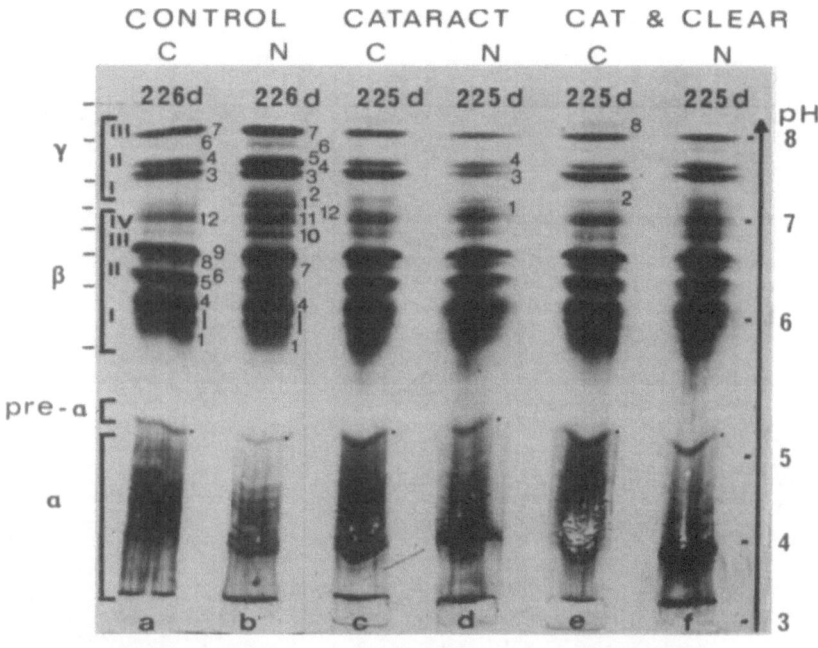

Fig. 3. Thin-layer isoelectric focusing patterns of the crystallins of the rat lens with triparanol-induced cataracts (c, d) with subsequent clearing (e, f) and of normal lenses (control: a, b). C = lens cortex, N = lens nucleus; d = age in days. The samples a-f amount to 400 μg of protein. For further information see the subscript to Figure 2.

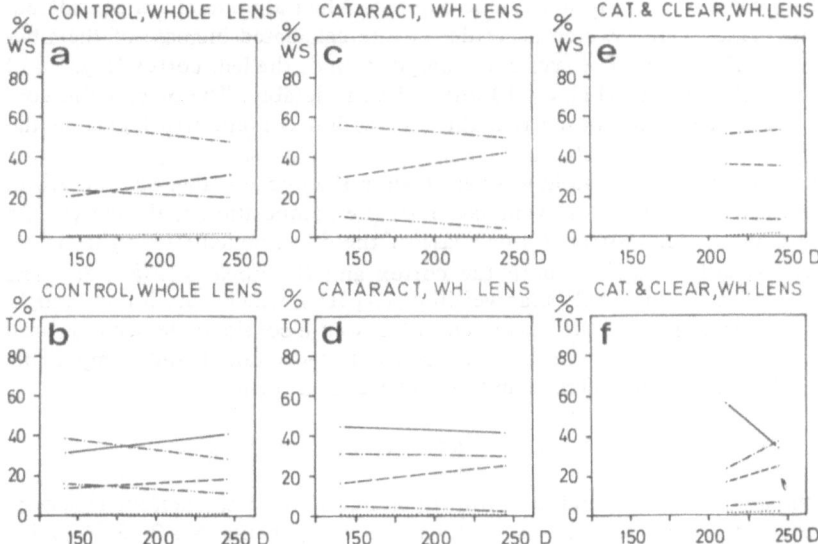

Fig. 4. Crystallin composition of the control whole rat lens compared to lenses which developed a cataract and those which cleared again after the cataract. ●———● = α-crystallin; ●—.—.—● = β-crystallins; ●—..—● = γ-crystallins; .... = pre α-crystallins; ●———● = albuminoid.

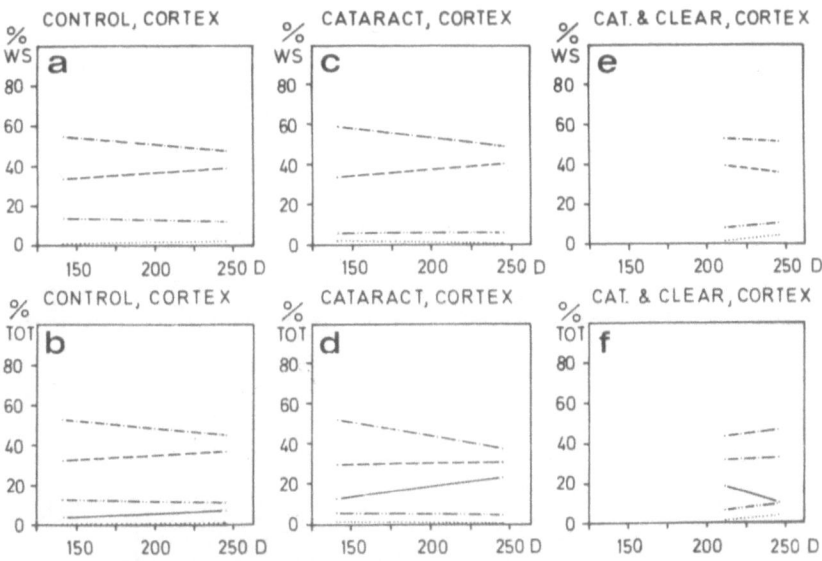

Fig. 5. Crystallin composition of the control lens cortex compared to the cortex of lenses which developed a cataract and those which cleared after the cataract. For further explanation see the subscript to Fig. 4.

the nucleus of ages from 122-226-day-old. When albuminoid is considered, these values were lowered according to the calculated increase of the albuminoid (Fig. 4-6b). The crystallin composition of the lens cortex (Fig. 5a, b) and of the nucleus (Fig. 6a, b) differed considerably. The α-crystallin content was ·higher in the cortex, the γ-crystallin content was higher in the nucleus, and the β-crystallin content was about the same (Fig. 5-6a, 9-10a). The content of albuminoid was very high in the nucleus (Fig. 6b) and low in the cortex (Fig. 5b). An examination of the composition of the β-crystallin components demonstrated a decrease of the β-components of higher molecular weight (β_{1-4}:I) of both the cortex and the nucleus (Fig. 7-8a). The β-crystallins of low molecular weight β_{10-12} :IV), which were found in highest concentrations in the lens nucleus, showed a considerable decrease with ageing (Fig. 8a). The content of the total γ-crystallins and components revealed a moderate decrease in the cortex and in the nucleus.

2. The cataractous lens (CAT)

Compared to the normal lens, the triparanol-induced cataractous lens demonstrated a disappearance of γ-crystallin components Nrs 2, 3, 6 and 7 (Fig. 2d) and a lower content of γ-crystallins in the cortex and the nucleus (Fig. 4-6c, d), but albuminoid in increasing amounts in the cortex and nucleus (Fig. 4-5d). In the cataractous lens nucleus the albuminoid reached a value of over 70% (Fig. 6d). The β-crystallins of high molecular weight β_{1-4}:I) showed a somewhat elevated level in the lens nucleus, but the rest of

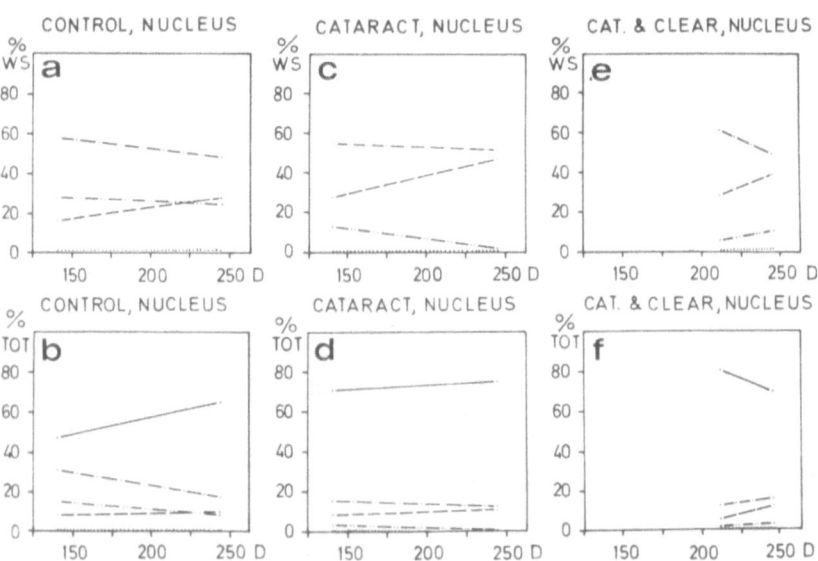

Fig. 6. Crystallin composition of the lens nucleus. For further explanations see the subscripts to Figs. 4 and 5.

the β-crystallin components were similar to the controls (Fig. 7-8c, d). The γ-crystallin components revealed a lower protein content than in the controls. In the nucleus, the components No. 3-6 (II) showed a sharp decrease with ageing (Fig. 10c, d), while in the cortex the lowered values were constant with ageing (Fig. 9c, d).

3. The cataractous lens that cleared again (CAT & CLR)

The clearing cataractous lens demonstrated an almost complete recovery of transparency, which was accompanied by an increase of pre-α-, α-, β- and γ-crystallin values and a decrease of the amount of albuminoid (Fig. 4-6f), as well in the cortex as in the nucleus. In figures 5f and 6f the percent total of albuminoid showed at 194 days a value corresponding to the cataractous cortex and nucleus, but there was thereupon up to 226 days a sharp decrease. The decrease in albuminoid was accompanied by an increase in soluble crystallins. This suggests a considerable stimulus of new synthesis of water-soluble crystallins and a certain decline of synthesis of albuminoid.

DISCUSSION

In the normal rat whole lens the β-crystallins of low molecular weight (β_{IV}) and the γ-crystallins decrease markedly with age (Fig. 4a; Bours, 1978), and simultaneously the amount of albuminoid increases with ageing (Fig. 4a, b; Bours, 1977, 1978). Part of this increase of the albuminoid moiety may be due to the decrease of the β_{IV}- and γ-crystallins. In the normal rat lens nucleus (Fig. 9a, b) the total amount of γ-crystallins and components is considerably higher than in the lens cortex (Fig. 10a, b). The γ-crystallins isolated from the lens nucleus and those isolated from the lens cortex vary in their distribution of components separated by isoelectric focusing (Fig. 2a, b, 2e, f, 3a, b). This phenomenon has also been observed in other species such as ox and dog (Bours & Hockwin, 1976, 1977).

In the cataractous lens the loss of γ-crystallins was even more pronounced (Fig. 9-10c, d) than in the controls (Bours et al., 1978). The cataractous lens that cleared again showed a recovery of the crystallin composition (Fig. 4-10f), which was also found in the previous study (Bours et al., 1978). In the clearing cataractous lens an increase of the dry weight (Fig. 1b) and of the soluble protein level (Fig. 1c) but a decrease of lens water was observed (Fig. 1f). Harris & Gruber (1969, 1972, 1973) and Rathbun et al. (1973) have also observed that the clearing of the triparanol cataracts represents a true reversal of the cataractous process, accompanied by an increase of the soluble protein level and dry weight, while the sodium concentration and the amount of lens water tended to return to normal values.

CONCLUSIONS

The phenomena observed may be explained as follows:
1. The normal ageing shows a difference in crystallin composition between

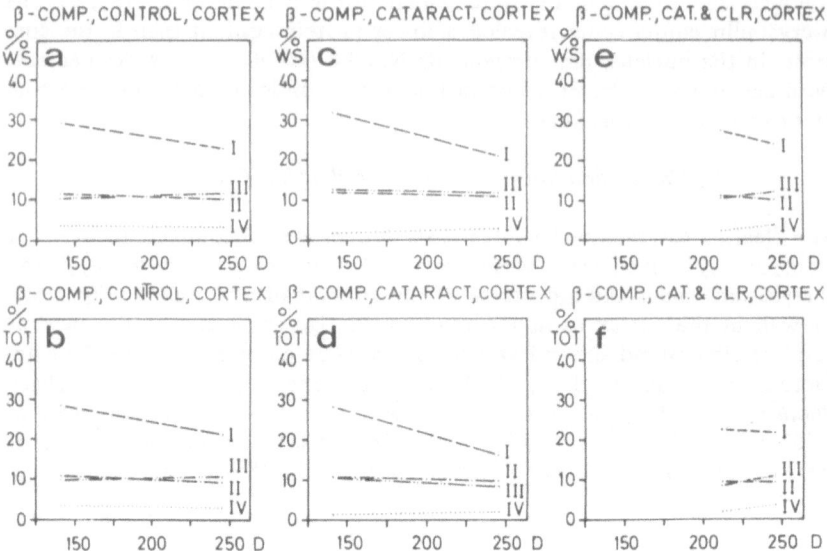

Fig. 7. *Composition of the β-crystallin components* of the control lens cortex compared to the cortex of lenses which developed a cataract and those which cleared after the cataract. I = β-components Nr. 1-4; II = β-components Nr. 5-7; III = β-components Nr. 8-10; IV = β-components Nr. 11-12.

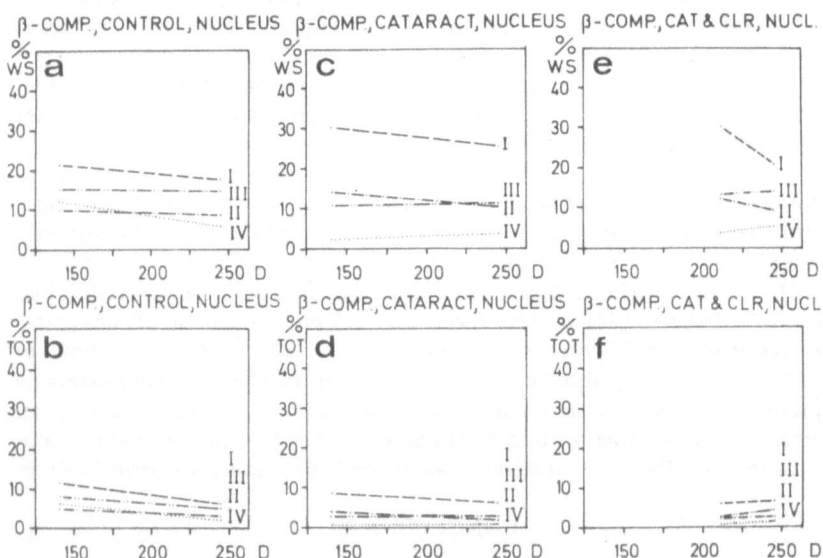

Fig. 8. *Composition of the β-crystallin components* of the lens nucleus. For further explanations see the subscript to Fig. 7.

60

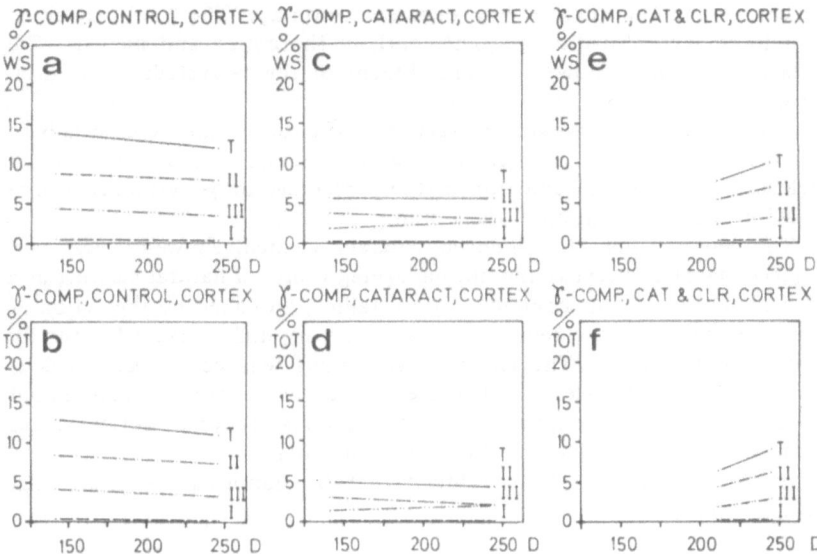

Fig. 9. *Composition of the γ-crystallin components* of the control lens cortex compared to the cortex of lenses which developed a cataract and those which cleared again after the cataract. T = total γ-crystallins; I = γ-components Nr. 1-2; II = γ-components Nr. 3-6; III = γ-components Nr. 7-9.

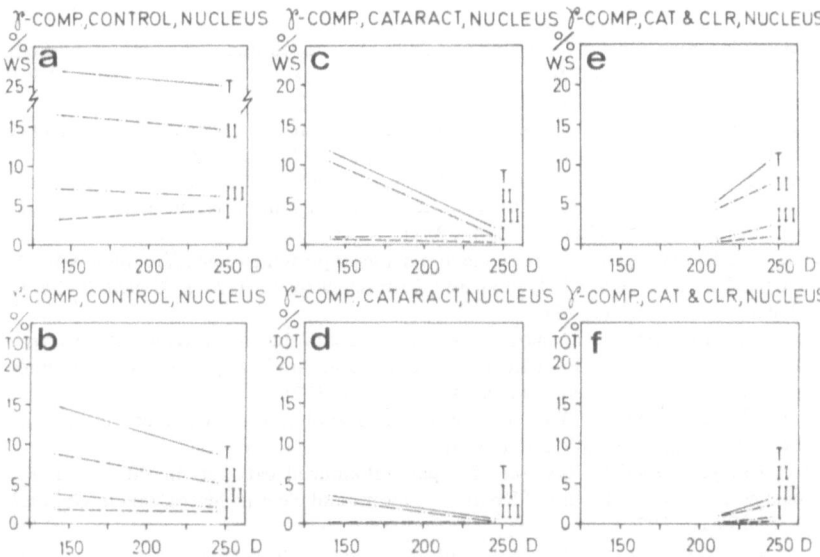

Fig. 10. *The composition of the γ-crystallin components of the lens nucleus.* For further explanations see the subscript to Fig. 9.

the cortex and the nucleus with dependence on age. The total percent of albuminoid increased during ageing, both in the cortex and nucleus. The normal ageing lens showed a diminishment of the γ-crystallin concentrations.

2. The lenses with provoked cataract and no clearing showed especially in the nucleus, a loss of β- and γ-crystallin components, and in both cortex and nucleus a considerable reduction in the percentage of γ-crystallins accompanied by an augmentation of the albuminoid level.

3. The lenses where the induced cataract cleared, showed a less pronounced damage, because the normal ageing caused a natural clearing at a moment where the low content of γ-crystallins, provoked by the action of triparanol, matched the reduced amount of γ-crystallin reached naturally during normal ageing. The clearing cataractous lens cortex and nucleus showed complete recovery, which is expressed as decrease of albuminoid and increase of water-soluble crystallins, and a restoration of normal values of lens wet and dry weight and the percent of water.

4. In this way it may be concluded that triparanol causes an artificial ageing of the lens.

ACKNOWLEDGMENTS

We are thankful to Mr Axel Ecker and Mr Helmut Lemoch for their skilful technical assistance, and to Mrs Elke Oellers for the photographic illustrations.

REFERENCES

Bours, J. The crystallins of the ageing lens from five species studied by various methods of thin-layer isoelectric focusing; in Radola & Graesslin Electrofocusing and isotachophoresis, pp. *303-312* (de Gruyter, Berlin, 1977).

Bours, J. Isoelectric focusing and isotachophoresis of rat lens crystallins in dependence on age. Interdiscipl. Topics Geront., vol 12, pp. *196-204* (Karger, Basel, 1978).

Bours, J., Gruber, L., Hockwin, O. and Harris, J. The crystallins of the rat lens with triparanol-induced cataracts, also related to ageing. Interdiscipl. Topics Geront., vol. 12, pp. *127-131* (Karger, Basel, 1978).

Bours, J. & Hockwin, O. Artunterschiede bei Linsenproteinen nach Trennung mit Isoelektrofokussierung auf Polyacrylamid-Dünnschichtplatten. *Berl. Münch. Tierärztl. Wschr.* 89: *417-422* (1976).

Bours, J. & Hockwin, O. Charakterisierung der wasserlöslichen Proteine der Linse mittels Immunologie und Isoelektrofokussierung und ihre Beziehungen zum Alterungsprozeß. *Klin. Monatbl. Augenheilk.* 170: *51-59* (1977).

Harris, J.E. & Gruber, L. The reversal of triparanol-induced cataracts in the rat. *Docum. Ophthal.* 26: *324-333* (1969).

Harris, J.E. & Gruber, L. Reversal of triparanol-induced cataracts in the rat. II. Exchange of ^{22}Na, ^{42}K, and ^{86}Rb in cataractous and clearing lenses. *Invest. Ophthal.* 11: *608-616* (1972).

Harris, J.E. & Gruber, L. The reversal of triparanol-induced cataracts in the rat. III. Amino acid content and uptake of ^{14}C α-AIB in cataractous and clearing lenses. *Invest. Ophthal.* 12: *385-388* (1973).

Rathbun, W.B., Harris, J.E., Vagstad, G. & Gruber, L. The reversal of triparanol-induced cataract in the rat. IV. Reduced sulfhydryl groups in soluble protein and glutathione. *Invest. Ophthal.* 12: *388-390* (1973).

Authors' address:
J. Bours,
Division of Biochemistry of the Eye,
Institute for Experimental Ophthalmology,
University of Bonn,
D-5300 Bonn-Venusberg, F.R.G.

Docum. Ophthal. Proc. Series, Vol. 18

INHIBITION OF SORBITOL PRODUCTION IN HUMAN LENSES BY AN ALDOSE REDUCTASE INHIBITOR

LEO T. CHYLACK, JR., HORACE F. HENRIQUES III
& WILLIAM H. TUNG

(Boston, Massachusetts) U.S.A.

ABSTRACT

Clear and cataractous non-diabetic, human lenses were obtained from eye bank eyes or at the time of routine cataract extraction. Fresh lenses were assayed for glucose, sorbitol, fructose, and aldose reductase and polyol dehydrogenase activities. A significant drop in aldose reductase actvity occurs during cataractogenesis. Clear and cataractous lenses were incubated in either 5.5 mM or 35.5 mM glucose medium with or without the aldose reductase inhibitor AY22,284 (1,3-dioxo-1H-benz-[de]-isoquinoline-2-(3H) acetic acid) present in a final concentration of 4×10^{-4} M. In the presence of high glucose, both the clear and cataractous lenses accumulate significant levels of sorbitol, fructose, and a high percentage gain sufficient water to rupture spontaneously. Due to the significant swelling of cataractous lenses in control medium, and the high rate of spontaneous rupture in high-glucose medium it was not possible to correlate the net sorbitol accumulation with the net change in wet weight. The presence of the aldose reductase inhibitor completely blocked net sorbitol accumulation and reduced fructose accumulation. This reduction occurred in the presence of high lenticular glucose levels and unchanged polyol dehydrogenase activity. The similarity of the human and animal lenticular responses to high glucose is striking (van Heyningen 1959a; Chylack & Kinoshita 1969). The relevance of this to 'senile' cataract formation in diabetics and the promise of aldose reductase inhibitors as a medical treatment for cataracts are discussed.

INTRODUCTION

In spite of the wealth of evidence documenting the relevance of sugar alcohol formation via the sorbitol pathway to cataractogenesis in animals (van Heyningen, 1959, 1956; Kinoshita, et al., 1962; Kinoshita & Merola, 1964; Chylack & Kinoshita, 1969), there is only one publication (Pirie & van Heyningen, 1964) showing elevated sorbitol levels in human diabetic lenses. However, much inferential data points to the existence of the sorbitol pathway in human lenses: (1) the acute cataract of the uncontrolled diabetic (O'Brien, et al., 1934; O'Brien & Allan, 1942), (2) the frequency with which uncontrolled diabetics experience change in refractive error (presumably due to

This work was supported by U.S.P.H.S. Research Grant No. AYO1276, Career Development Award EY00034, the Brigham Surgical Group Foundation and the Cooperative Cataract Research Group.

osmotically induced changes in lens volume as sorbitol accumulated (Granstrom 1933) (3) and more recently, the reversible cataract in a diabetic patient with wide fluctuations in blood sugar (Epstein 1976).

The recent demonstrations that aldose reductase inhibitors are capable of preventing sugar cataract formation in animals (Chylack & Kinoshita 1969; Dvornik, et al 1973) and the exciting discovery by Varma that the bioflavonoids are potent, non-toxic inhibitors of aldose reductase (Varma & Kinoshita 1976; Varma et al. 1977) add to the optimism that a medical 'cure' for diabetic cataracts may soon be available. These discoveries make it mandatory to conclusively show that the human lens is capable of producing sorbitol in the presence of high glucose, and, of equal importance, that the human lens is responsive to an aldose reductase inhibitor. This study was done with these goals in mind.

METHODS

Non-diabetic, human lenses were obtained from the New England Eye Bank, usually within 36 hours of death, and from patients undergoing routine intra-capsular cataract extraction at the Massachusetts Eye & Ear Infirmary. Cataracts were gently irrigated from the tip of the cryoprobe with Balanced Salt Solution (Alcon Laboratories, Fort Worth, Texas), immediately after extraction. They were photographed and classified according to the method of Chylack (1978) and weighed prior to incubation. The incubation medium contained TC-199 without phenol red (GIBCO No. 115, HS, Grand Island, N.Y.) with final concentrations of bicarbonate (34 mM); Ca^{++} (2.5 mM); and glucose (35.5 mM, experimental or 5.5 mM, control). In the control medium, 15 mM NaCl is added so that the final tonicity (290 ± 2 m Osm/l) is the same as in the experimental medium (Chylack & Kinoshita 1969).

All lenses were incubated for 24 hrs. at 37.5°C in 12 ml of control or experimental medium plus 0.6 ml of fetal calf serum (GIBCO No. 614) in 10 x 35 mm plastic Petri dishes (Falcon Plastics, Oxnard, California) (Chylack 1975). At the end of the incubation period, each lens was examined; if ruptured, it was discarded. If intact, it was rephotographed, weighed and homogenized in 3.0 ml of 0.065 M phosphate buffer, pH 6.8, in a ground glass homogenizer (Tenbroeck, Vitro, VWR Scientific, Newton Upper Falls, Mass; Catalog No. 62400-493). 0.5 ml of the homogenate was removed and centrifuged at 27,000 g for 15 min. at 4°C in a Sorvall RC-5 Superspeed Regrigerated Centrifuge (Dupont Instruments, Newton, Conn. 06470). The supernatant was assayed for aldose reductase activity (Hayman, et al. 1966) and protein (Lowry, et al. 1951). To the remainder of the lens homogenate was added 0.625 ml of 50% trichloracetic acid. After homogenization and centrifugation, the supernatant was assayed for glucose, sorbitol and fructose. Glucose was measured enzymatically with the Sigma Diagnostic Kit No. 510 (Sigma Chemical Co., St., Louis, MO). Hexitols were measured by the procedure of West & Rapoport (1949). Fructose was measured with the technique of Roe (1934). The aldose reductase inhibitor, AY22, 284 (Ayerst Pharmaceuticals, Montreal, Quebec, Canada) was prepared fresh weekly as a

4×10^{-3}M solution. The final concentration in the medium was 4×10^{-4}M (Varma & Kinoshita 1976). A solution without inhibitor was prepared in a similar fashion for lenses in control media.

Statistical analysis of data was performed on an HP-97 calculator (Hewlett Packard, Corvallis, Oregon) using the mean and standard deviation functions and program tape ST1-15A, 't-statistics'.

RESULTS

1. Adequacy of Incubation System

While this, or a similar incubation system, has been used successfully in several studies employing animals lenses (Chylack & Kinoshita 1969; Chylack 1975), this was the first time human lens incubations were attempted It was difficult to assess the adequacy of the incubation system with human lenses, since it was impossible to compare paired fresh unincubated and incubated human lenses. Only rarely do clear, paired eye bank lenses become available. Paired identical cataracts are also not available. Therefore, parameters derived from a single lens incubation were utilized to evaluate our incubation system. Clear lenses in contol medium (5.5 mM glucose) remained clear for 48 hrs.; they also experienced only a 6.5% increase in wet weight. Cataractous lenses from eye bank eyes, as well as surgical specimens, swelled in control medium gaining 19 and 24% in wet weight respectively. Surgical specimens all were traumatized by the cryoprobe and might be expected to swell in much the same way as an injured, incubated, animal

Table 1. Cataracts classified according to (Chylack, 1978). Opacification was noted in the following zones: CXE: equatorial cortex; CXA: anterior cortex; SCP: subcapsular posterior zone; SCA: subcapsular anterior zone; N: nuclear; M: mature.

Major Cataract Classification					No. Lenses
	CXE,	SCP,	N		97
	CXE,		N		52
CXA,	CXE,	SCP,	N		52
				M	46
			N		40
		SCP,	N		39
	CXE,	SCP			36
	CXE,	SCP,	N	SCA	35
CXA					33
		Other			280
					—
		TOTAL			710

67

lens. The preservation of clarity and small change in wet weight of clear human lenses indicated that this system was adequate for our purposes. The amount of information to be gained from wet weight changes in cataractous lenses is very limited.

2. Cataract Populations Studied

750 human cataracts have been classified, to date, at the Massachusetts Eye & Ear Infirmary. The most frequent types of cataracts are listed in Table 1. The populations of surgical cataracts (with and without aldose reductase inhibitor) were not significantly different with regard to age (See Table 2) or cataract type and were similar to the total population in the distribution of cataract types. The frequency of mature and advanced cataracts is definitely less in the eye bank cataract population; this is not surprising in view of the lower mean age of the eye bank population. Clear eye bank lenses were obtained from a younger population. In spite of the differences, statistics

Table 2. Mean age ± standard deviation of lenses used in this study. The number of lenses in each group is bracketed. E.B. = eye bank. Surg. = surgical specimen.

	ARI	AGE (yrs)
FRESH(E.B.)	–	41 ± 20 (18)
		p = 1.00
Cataract(E.B.)	–	68 11 (6)
		p = 1.00
Cataract(surg)	–	72 11 (44)
		p = 1.00
Cataract(surg)	+	75 ± 9 (39)

Table 3. Percent change in wet weight of lenses incubated in low and high glucose medium ± standard deviation. Number of lenses studied is bracketed. E.B. = eye bank. Surg. = surgical specimen.

		% CHANGE IN WET WEIGHT		
INCUBATED	ARI	5.5.mM G	P	35.5 mM G
Clear	–	+ 6.5 ± 12.1 (6)	0.85	+ 8.7 ± 8.4 (8)
		p = 1.0		p = 1.00
Cataract(E.B.)	–	+19.1 ± 4.6 (2)	0.33	+ 8.6 ± 6.7 (7)
		p = 1.0		p = 1.0
Cataract(surg)	–	+24.4 ± 21.2 (30)	0.12	+26.6 ± 15.2 (44)
		p = 1.0		p = 1.0
Cataract(surg)	+	+26.0 ± 6.0 (2)	0.79	+27.1 ± 16.8 (39)

suggest that the mean ages of each population are insignificantly different. This will facilitate comparison within the 5.5 mM and 35.5 mM glucose groups.

3. Changes in Wet Weight in 35.5 mM Glucose Medium

Clear lenses incubated in 35.5 mM glucose medium were observed to swell more than lenses in 5.5 mM glucose medium. Frequently, separation of the epithelium from the underlying cortex was observed. That this occurred more strikingly in high than low glucose medium was our strong visual impression, but the statistical significance of the weight change under these conditions is not clear cut (See Table 3). The incidence of lenses swelling sufficiently to rupture spontaneously *in vitro* was much higher in the surgical cataracts in high glucose medium (See Table 4). Our inability to demonstrate a statistically significant weight gain in our high-glucose lenses may

Table 4. Percentage spontaneous rupture of lenses incubated in low and high glucose medium.

INCUBATED	ARI	TOTAL INCUBATED POPULATION MEDIUM	%RUPTURED LENSES	
Clear	–	35.5 mM G	2/22 = 1/11	9%
Cataract(E.B.)	–	,,	2/22 = 1/11	9%
Cataract(surg)	–	,,	10/22 = 5/11	45%
Cataract(surg)	+	,,	6/22 = 3/11	27%
Cataract(surg)	–	5.5 mM G	2/22 = 1/11	9%

Table 5. Sorbitol levels in lenses incubated in low and high glucose medium ± standard deviation. Number of lenses studies is bracketed. E.B. = eye bank. Surg. = surgical specimen.

FRESH			SORBITOL Micromoles/Lens	
Clear			0.27 ± 0.16 (7)	
			$p > 1.0$	
Cataract(surg)			0.32 ± 0.18 (21)	
INCUBATED	*ARI*	*5.5 mM G*	*p*	*35.5 mM G*
Clear	–	0.46 ± 0.28 (6)	<0.001	1.27 ± 0.47 (8)
		$p < 0.70$		$p < 0.50$
Cataract(E.B.)	–	0.30 (1)	<0.13	0.87 ± 0.78 (6)
		$p = 1.0$		$p < 0.50$
Cataract(surg)	–	0.32 ± 0.20 (24)	<0.001	0.62 ± 0.25 (35)
		$p = 1.0$		$p < .001$
Cataract(surg)	+	0.31 ± 0.03 (2)	<0.71	0.33 ± 0.19 (38)

in part have been due to the high rate of spontaneous lens rupture. This would select out of the high-glucose population those lenses which would most clearly demonstrate the swelling. These observations suggest that: (1) the human lens is responding to a glucose load in much the same way as the animal lens (Chylack & Kinoshita 1969), and (2) that cataract surgery damages the lens and makes it less resistant to osmotic stress.

4. Sorbitol Accumulation

The sorbitol concentrations in the fresh, clear and cataractous lenses are not significantly different (0.27-.32 μmoles/lens). (See Table 5).

Incubation in 5.5 mM glucose medium leads to a slight increase in sorbitol level in the clear, but not in the cataractous lens. However, in 35.5 mM glucose, the sorbitol level increases to 1.27 μmoles/lens, a net increase of approximately 100%. In the cataractous lenses, the net accumulation is even greater. It has not been possible to correlate the net changes in sorbitol with the net changes in wet weight, due to the lack of paired identical lenses and to the wide variability in amount of swelling in control medium. However, it is clear that the human lens is capable of producing significant amounts of sorbitol in response to a high glucose load.

5. Aldose Reductase Activity

There is a highly significant drop in aldose reductase activity as cataract formation occurs (See Table 6). There is a slight, but equally significant, further reduction when surgically removed cataracts are incubated in high glucose medium. It is possible that this merely reflects the osmotic damage to aldose reductase-containing fibers.

Table 6. Aldose reductase activity in lenses incubated in low and high glucose medium ± standard deviation. Number of lenses studied is bracketed. E.B. = eye bank. Surg. = surgical specimen.

FRESH			ALDOSE REDUCTASE ACTIVITY ($\Delta OD_{340} \times 1000/5$ *min/mg protein*)	
Clear			7.12 ± 1.57 (6)	
			$p < 0.001$	
Cataract(surg)			3.84 ± 1.16 (8)	
INCUBATED	*ARI*	*5.5 mM G*	*p*	*35.5 mM G*
Clear	—	5.5 ± 3.8 (6)	0.46	6.1 ± 2.5 (8)
		$p < 0.20$		$p < 0.02$
Cataract(E.B.)	—	9.2 ± 3.5 (2)	0.35	3.9 ± 1.5 (7)
		$p < 0.30$		$p < 0.08$
Cataract(surg)	—	4.4 ± 1.9 (24)	0.001	3.0 ± 1.8 (39)
		$p < 0.04$		$p < 0.001$
Cataract(surg)	+	0.7 ± 0.2 (2)	0.08	1.5 ± 1.3 (37)

6. Fructose Levels

Clear and cataractous fresh human lenses have approximately the same fructose level (.15-.19 μmoles/lens) See Table 7. Incubation in high glucose medium leads to a net increase of approximately 36%. That this increase is less than the increase in sorbitol content is to be expected since fructose is fully diffusible through the cell membrane. It is interesting to note in Table 8 that the polyol dehydrogenase activity is highest in clear incubated lenses; also, it is in these lenses that the highest fructose levels are found. The activity of this enzyme is preserved even in cataractous lenses. It is not possible to say from these few experiments if incubation conditions, per se, induce greater polyol dehydrogenase activity.

7. Effects of Aldose Reductase Inhibitor AY22,284

The effects of including 4×10^{-4} M (1,3-dioxo-1H-benz[de]-isoquinoline-2-(3H) acetic acid), an aldose reductase inhibitor commonly known as AY22,284, in the incubation media is clearly shown in Tables 4-8. There is a striking reduction in the number of lenses rupturing spontaneously in high glucose medium. This is not due to a difference in the distribution of cataract types within the two populations of surgical cataracts. There is a highly significant decrease in the aldose reductase activity in cataractous lenses incubated with the inhibitor. Similar decreases were seen with enzyme prepared from clear, fresh lenses. Consistent with this is an equally significant drop in the net sorbitol accumulation. In fact, the production of sorbitol is almost totally blocked. That this difference is not due to a block in glucose entry into the lens is shown in Table 9. It is clear that the glucose levels in lenses with and without the aldose reductase inhibitor are insignificantly

Table 7. Fructose levels in lenses incubated in low and high glucose medium ± standard deviation. Number of lenses studied is bracketed E.B. = eye bank. Surg. = surgical specimen.

FRESH			FRUCTOSE LEVEL Micromoles/Lens	
Clear			0.19 ± 0.08 (7) p < 0.70	
Cataract(surg)			0.15 ± 0.12 (17)	
INCUBATED	*ARI*	*5.5 mM G*	*p*	*35.5 mM G*
Clear	–	0.23 ± 0.16 (6) p = 1.00	<0.04	0.49 ± 0.09 (8) p < 0.10
Cataract(E.B.)	–	0.22 (1) p < 0.04	<0.04	0.35 ± 0.11 (6) p < 0.70
Cataract(surg)	–	0.10 ± 0.04 (24) p < 0.01	<0.001	0.33 ± 0.18 (36) p < 0.40
Cataract(surg)	+	0.10 ± 0.00 (2)	<0.43	0.32 ± 0.15 (38)

different. The results in Table 8 show no difference in the polyol dehydrogenase activity in lenses incubated with and without AY22,284, so it is unlikely that altered polyol dehydrogenase activity is the basis for the difference in sorbitol level. The net fructose level also decreases in the presence of the inhibitor, but these data are based on a few lens pairs.

It is disappointing to have been unable to show a change in wet weight consistent with the decreased sorbitol accumulation. However, it is not the lack of such an effect that is responsible, rather, we believe, it is an effect not demonstrable with cataractous lenses. The membrane damage is sufficiently great to preclude the demonstration of small, osmotically induced, shifts in lens water.

Table 8. Mean polyol dehydrogenase activity in lenses incubated in 35.5 mM glucose medium ± standard deviation. Number of lenses studied is bracketed. E.B. = eye bank. Surg. = surgical specimen.

FRESH		POLYOL DEHYDROGENASE ACTIVITY $(\Delta OD_{340}X1000/5''/ml)$
Clear		75.3 ± 2.7 (2)
		p = 1.00
Cataract		74.0 ± 5.6 (2)
INCUBATED	ARI	
Clear	–	106.6 ± 13.7 (2)
Cataract(E.B.)	–	–
Cataract(surg)	–	84.9 ± 14.2 (3)
		p = 1.00
Cataract(surg)	+	84.3 ± 16.9 (3)

Table 9. Glucose levels in lenses incubated in low and high glucose medium ± standard deviation. Number of lenses studied is bracketed. E.B. = eye bank. Surg. = surgical specimen. The glucose level in control lenses was too low to assay with our method; therefore 0 implies no detectable glucose.

FRESH			GLUCOSE LEVEL Micromoles/lens		
Clear			0.0 (5)		
			p = 1.00		
Cataract			0.0 (1)		
INCUBATED	ARI	5.5 mM G	p		35.5 mM G
Clear	–	0 (2)	<0.001		1.20 ± 0.02 (5)
					p = 1.00
Cataract(E.B.)	–	( )	–		2.03 ± 1.16 (5)
					p = 1.00
Cataract(surg)	–	0 (3)	0.001		4.13 1.84 (27)
		p = 1.00			p = 1.00
Cataract(surg)	+	0 (3)	0.001		4.01 1.76 (30)

DISCUSSION

It has been most encouraging to document the similar responses of human and animal lenses to high glucose and to an aldose reductase inhibitor. That the 'sugar alcohol theory' of cataractogenesis may be relevant to human cataract formation is strengthened by the results of this study. However, we have not demonstrated cataract formation in response to sorbitol accumulation as was done approximately ten years ago by Chylack & Kinoshita (1969) in rabbit lens. Rather, we have shown that the same mechanisms exist in the human lens that have been studied in several different animal lenses. Many lenses in 35.5 mM glucose were observed to swell markedly while others swelled no more than control lenses. The frequency of spontaneous lens rupture in high-glucose lenses is convincing proof of the adverse potential of this osmotic stress. While it is tempting to attribute this swelling solely to intralenticular sorbitol accumulation, our data do not support this strong an association between net (sorbitol plus fructose) accumulation and wet weight gain. The net accumulation of 0.81 μmoles sorbitol and 0.26 μmoles fructose per lens would equal 1.07 μmoles (or 1.07 μosmoles)/ lens. It is obvious that this change in osmolarity is insufficient to account for lens rupture. In our study, levels of sorbitol and fructose are quite similar to those observed by Pirie & van Heyningen (1964) in cataractous lenses extracted from diabetics. They found an inverse correlation between glucose and inositol in cataractous lenses from diabetics and concluded that 'the cataractous lens is no longer able to maintain the concentration gradients between lens fiber and aqueous humor'. Our data, showing a declining sorbitol level as cataract maturation progresses, certainly support this proposal. The highest net sorbitol levels were observed in the clear human lenses obtained from eye bank eyes. Even in these lenses, fiber membranes may become more permeable than normal during the interval between the patient's death and lens extraction. Therefore, it is not unreasonable to expect higher net sorbitol accumulation *in vivo* in young diabetics. If most of the sorbitol is formed in the superficial zones of the lens (where glucose concentration and aldose reductase activity are highest) the osmotic stress may be exerted more forcefully in one region of the lens than would be expected if one assumed a uniform distribution of sorbitol within the lens.

The introduction of insulin and oral hypoglycemic agents has greatly reduced the frequency with which extremely high blood sugars are found. However, fairly wide swings of blood sugar still occur even in patients experiencing 'good control' of blood sugar on these therapeutic agents. Both rapidly changing glucose levels *and* intracellular sorbitol accumulation can exert osmotic stress on lens fibers, and these, in combination, may be sufficient to cause transient opacification of zones of the crystalline lens. The opportunity to eliminate that component of osmotic stress due to sorbitol accumulation, by using an aldose reductase inhibitor such as AY22,284 or the more recently introduced bioflavonoids (Varma 1976, 1977), is one of great potential benefit. By eliminating one cataractogenic process, the overall rate of cataract production and/or maturation may be slowed or stopped completely. Several studies summarized in an excellent recent review article (Hockwin & Koch 1975) have shown the cataractous process to be a cumulative one involving many sub-threshold cataractogenic processes. Interrupting one or more of these in experimental cataracts in animals, has interrupted the cataractogenic process. It is hoped that an aldose reductase inhibitor used in human diabetics may similarly interrupt or delay the cataractogenic process.

ACKNOWLEDGEMENTS

The invaluable assistance of Dr. Lois Smith, Mr. John Downing, Mr. Hugo Cerri, Ms. Anne Sebestyen, Mr. Albert Kalustian and Ms. Kathryn Allen is gratefully acknowledged. The splendid cooperation of surgeons and operating room nurses at the Massachusetts Eye & Ear Infirmary contributed significantly to the success of this study. The constructive criticism offered by Drs. Judith Jedziniak-MacGregor and Hong-Ming Cheng during the course of this research has been greatly appreciated.

REFERENCES

Chylack, L.T., Jr.: Classification of human cataracts. *Archs. Ophthal.* (1978) (In Press).

Chylack, L.T., Jr. & Kinoshita, J.H. A biochemical evaluation of a cataract induced in a high-glucose medium. *Invest. Ophthal.* 8: *401-412* (1969).

Chylack, L.T., Jr. Mechanism of 'hypoglycemic' cataract formation in the rat lens. I. The role of hexokinase instability. *Invest. Ophthal.* 14: *746-755* (1975).

Dvornik, D., Simmard-Duquesene, N., Krami, M., Sestang, K., Gabbay, K.H. & Kinoshita, J.H. Polyol accumulation in galactosemic and diabetic rats: Control an aldose reductase inhibitor. *Science, N.Y.* 182: *1146-1148* (1973).

Epstein, D.L. Reversible unilateral lens opacities in a diabetic patient. *Archs. Ophthal.* 94: *461-463* (1976).

Granstrom, K.D. Reflaktionsverauderingen bei diabetes mellitus. *Acta Ophthal.* 11: *1-160* (1933).

Hayman, S., Lou, M.F., Merola, L.O. & Kinoshita, J.H. Aldose reductase activity in the lens and other tissues. *Biochim. biophys. Acta* 128: *474-482* (1966).

Hockwin, O. & Koch, H.R. Combined noxius influence in Cataract and Abnormalities of the lens. (ed. Bellows, J.G.) Grune and Stratton, New York, 1975, pp. *243-254*.

Kinoshita, J.H., Merola, L.O. & Dikmak, E. Osmotic changes in experimental galactose cataracts. *Expl. Eye Res.* 1: *405-410* (1962).

Kinoshita, J.H. & Merola, L.O. Hydration of the lens during the development of galactose cataract. *Invest. Ophthal.* 3: *577-584* (1964).

Kuck, J.F., Jr. Sorbitol pathway metabolites in the diabetic rabbit lens. *Invest. Ophthal.* 5: *65-74* (1966).

Lowry, O.H., Rosebrough, N.J., Farr, A.L. & Randall, R.J. Protein measurement with the Folin-phenol reagent. *J. biol. Chem.* 193: *265-275* (1951).

O'Brien, C.S., Molsberry, J.M. & Allen, J.H. Diabetic cataract incidence and morphology in 126 young diabetic patients. *J. Am. med. Ass.* 103: *892-897* (1934).

O'Brien, C.S. & Allen, J.H. Ocular changes in young diabetic patients. *J. Am. med. Ass.* 120: *190-192* (1942).

Pirie, A. & van Heyningen, R. The effect of diabetes on the content of sorbitol, glucose, fructose and inositol in the human lens. *Expl. Eye Res.* 3: *124-131* (1964).

Roe, J.H. A colorimetric method for the determination of fructose in blood and urine. *J. biol. Chem.* 107: *15-22* (1934).

van Heyingen, R. Formation of polyols by the lens of the rat with 'sugar' cataract. *Nature* 184: *194-195* (1959a).

van Heyningen, R. Metabolism of xylose by the lens. *Biochem. J.* 73: *197-207* (1959b).

Varma, S.D. & Kinoshita, J.H. Sorbitol pathway in diabetic and galactosemic rat lens. *Biochim. biophys. Acta* 338: *632-640* (1974).

Varma, S.D. & Kinoshita, J.H. Inhibition of lens aldose reductase by flavonoids – their possible role in the prevention of diabetic cataracts. *Biochem. Pharmac.* 25: *2505-2513* (1976).

Varma, S.D., Mizuno, A. & Kinoshita, J.H. Diabetic cataracts and flavonoids. *Science* 195: *205-206* (1977).

West, C.D. & Rapoport, S. Modification of colorimetric method for determination of mannitol and sorbitol in plasma and urine. *Proc. Soc. exp. Biol. Med.* 70: *141-146* (1949).

Authors' address:
Howe Laboratory of Ophthalmology
Harvard Medical School
and the Massachusetts Eye & Ear Infirmary
Boston, Massachusetts, USA

ALTERATION OF LENS TONICITY BY LOW TEMPERATURE AND THE EFFECT OF INHIBITORS ON OSMOTIC WATER TRANSPORT

W.L. FOWLKS

(Minneapolis, U.S.A.)

ABSTRACT

Osmotic water transfer, between excised rabbit lenses and an incubation medium of constant ionic concentration but different osmotic pressures, is altered by a temperature change even when lens permeable solutes in the medium and lens have equal concentrations, the isotonic point changes from 273 mOsmolal at 35°C to 343 mOsmolal at 0°C. Thus in vivo at steady state, the lens is maintained approximately 40 mOsmolal hypertonic to serum. Changes in composition of the incubation medium had no measurable effect on the osmotic exchange of water at either temperature. Increasing or decreasing K^+ concentration did not affect the uptake of water at 0°C, thus, hydration at low temperature is not due to an approach to Donnan equilibrium. Ouabain 7×10^{-4} M, did not affect osmotic water exchange at 35°C, but at 35°C, F^- 20 mM, or oxalate, 10 mM, had the same affect as the 0°C temperature. Calcium free medium with EDTA, 10 mM, had no significant effect on osmotic water exchange at 35°C. The hypertonic (compared to serum) lens secretes a hypotonic solution even when cation transport is completely inhibited.

INTRODUCTION

Transport of water, not mediated directly by the transport of any known solute, has been shown in insects (Beament, 1964) and in at least one plant species (Ginsburg & Ginzburg, 1971). House (1974, p. 285) suggests that recent findings of hypotonic amnionic fluid bathing mammalian embryos at early stages of development may also imply transport of water not involving solute transport.

Harris (1966) hypothesized that the water balance of the lens is closely associated with its sodium ion content although he also noted that the water balance of the lens (both rat and rabbit) is not affected significantly by concentrations of ouabain which severely inhibit the transport of cations and other substances. Cotlier, et al. (1968) concluded that the lens is a 'perfect osmometer'. Patterson & Fournier (1976) observed that isolated rat lenses incubated in hypotonic media (149-296 mOsmol) first swelled then returned to their normal volume during the next two days. Fowlks (1973a) reported that the normal rabbit lens will dehydrate itself in silicone oil and that the fluid secreted is hypotonic to serum (Fowlks, 1973b).

METHODS

The lenses used in these experiments were obtained from 1.5-2.0 kg, New Zealand Giant strain, albino rabbits. Lenses were excised as soon post mortem as possible by the method previously reported (Fowlks, 1973a). The first lens excised from one rabbit was used as a control. The second lens was used for the experiment. Control lenses were freed immediately after excision of excess fluids and vitreous body by rolling them on hardened filter paper barely dampened with 0.9% saline. They were then rapidly weighed into a silica crucible and dried to constant weight in an oven ($100°C \pm 1°C$, approximately 48 hrs). The experimental lenses were only freed of most of the vitreous body before incubation. After incubation, they were freed of surface fluids and tissues and analyzed by the same method used for their paired control. Sodium and potassium content of some of the dried lenses were determined as reported by Harris (1966).

Four different incubation media were used (Table 1). The isocomposite medium (ICM) contained most of the low molecular weight solutes which have been reported to be present in the rabbit lens (Prince & Eglitis, 1964; Reddy & Kinsey, 1962 and 1963; van Heyningen, 1962) and at the same concentrations. The amino acid medium (AAM) contains a set of amino acids which have been reported to be transported into the lens by the different amino acid transport systems. This solution also contained inorganic constituents at intralenticular concentrations. An inorganic medium (IOM) containing only the inorganic constituents of ICM was also used in some experiments. The osmolarity of all solutions was adjusted by addition of raffinose and the pH was adjusted to 7.3-7.4 by bubbling a gas mixture containing 5% CO_2 and 95% O_2 unless otherwise stated.

No more than four lenses were incubated sequentially in a 10 ml aliquot of the medium used. Incubation times were 30 min except one set of 1 hr. The medium was stirred with a magnetic stirrer and its temperature controlled by a water bath. During incubation the lenses were supported on the nylon grid of an acrylic plastic device designed to allow the stirred medium to flow over and around the lens.

The osmolality of the medium used was measured immediately at the conclusion of an experiment by comparison with NaCl standard solutions using a Mechrolab 302A vapor pressure osmometer at $37°C$ with a 200 milliosmolal (mOsmolal) standard solution (containing 6.25g NaCl/Kg H_2O) in the sample chamber of the instrument and on the reference probe. The other standard solutions of NaCl used contained sufficient excess NaCl to compensate for the lowered thermodynamic activity of NaCl at the concentration used, i.e. the 300 mOsmolal standard solution contained 9.46g NaCl/Kg H_2O. The osmometer was standardized before and after each measurement of the osmolality of an incubation medium.

The differences (experimental minus control) in weight of water, Δw, and in the dry weight, Δd, were calculated. If Δd differed more than 2 mg, the data were not used. The percent change in weight of water was calculated by: $\%\Delta w = (\Delta w/w) 100$ w = water (g) of the control lens. The data for each lens was submitted to a computer for calculation and plot of the linear regression line and to plot the data points.

Oxygen uptake at 5°C and at 35°C of freshly excised rabbit lenses was measured in 4 ml of modified Tyrode's medium, Table 1, using a model 53 biological oxygen monitor (Yellow Springs Industries). The plexiglas plunger, which supported the Clark electrode and sealed the test chamber from

Table 1. Composition of the media used.

Constituent**	Isocomposite Medium	Amino acid Medium	Inorganic Medium	Modified Tyrode's
Na$^+$	23	23	25.1	151
K$^+$	121	121	121	4.9
Ca^{++}	0.69	0.69	0.69	3.6
Mg^{++}	0.37	0.37	0.37	1.0
Cl$^-$	14.8	14.8	14.8	134
H$_2$PO$_4^-$	1.5	1.5	1.5	0.55
HCO$_3^-$	130	130	132	30.6
D-Glucose	–	–	–	8.33*
D-Glucose-6PO$_4$	29.81*	–		
L-Ascorbate	19.94*	–		
Glutathione	17.81*	–		
Inositol	12.46*	–		
Taurine	6.85	6.85		
Urea	5.98	–		
L-Glutamic Acid	5.83	5.83		
L-Alanine	2.54	2.54		
L-Glutamine	1.97*	–		
Glycine	1.79	1.79		
L-Serine	1.42	–		
L-Proline	1.05	1.05		
L-Tyrosine	0.88	–		
L-Asparagine	0.66*	–		
L-Valine	0.66	–		
L-Lysine	0.54	0.54		
L-β-Alanine	0.53	–		
L-Threonine	0.51	–		
L-Phenylalanine	0.41	–		
L-Histidine	0.35	0.35		
L-Leucine	0.34	0.34		
L-Arginine	0.33*			
L-Isoleucine	0.22			
L-Methionine	0.16*			
Lactate	0.09*			
Raffinose	Variable to adjust osmolality.*			

* These constituents were weighed into a sterile solution of the other constituents. After the solids had dissolved the solution was bubbled with 95% O$_2$, 5% CO$_2$ mixture until pH = 7.3 – 7.4 unless noted otherwise.
** milliatoms/Kg/H$_2$O for single element ions, mM/Kg for all others.

atmospheric O_2, was modified by addition of a plexiglas extension and a nylon filament grid to support the lens near the electrode and allow the magnetic stirrer in the test chamber to circulate fluid over and around the lens. The medium in the test chamber was equilibrated with gas (5% CO_2, 95% O_2) prior to addition of the lens.

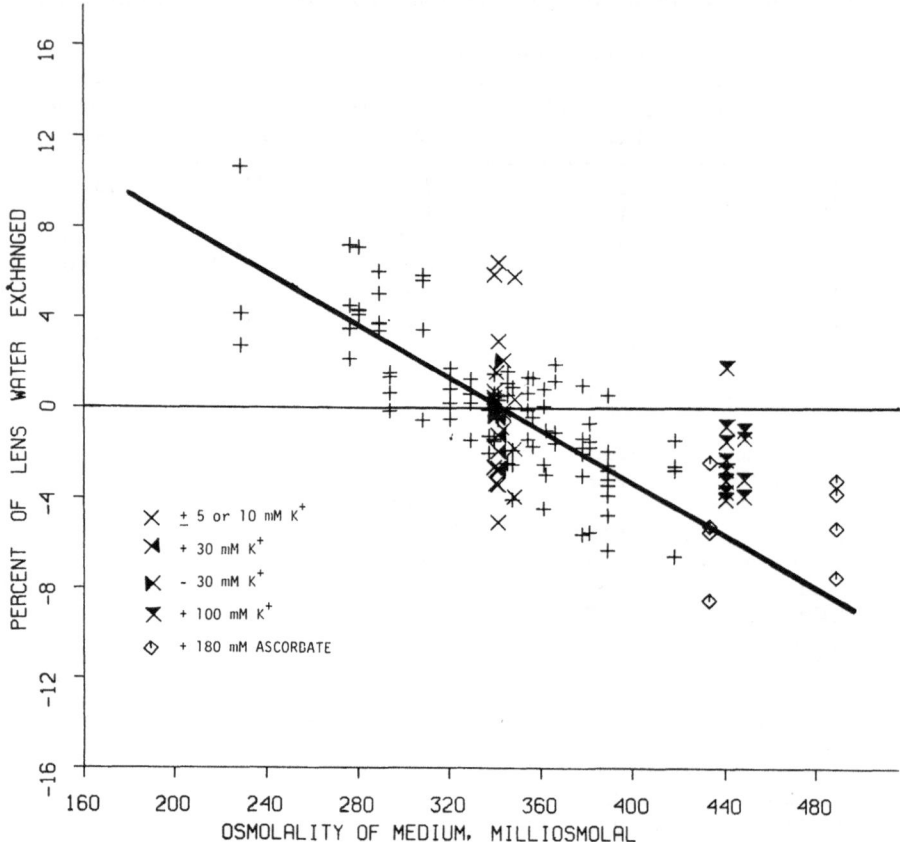

Fig. 1. The heavy line is the linear regression line for the data from 92 lenses depicted by + with an isotonic point at 343 mOsmolal. Note that these data, +, appear to be uniformly and randomly distributed about the line even though they are data from experiments done either in ICM, AAM, IOM or modified Tyrodes at 0°C for 30 min and the 23 lenses incubated for 60 min (Table II). In none of these media do a preponderance of the data at any particular osmolality range lie either above or below the line as is evident from examination of the data in Table II and III. The mean for all the data points from 339 to 348 mOsmolal is −0.28 ± 5.85 (n = 40). Note that of the 100 mM excess K⁺ data and 180 mM ascorbate data only one point lies further above the line than the highest points near the isotonic point. The K⁺ data is a test of the role of Donnan equilibrium in water uptake by the lens at 0°C. The excess ascorbate experiments were the result of an arithmetical error in calculating the amount of ascorbate to use.

80

RESULTS

The lenses from 24 animals were prepared for analysis and analyzed for water and dry weight as reported in the methods section. The first lens excised was obtained from an eye which was randomly chosen from a pair of eyes from one animal. The mean difference in weight of water found was 0.90 mg (± 3.93, standard deviation of the mean). The difference in dry weight was −0.10 mg (± 0.56). In a retrospective study of the lens pairs of 180 animals it was found that only 3.3 percent of the animals had a difference in dry weight of their lenses in excess of 2.5 mg. Thus it appears that one lens from an animal is a satisfactory control lens for the experiments reported herein.

The results of incubation at 0°C in media of different compositions and osmolalities of the lenses from 92 rabbits are shown in Fig. 1. From the slope and y-intercept of the linear regression line, Table II, it appears that the isotonic point, i.e. the osmolality of the incubation medium at which no change in weight of water of the experimental lens occurred, is at or near 343 mOsmolal. The regression data from experiments done in various solutions are reported in Table II. From these data it appears that the composition of the solution used for the incubations or time had little effect on the direction of net exchange, or on the exchange rate for water between the lens and its surrounding aqueous medium. From the 60 min data it appears that the process being measured, i.e. a rapid net exchange of water, is more than 95% complete by 30 min. The isotonic point calculated from the 60 min data is 348 mOsmolal. The calculated isotonic point in AAM at 0°C is 339 mOsmolal.

The experiments done at 0°C in ICM (approximately 340 mOsmolal), with the cation concentration altered either by adding or by omitting 5, 10, or 30 mM of $KHCO_3$, gave the results shown in Table III. The movement of water between the lens and the medium was not in the direction predicted by Donnan equilibrium theory except for the ± 5 mM cation concentrations differences. The data points for the three experiments in which a 100 mM excess of K^+ was added to the medium were well within the experimental error of the method. This is also true for the data points for excess ascorbate (− 180 mM) since they appear to fit the plotted linear regression line even better than the data points for 100 mM K^+ excess.

The results from 30 min incubation experiments (52 lenses) at 35°C in AAM, IOM or modified Tyrode's medium are shown in Fig. 2. It appears that the isotonic point at 35°C is at or near 273 mOsmolal. Additional data using media without Ca^{++} and with 10 mM EDTA at 35°C are also plotted in Fig. 2. It is apparent that, within the experimental error of this method, all the data points shown in Fig. 2 fit the linear regression line. Thus it appears from these data that, at equal osmolalities, the net osmotic exchange of water is different at 0°C than at 35°C. The data also suggest that the difference in the results obtained was not due to the differences in solute composition of the media used nor was it affected by a lack of Ca^{++}.

The results of incubation (30 min at 35°C) in AAM to which ouabain at

Table 2. Linear regression data.

MEDIUM	TIME	NO. LENSES	Y-INTERCEPT AND s.d.	SLOPE AND s.d.	RHO	MEAN RESIDUAL	ISOTONIC POINT
				0° C			
ICM	30	40	16.394 ± 2.084	−0.0480 ± 0.0059	0.798	2.119	342
ICM	60	23	20.846 ± 3.559	−0.0599 ± 0.0102	0.790	2.300	348
AAM	30	21	14.353 ± 2.171	−0.0424 ± 0.0061	0.846	1.571	339
ALL 0°C DATA*		92	20.018 ± 1.624	−0.0584 ± 0.0047	0.793	1.921	343
				35° C			
AAM & AAM&	30	27	19.537 ± 3.035	−0.0696 ± 0.0090	0.839	2.175	281
OUABAIN	30	24	22.351 ± 5.764	−0.0800 ± 0.0186	0.677	3.121	280
INORG.	30	33	12.737 ± 1.361	−0.0478 ± 0.0041	0.853	1.428	267
ALL35° DATA**	30	74	16.987 ± 1.752	−0.0622 ± 0.051	0.802	1.789	273

* Except with altered K^+
** Except Ca^{++} free, Ouabain, F^- or Oxalate

Table 3. Test for Donnan equilibrium effect.

CHANGE IN MEDIUM	NO. LENSES (n)	MEDIUM mOSMOLAL	MEAN* RESIDUAL	SUM OF RES. SQUARED	SSR/n
		0° DATA			
+100 mM K$^+$	4	440	2.245	52.78	13.20
”	4	440	3.691	80.31	20.08
”	4	448	3.806	63.92	15.98
+5mM K$^+$	4	339	0.917	40.91	10.23
−5mM K$^+$	4	340	−0.611	14.70	3.68
+10mM K$^+$	4	348	0.444	53.45	13.36
−10mM K$^+$	4	341	0.292	83.63	20.91
+30mM K$^+$	4	341	−2.396	25.51	6.38
−30mM K$^+$	4	343	0.237	5.50	1.37
+180mM ascorbate	4	433	−0.164	20.78	5.19
”	4	489	3.60	62.99	15.75

* compared to 0° regression line

83

7×10^{-4} M was added are shown in Fig. 3. The linear regression line for the lens incubation experiments without ouabain is also shown. The slope, y-intercept, and isotonic point of this regression line may be compared to the respective values for the line shown in Fig. 2 by examination of Table II. There is no significant difference between these two lines. It is also obvious that in these experiments there was no detectable effect of ouabain on net water exchange between the lens and the medium. However, the effect of fluoride or oxalate on net water exchange is somewhat different. The data points for experiments in which fluoride ion at 20 mM or oxalate at 10 mM was added to AAM or IOM are also plotted in Fig. 3. These data points, as a group, do not appear to belong to the population of other data points (amino acid media ± ouabain) which are plotted in Fig. 3. Rather the data

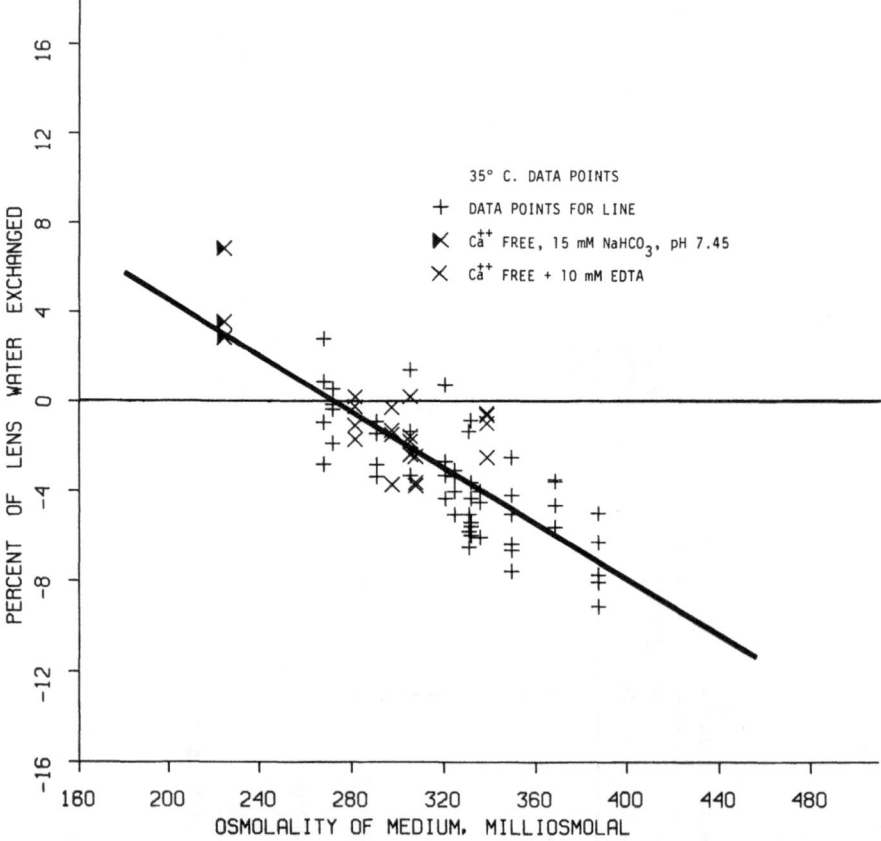

Fig. 2. The 52 data points indicated by + are from experiments done in AAM, IOM or modified Tyrode's medium. The 19 data points from experiments done in AAM or IOM without Ca^{++} and with 10 mM EDTA indicated by x appear to fit the line about as well as the data used to calculate it.

84

points from the fluoride and oxalate experiments appear to fit better the linear regression line of the data obtained at 0°C. Thus it appears that these metabolic inhibitors, both of which reduce ATP production, have an effect on net water exchange similar to the effect of 0°C temperature.

In all the experiments, except those using ouabain, there was no significant difference in the sum of the concentration of the monovalent cations ($[K^+] + [Na^+]$), when this value for the experimental lens was subtracted from the same value for the control lens. But it was noted that lenses which were

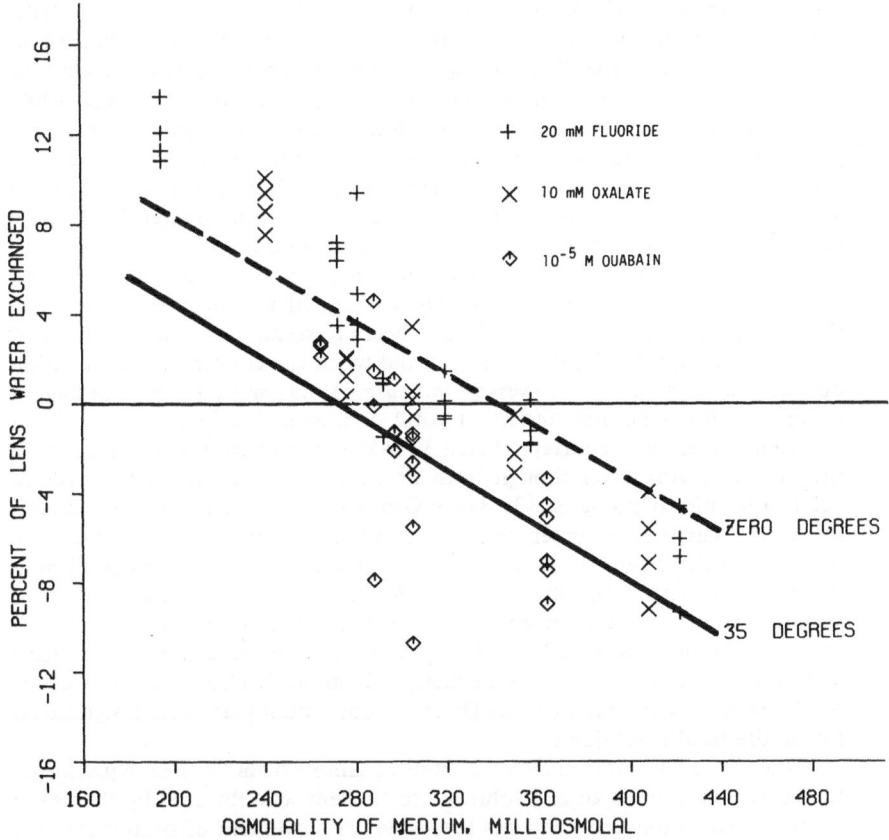

Fig. 3. The linear regression line for 0°C data of Fig. 1, dashed line, and the linear regression line for the 35°C data of Fig. 2, solid line, are shown together with data points of experiments done at 35°C with the indicated inhibitors in AAM. Note that the ouabain data points fall within the envelope of plus and minus values for the 35°C data in Fig. 2 while both the F⁻ and oxalate data points are fit better by the 0°C line. The horizontal difference between the two lines, 70 mOsmolal, is significantly greater than zero, $p < 0.05$. The correct Ouabain concentration is 7×10^{-4} M.

incubated in media with high K^+ concentration had slightly higher K^+ content than the control lenses. Rabbit lenses incubated in modified Tyrode's at 5°C had a mean O_2 uptake rate of 0.11 ± 0.035 $\mu M/h/cm^2$ of anterior surface (8 lenses) which is 43 percent of the oxygen uptake rate measured at 35°C, 0.26 ± 0.054 $\mu M/h/cm^2$ (6 lenses).

DISCUSSION

It has generally been assumed (Dick, 1966, Stein, 1967) that the observed hydration of animal tissues or eggs following application of metabolic poisons (Robinson, 1960) or the hydration of the lens incubated at 0°C or with metabolic poisons, is due solely to an approach to true Donnan equilibrium (Harris, 1966). At true Donnan equilibrium the concentration of counter ions, cations, except H^+, is higher on the protein side of the membrane, while the anion concentration and hydrogen ion concentration are higher on the protein-free side of the membrane. Thus if water influx into the lens resulted from an ion influx needed to reach Donnan equilibrium, this effect on the net water exchange in these experiments could be counteracted by a *reduction* in cation concentration in the solution bathing the lens by an amount approximately equal to the colloid osmotic pressure of the lens proteins. Thus with 30 mM *less* cation ($KHCO_3$ content of the medium reduced) in the outside medium there should have been *no uptake* of water by the lens while a *larger* uptake should have occurred when the concentration of cation outside was *increased*. An average *increase* of 0.31 mg H_2O/lens (4 lenses) occurred with a 30 mM *deficit* of total cations and a *loss* of 4.04 mg of H_2O/lens (4 lenses) occurred when a 30 mM *excess* of cations was present in the outside media even though both of these experiments used a medium nearly isotonic to the lens, 339-348 mOsmolal, at 0°C. Thus in these experiments the changes in water content found in the experimental lens were opposite to the effect on water exchange predicted by Donnan equilibrium theory. Even with a 100 mM excess of K^+ in the outside medium there was an insignificant effect on water exchange which clearly shows that too little solute could move down a 100 mM concentration gradient in 30 min to have a measurable effect on water exchange. Thus, it is clear from the above results that the approach to true Donnan equilibrium played an insignificant role in the results obtained.

Other than the movement of cations or anions from Donnan equilibrium forces, the movement of any solutes into the lens was obviated by the use of media which eliminated gradients favorable for movement of solutes into the lens. The 30 min experimental time was chosen so that during the incubation period sufficient net water exchange might occur to be detectable by the analytical method employed but, considering the permeability and diffusion coefficients of tissue solutes compared to these values for water (Stein, 1967; House, 1974), it would be highly improbable that sufficient solute movement would occur for analytical detection of the amount of water which should accompany that solute to equate osmolality. Because solute movement was totally obviated in the experiments using ICM at 0°C, it is clear that only water was exchanged to give the results obtained. Thus finding an isotonic point from the experiment at 0°C which is approximately 40 mOsmolal hypertonic to serum means that these lenses were also hypertonic. Thus the lens maintains its water at a lower chemical potential than the water of the intraocular fluids. We have no reason to ascribe this difference in the chemical potential of water to the decrease in temperature from 35°C to 0°C. The reduction in the chemical potential of water due to a reduction in temperature must be equal both in the lens and in the medium.

The concept of an osmotic steady state implies that the total efflux of all solutes, in terms of $Osmols/cm^2/sec$, must exactly equal the total influx of all solutes in the same units. If this condition were not met, then osmotically active solutes would either accumulate inside the lens or would be lost from the lens and osmotic theory then demands that water exchange must occur in a direction to equalize the chemical potential of water inside the lens with the chemical potential of water of the outside medium. However, it is also obvious that, if a mechanism exists in the lens for the transport of water independent of solute transport and if such a transport mechanism operates in the lens to outside direction, then the lens could be maintained in a hypertonic condition until the rate of that transport mechanism was reduced. One of the effects of lowered temperature is to lower the supply of metabolic energy. Thus water uptake by the lens incubated at 0°C in medium apparently isotonic to the lens at 35°C and isocomposite with intralenticular fluids should occur if the transport of water from a hypertonic lens required metabolic energy.

The demonstration from the experiments reported herein, that any net water exchange between the lens and an incubation medium which occurred during the first 30 minutes of incubation is not due to an approach to true Donnan equilibrium and indeed is apparently independent of the solute composition of the media employed also means that solute movements of any kind played an insignificant role in the results obtained. Even media devoid of calcium ion, which reportedly should increase the permeability of lens membranes (Harris & Nordquist, 1954, Thoft & Kinoshita, 1965) to salts and water and thus increase water exchange fluxes, had no detectable effect on net water exchange in the experiments reported here implying no effect on the rate of water exchange.

In the experiments with ouabain, the concentration used was sufficient to severely inhibit cation transport (Harris & Becker, 1965; Kinsey & Reddy, 1965) and also to severely inhibit transport of amino acids (Kinsey & Reddy, 1963; Cotlier & Beaty, 1967), taurine (Reddy, 1970), and inositol (Cotlier, 1970; Varma et al., 1970). No effect on net water exchange during incubations at 35°C for 30 minutes was noted in the experiments with ouabain in the medium. However, addition of either 20 mM F^- or of 10 mM oxalate to AAM or IOM altered appreciably the net water exchange during a 30 minute incubation at 35°C. These data lead to the conclusion that a transport mechanism for water which is independent of cation movement probably exists in the rabbit lens and that this transport mechanism requires a continuous supply of metabolic energy and requires some substance or effect resulting from the metabolism. Thus, an hypothesis that the rabbit lens maintains its water balance as a result of transport of water by a mechanism which is independent of transport of lens solutes is tenable on the basis of the above evidence.

The isotonic point for lenses incubated in various media at 37°C is apparently at or near 273 mOsmolal (40 mOsmolal hypotonic to average serum). The experiments reported herein clearly demonstrate that a change in temperature from 35°C to 0°C results in an apparent change in the isotonic point of the lens from 273 mOsmolal to 343 mOsmolal, an increase of 70 mOsmolal. This difference is too large to be due to experimental error given the correlation coefficient, rho, and the variances of the data at 0°C and 35°C. Because osmotic pressure is independent of temperature this difference cannot be due just to the change of temperature. It does, however, correlate well with the observation that in silicone oil, fluid secretion from the anterior surface of the lens ceases at temperatures below 15°C and that the fluid secreted by the lens is hypotonic to serum (Fowlks, 1973b). Because the lens is secreting a fluid in experiments done at 35°C it is obvious that there should be no net influx of water into the lens unless the osmotic pressure of the incubation medium at 35°C is less than the osmotic pressure of the secreted fluid and vice versa for net efflux. The observed osmotic pressure of the fluid secreted from the anterior surface of the lens dehydrating itself in silicone oil was 262 ± 16.5 mOsmolal (Fowlks, 1973b). Thus unless the lens also secretes a fluid from the posterior surface which is hypertonic to 262 mOsmolal, one should expect to observe that at 35°C, the lens appears to be hypotonic to serum and aqueous humor. The fluid secreted by the isolated lens in silicone oil (Fowlks, 1973a) resulted in a net dehydration of the lens which must have caused an increase in the intralenticular osmotic pressure of about 30 mOsmolal thus one should expect to find that the lens secretes *in vivo* a solution with osmolality less than 262 mOsmolal. Indeed it has been recently reported (Fowlks, et al., 1978) that the vitreous humor of the rabbit has a large radially oriented osmotic pressure gradient with a retrolental osmotic pressure 50 mOsmolal hypotonic to serum. The retrolental vitreous humor *in vivo* could not have a steady state value lower than serum unless the lens secreted a fluid which is isotonic to the adjacent vitreous humor. At steady state the fluid imbibed by the lens must have an osmotic pressure equal to the osmotic pressure of the fluid secreted otherwise the lens could not be at steady state with regard to its solutes and water.

ACKNOWLEDGMENT

Many thanks are due Caroline McDonald and Jacqueline Wright who assisted with these experiments. My special thanks to Professor John E. Harris who provided me the opportunity to carry out these and other studies. This work was supported in part by NIH Grant NB-01979; an anonymous donor, and from other funds provided by the Department of Ophthalmology at the University of Minnesota.

REFERENCES

Beament, J.W.L. The active transport and passive movement of water in insects. *Adv. Insect. Physiol.* 2: *67-129* (1964).

Cotlier, E. Myo-inositol: active transport by the crystalline lens. *Invest. Ophthal.* 9: *681-691* (1970).

Cotlier, E., Kwan, B. & Beaty, C. The lens as an osmometer and the effect of medium osmolality on water transport, ^{86}Rb efflux and ^{86}Rb transport by the lens. *Biochim. biophys. Acta* 150: *705-722* (1968).

Cotlier, E. & Beaty, C. The role of Na$^+$ions in the transport of α-aminoisobutyric acid and other amino acids into the lens. *Invest. Ophthal.* 6: *64-75* (1967).

Dick, D.A.T. Cell Water, Butterworths Inc., Washington, D.C. (1966) pp. *38-111*.

Fowlks, W.L. Demonstration of a net movement of water through the lens. *Experientia.* 29: *548-549* (1973a).

Fowlks, W.L. Osmotic relations between fluids of the rabbit eye. *Proc. Soc. exp. Biol. Med.* 143: *1176-1179* (1973b).

Fowlks, W.L., Conway, J.H. & Wedekind, T.D. Solute and Osmotic gradients in the rabbit's ocular vitreous body. *Fed. Proc. Feda. Am. Socs. exp. Biol.* 37: *623* (1978).

Ginsburg, H. & Ginzburg, B.Z. Evidence for active water transport in a corn root preparation. *J. Membr. Biol.* 4: *29-41* (1971).

Harris, J.E. The temperature-reversible cation shift of the lens. *Trans. Am. Ophthal. Soc.* 64: *675-699* (1966).

Harris, J.E. & Becker, B. Cation transport of the lens. *Invest. Ophthal.* 4: *709-722* (1965).

Harris, J.E. & Nordquist, L.T. Factors effecting the cation and water balance of the lens. *Acta XVII Conc. Ophthal.* 1: *1002-1012* (1954).

House, C.R. Water transport in cells and tissues. Edw. Arnold Ltd, London (1974) pp. *152-390*.

Kass, M.Z. & Green, H. Osmotic pressure measurement of intraocular fluids by an improved cryoscopic method. *Am. J. Ophthal.* 48 pt. II: *33-46* (1959).

Kinsey, V.E. & Reddy, D.V.N. Studies of the crystalline lens X. Transport of amino acids. *Invest. Ophthal.* 2: *229-236* (1963).

Kinsey, V.E. & Reddy, D.V.N. Studies on the crystalline lens XI. The relative role of the epithelium and capsule in transport. *Invest. Ophthal.* 4: *104-116* (1965).

Patterson, J.W. & Fournier, D.J. The effect of tonicity on lens volume. *Invest. Ophthal.* 15: *866-869* (1976).

Prince, J.H. & Eglitis, I. Lens and ligaments, in The Rabbit in Eye Research. (ed. Prince, J.H.). Chas. C. Thomas. Pub. Springfield, *342* (1964).

Reddy, D.V.N. Studies on the intraocular transport of taurine. *Invest. Ophthal.* 9: *206-219* (1970).

Reddy, D.V.N. & Kinsey, V.E. Studies on the crystalline lens IX. Quantitative analysis of free amino acids and related compounds. *Invest. Ophthal.* 1: *635-641* (1962).

Reddy, D.V.N. & Kinsey, V.E. Transport of amino acids into intraocular fluids and lens in diabetic animals. *Invest. Ophthal.* 2: *237-242* (1963).

Robinson, J.R. Metabolism of intracellular water. *Physiol. Rev.* 40: *112-149* (1960).

Stein, W.D. The Movement of Molecules Across Cell Membranes. Academic Press, N.Y. 1967, pp. *74-210*.

Thoft, R.A. & Kinoshita, J.H. The effect of calcium on rat lens permeability. *Invest. Ophthal.* 4: *122-128* (1965).

Van Heyningen, R. The lens, in The Eye. Vol. 1, (ed. Davson, H.) Academic Press, N.Y. 1962 pp. *231-287*.

Varma, S.D., Chakrapani, B. & Reddy, V.N. Intraocular transport of myoinositol. Accumulation in the rabbit lens *in vitro*. *Invest. Ophthal.* 9: *794-800* (1970).

Author's address:
Department of Ophthalmology
University of Minnesota Medical School
Box 387 Mayo Building
Minneapolis, MN 55455 USA

90

Docum. Ophthal. Proc. Series, Vol. 18

A PRELIMINARY STUDY OF THE DYNAMIC ASPECTS OF AGE DEPENDENT CHANGES IN THE ABUNDANCES OF HUMAN LENS POLYPEPTIDES

WILLIAM H. GARNER & ABRAHAM SPECTOR

(New York, U.S.A.)

ABSTRACT

Growth of normal human lenses is maintained at a relatively constant rate of 0.4 mg per year after the first years of life. Water insoluble material increases at a similar constant rate, while the amount of water soluble components remains constant. Early growth stages are reflected by significant changes in relative abundance of all the major subunits in these fractions. However, from approximately age 40, the relative concentrations of the different subunits of lens proteins are fairly constant, except for a continued marked decrease in the 20,000 and increase in the 10,000 dalton water insoluble components. The relative stability in the concentrations of the polypeptides suggests that the rates of synthesis are comparable to the rates of degradation and/or insolubilization. The 10,000 dalton polypeptide is the result of degradation, probably of both soluble and insoluble 20,000 dalton components, which appears to be more rapid in the water insoluble fraction.

The 43,000 dalton polypeptide is found in the water insoluble fraction of all ages; in the water soluble fraction, it only appears after the first few years of life, increasing until approximately age 30 at which time it is equivalent to that found in the insoluble fraction.

Amino acid incorporation studies confirm the conclusion that the 43,000 dalton polypeptide is directly synthesized and the 10,000 dalton component arises by post-translational degradation. Ouabain causes differential inhibition, blocking almost completely the synthesis of polypeptides equal to or greater than 27,000 daltons. The decrease with aging of overall protein synthesis appears to occur at a uniform rate in the soluble cortical region at least in the 26 to 52 year-old age group.

INTRODUCTION

The earlier view that the lens is a simple ametabolic tissue was altered by the work of Harris & Gehrsitz (1951, 1953), Merriam & Kinsey (1950a, b) and others (van Heyningen, 1969). The lens has been shown to be a complex tissue with multifaceted metabolic activities. Although many of these metabolic pathways have been studied in detail, little is known concerning the dynamic aspects of lens protein metabolism. The structural proteins have been usually defined in young lenses and little protein synthesis has been detected in the nuclear region. (Wannemacher & Spector, 1968). The synthesis of γ-crystallin in animal lenses is markedly decreased shortly after birth (Harding & Dilley, 1976). However, the impact of age upon the relative abundance of proteins in a long-lived species such as man has received little attention.

The properties of lens proteins change as the lens ages. This has been shown for human lens α-crystallin (Roy & Spector, 1976). In young lenses, this protein is fairly homogeneous in aggregate size and is composed of three differently charged polypeptides: two A-chains and one B-chain. With aging, a broad range of macromolecular aggregates is formed and the complexity of the polypeptide subunit makeup increases. In old lenses, six A-chains and five B-chains with varying charge distribution have been found, further complicating the relating of a particular macromolecular species to one of the structural protein groups found in younger lens.

In aging, soluble proteins are apparently converted to insoluble components. In order to solubilize these insoluble components, their integrity must generally be destroyed. Although study of the intact macromolecules is not usually possible, variations in the abundance of the constituent polypeptides may be studied. This communication reports the effects of aging upon the relative abundance of the water-soluble and water-insoluble human lens fractions, the distribution of the major polypeptides within these fractions, and their synthesis. Recently Piatigorsky reported that the relative polypeptide synthesis of ouabain-treated normal mice lenses mimicks the labeled amino acid uptake patterns of Nakano mice (Piatigorsky, Fukui & Kinoshita, 1978). Such observations as well as studies with cultured embryonic chick lenses (Sinohara & Piatigorsky, 1977) suggest changes in sodium-potassium concentrations which produce a differential effect upon protein synthesis. Therefore an initial study on the effect of ouabain on the human lens system is also reported herein.

MATERIALS AND METHODS

Dry weights. The human lenses were freshly obtained and stored at $-80°$ prior to use. The water-soluble fraction was defined as the 60,000 g supernatant obtained from individual homogenized lenses (Roy & Spector, 1976). The water-insoluble fraction represented the pellet obtained from the above centrifugation. The water-soluble fraction was dialyzed against deionized water before drying. Both fractions were transferred to preweighed vials and then lyophilized for 72 hours.

Subunit distribution. The dried material from selected samples from the above age groups were taken from both the water-soluble and water-insoluble fractions and analyzed by 0.1% SDS polyacrylamide gel electrophoresis in the precence of 1% mercaptoethanol according to the method of Weber & Osborn (1969). The gels were stained with Coomassie Blue and after sufficient destaining (absorbance max. $\simeq$ 2.0) were scanned at 590 nm with a Gilford gel scanner interfaced with a DEC minicomputer for the purpose of integrating selected peak areas representing polypeptides of different molecular weights. The sum of the total areas from the different sized subunits examined were subsequently normalized to 100% in order to minimize the gel background. Material at the upper gel interface was excluded from direct measurement for technical reasons, and therefore was not considered in this report.

Incorporation of [^3H] amino acids. Three sets of paired human lenses (26, 44 and 52 years) were obtained 6 hours after death. Organ cultures, in the presence of uniformly labelled [^3H] amino acids (NEN-250), were performed with TC 199 media essentially according to the procedure of Merola, Kern & Kinoshita (1960). One lens from each set was incubated in the presence of 10^{-4}M ouabain. After 44 hours all lenses were placed in fresh TC 199 solution for approximately one hour. This wash procedure was repeated and then the lenses were frozen at $-80°$. The cortical region (40% by weight of the total lens) was separated from the corresponding nuclear region with a trephine. The water-soluble and water-insoluble fractions were isolated according to the procedure already described above, except that prior to dialysis the water-insoluble fraction was dissolved in 8 M urea to remove potentially trapped [^3H]-amino acids. Preparative 0.1%SDS polyacrylamide gels were run to determine the distribution of label within given molecular weight species. The gels were divided into uniform 1.7 mm divisions after staining and were oxidized with hydrogen peroxide at $80°$ prior to counting in Aquasol-2®.

RESULTS AND DISCUSSION

The dry weight data for individual normal lenses are shown in Fig. 1. The total weight (water-soluble plus water-insoluble fractions) of the lenses shows an apparent constant linear increase of 0.4 mg per year after an early period of rapid growth. This increase in weight parallels the increase in the water-insoluble fraction so that in normal developing lenses, the water-soluble fraction seems to remain quite constant at 30 mg. From birth to approximately age 70 the water-insoluble fraction thus increases from 1% to 50%, respectively.

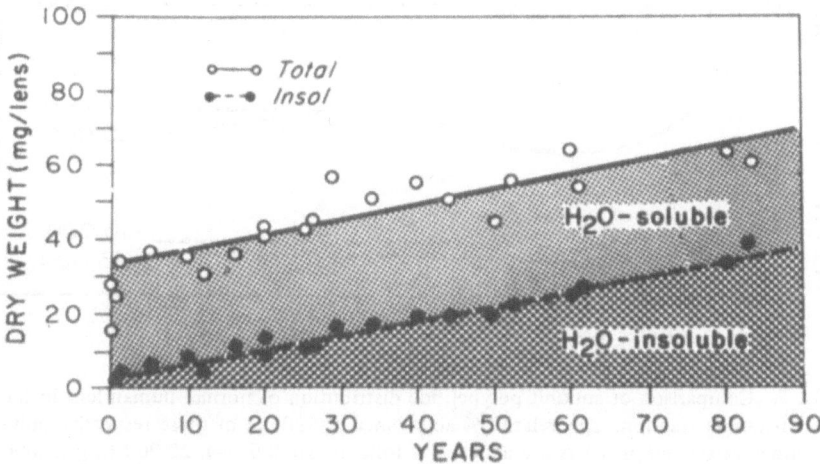

Fig. 1. Normal lens growth. A plot of total lens dry weight (mg/lens) versus age for the total water-soluble plus water-insoluble fractions (o—o) and the water-insoluble fractions (●—●).

Since both the water-soluble and insoluble fractions contain mostly protein, the percent distribution of the major polypeptides constituting these fractions was investigated with respect to age. Such data should indicate whether the relative abundances of specific polypeptides vary with age. The results are shown in Figs. 2 and 3. The data suggest that there are three relatively defined periods into which the lens can be divided: an early period encompassing the first few years of life ($\simeq$ 5 years) in which dramatic changes in relative abundance of the polypeptides occur; a second stage ranging from approximately 10 years to 40 years of age in which gradual changes in composition are observed; and finally, a third period encompassing later life where with a few exceptions the relative polypeptide abundances remain fairly constant. The first period reflects sharply different rates of polypeptide synthesis, little degradation, and a marked increase in the total dry weight of the lens. In this stage the insoluble protein probably represents primarily membrane components and comprises only a few percent of the total protein. Most of the components observed in this fraction during this period perhaps may result from contamination of the soluble fraction. There is one notable exception to the above conclusion. The 43,000 dalton polypeptide, while not present in the soluble fraction, is present in the insoluble fraction with approximately the same abundance as in older lenses. During this early period, there is a precipitous decrease in the

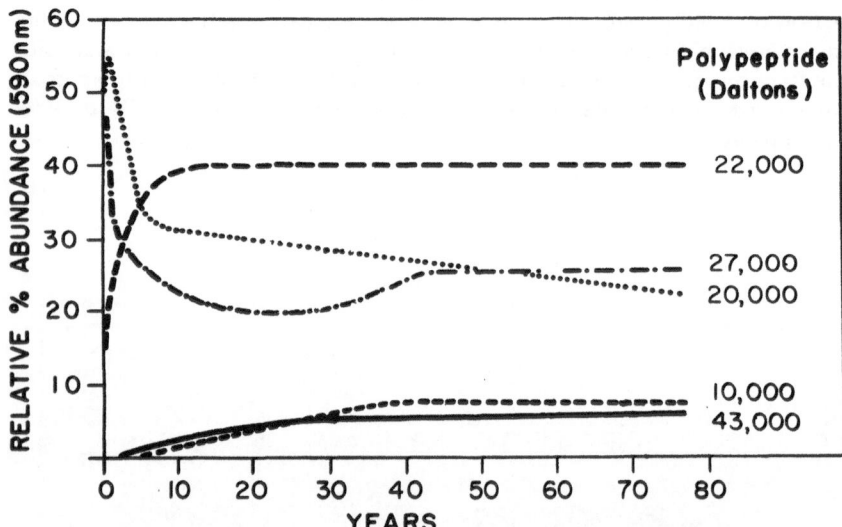

Fig. 2. Comparison of subunit polypeptide distribution of normal human lens in the water-soluble fraction. The relative % abundance at 590 nm of these respective polypeptides versus age in years are denoted as follows: 10,000 (—); 20,000 (...); 22,000 (— —). 27,000 (-··-); and 43,000 (——). The lines represent the best fit to the overall experimental data with approximately ± 10% error; therefore, the total % at given ages do not always total 100.

abundance of the 27,000 and 20,000 dalton polypeptides and an even more rapid increase in the 22,000 dalton component.

In the second and third stages, the total soluble protein in the lens appears to remain constant reflecting an equilibrium between synthesis and degradation. The variation in the abundance of the polypeptides reflects the relative rates of synthesis, insolubilization and degradation to lower molecular weight species of each size class of polypeptides. During the second stage the 10,000 and 43,000 dalton polypeptides gradually appear in the soluble fraction, continuing to increase until approximately 25 to 40 years of age respectively. The absence of the 43,000 dalton polypeptide in the soluble fraction of the young lens and its atypical chemical properties suggests that it may be an extrinsic membrane protein. Its gradual appearance in the soluble fraction perhaps is due to changes in the concentration and structure of the membrane, thus causing the release of this polypeptide from the insoluble membrane matrix during homogenization of lenses older than a few years. This viewpoint is supported by recent observations of Mostafapour & Reddy (1978) who found that, if the soluble lens protein was released by osmotic shock, the 43,000 dalton component could not be detected in the soluble phase.

The 10,000 dalton fraction is apparently the result of post-translational reaction, since it is absent in both soluble and insoluble fractions in the very young lens. Also it has recently been shown that the 10,000 dalton component is derived from the A-chain of α-crystallin (Roy & Spector, 1978).

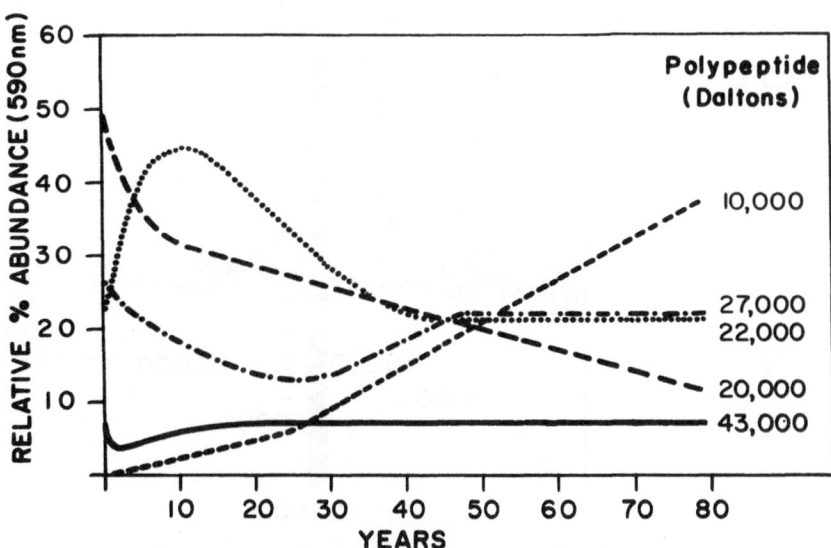

Fig. 3. Comparison of subunit polypeptide distribution of normal human lens in the water-insoluble fraction. The relative % abundance at 590 nm of the respective polypeptides versus age in years are denoted as follows: 10,000 (–); 20,000 (— —); 22,000 (...); 27,000 (---); and 43,000 (——). See last note in Fig. 2.

Toward the end of the second stage, there is a marked increase in the rate of accumulation of this component in the insoluble fraction which continues through the remainder of the aging process. These results suggest that the insolubilized 20,000 dalton polypeptide may be a direct precursor to this latter species. Evidence based on D/L aspartic acid abundance reported elsewhere also indicate that this increased rate of formation of the 10,000 dalton polypeptide may be due to degradation of already insolubilized material (Masters, Bada & Zigler, 1978; Garner & Spector, 1978). Aside from the continuing decrease in the abundance of the 20,000 dalton compo-

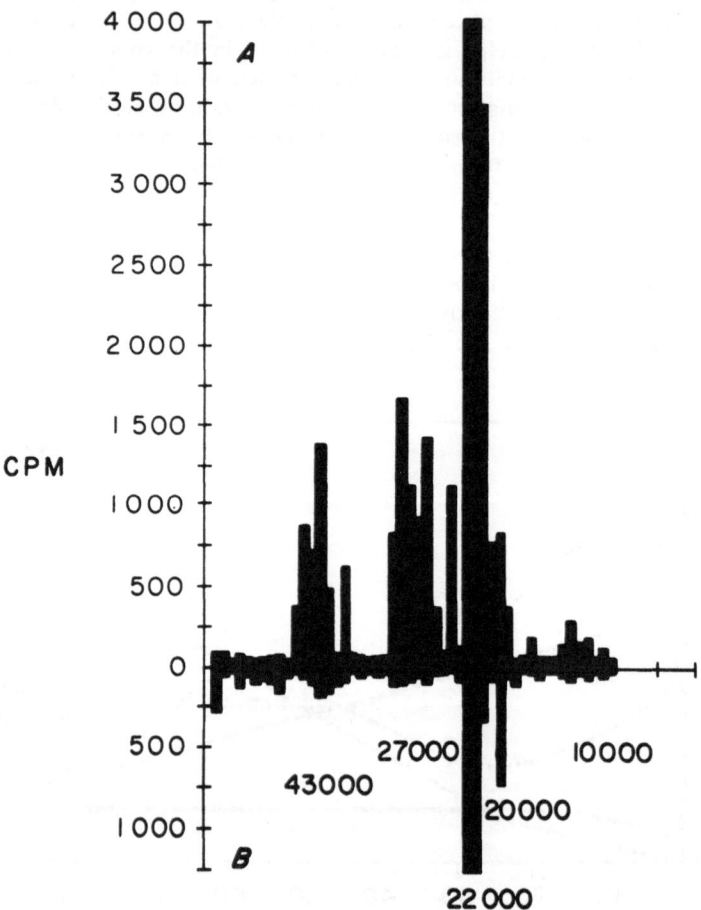

Fig. 4. Incorporation of [³H] amino acids into the water-soluble cortical region of a 26 year old lens during organ culture. Part A denotes the cpm versus gel position (1.7 mm slice) without ouabain. Part B denotes the cpm versus gel position with ouabain treatment. The approximate molecular weights are indicated. The cpm are based upon combined gels containing 6 mg.

nent and the aforementioned increase in the 10,000 dalton component, all other polypeptides in the insoluble fraction appear to remain remarkably constant in the third period. In the soluble fraction, there is a relatively stable set of abundances for the polypeptides with the exception of the 20,000 dalton component which gradually decreases and a slight increase in the 27,000 dalton fraction. The constant level of the 10,000 dalton soluble component suggests that the rate of formation and possibly insolubilization or further degradation are relatively constant. The actual situation can be examined more critically by considering the apparent rates of appearance of the 10,000 dalton polypeptide and the disappearance of the 20,000 dalton component. The soluble 20,000 dalton polypeptide decreases at 0.13%/yr and its insoluble counterpart at 0.29%/yr, giving a total degradation rate of 0.42% per year. The combination of insolubilization of the 10,000 dalton component plus its formation in the insoluble fraction represent a rate of 0.58%/yr. Such data are in reasonably good agreement and suggest that it is unlikely in normal lenses that there is a significant loss of this polypeptide by diffusion from the tissue.

The overall results suggest a number of important conclusions: (1) the 10,000 dalton polypeptide in the insoluble fraction probably arises from both the soluble 10,000 dalton polypeptide pool and from degradation of the insoluble 20,000 dalton component; (2) the 43,000 dalton component is synthesized *de novo* and is not the result of post-translational reaction; and (3) the relative rates of synthesis of the soluble polypeptides other than the 20,000 dalton component is balanced by degradation and insolubilization.

Further information about synthesis of the lens subunits can be obtained by incorporation studies of labelled amino acids in lens organ culture: (1) which subunits arise by post-translational mechanisms; (2) what is the change in the rate of protein synthesis with age; (3) is there a differential polypeptide synthesis brought about by alterations in cellular environment caused by the presence of ouabain? A representative experiment with a 26 year old lens from which the water-soluble cortical fraction was isolated,

Table 1. Incorporation of [³H]-Amino Acids into Human Lens Proteins

Ages	Ouabain	H₂O-Soluble*		H₂O-Insoluble*	
		Cortex	Nuclear	Cortex	Nuclear
26	−	50176	10354	16743	2601
	+	8968	4795	5438	1509
44	−	41051	21950	17285	3408
	+	15435	4977	8922	1230
52	−	28043	13671	10568	2360
	+	13769	9069	8748	1422

* Expressed as cpm/mg. See text for further information

gave information pertaining to both the former and latter questions (Fig. 4). From the results show in Part A, Fig. 4, it is suggestive that only the 10,000 dalton polypeptide arises post-translationally. Only this polypeptide has incorporated little radioactivity, thus further supporting the prior conclusion concerning the origin of the component and answering the first query. Question 3 is answered by Part B in Fig. 4. By altering the cation environment by treatment of the lens with 10^{-4}M ouabain during the culture period, it is apparent that the larger polypeptides greater or equal to 27,000 are almost completely inhibited while less extensive inhibition is observed in the 22,000 dalton range and with possibly the least inhibition being found in the 20,000 range. The second question is answered by comparison of incorporation of amino acids into various aged human lenses. These results are shown in Table 1. The table lists the cpm of incorporated amino acids per mg of the water-soluble and water-insoluble fractions in each of the three sets of lenses. Since the nuclear region represents 60% of the total lens weight in these experiments somewhat more incorporation was found than previously reported for calf lenses by Wannemacher & Spector (1968). The effect of 10^{-4} M ouabain is also shown. From this somewhat limited data, the rate of protein synthesis between the ages of 26 and 52 years can be assumed to decrease rather linearly in the soluble cortical region of approximately 1 percent per year. In addition, the inhabition of protein synthesis produced by ouabain is definitely more pronounced in the cortical region of younger lenses. Associated with these molecular changes was noted progressive relative swelling of the lens, probably caused by a number of factors, in the following order: $26 > 44 > 52$ years.

ACKNOWLEDGMENTS

The skilled assistance of Ms. Sabrina Lerman is gratefully noted. We thank Drs. Lu-Ku Li, M. Flood, S. Garcia-Castineiras, M. Garner, D. Roy and J. Dillon for help and discussion. This work was supported by grants from the National Eye Institute, National Institutes of Health.

REFERENCES

Garner, W.H. & A. Spector. Racemization in human lens: evidence of rapid insolubilization of particular polypeptides in cataract formation. *Proc. natn. Acad. Sci.* USA: in press (1978).

Harding, J.J. & K.J. Dilley. Structural proteins of the mammalian lens: a review with emphasis on changes in development, aging and cataract. *Expl. Eye Res.* 22: *1-73* (1976).

Harris, J.E. & L.B. Gehrsitz. Significance of changes in potassium and sodium content of the lens. A mechanism for lenticular intumescence. *Am. J. Ophthal.* 34 part II: *131-138* (1951).

Harris, J.E., L.B. Gehrsitz & L.T. Nordquist. The in vitro reversal of the lenticular cation shift induced by cold or calcium deficiency. *Am. J. Ophthal.* 36 part II: *39-49*, (1953).

Masters, P.M., J.L. Bada & J.S. Zigler, Jr. Aspartic acid racemization in heavy molecular weight crystallins and water-insoluble protein from normal lenses and cataracts. *Proc. natn. Acad. Sci. USA* 75: *1204-1208* (1978).

Merola, L.O., H.L. Kern & J.H. Kinoshita. The effect of calcium on the cations of calf lens. *A.M.A. Archs. Ophthal.* 63: *1830-1835* (1960).

Merriam, F.C. & V.E. Kinsey. Studies on the crystalline lens. I: Technic for in vitro culture of crystalline lenses and observations on metabolism of the lens *A.M.A. Archs. Ophthal.* 43: *979-988* (1950a).

Merriam, F.C. & V.E. Kinsey. Studies on the Crystalline lens. III: Incorporation of glycine and serine in proteins of lenses cultured in vitro. *A.M.A. Archs. Ophthal.* 44: *651-658* (1950b).

Mostafapour, M.K. & V.N. Reddy. Personal communication.

Piatigorsky, J., H.N. Fukui & J.H. Kinoshita. Differential synthesis, degradation and leakage of protein in an inherited cataract and in the normal lens cultured with ouabain. *Nature*: in press (1978).

Roy, D. & A. Spector. High molecular weight protein from human lenses. *Expl. Eye Res.* 22: *273-279* (1976).

Roy, D. & A. Spector. Human alpha crystallin. III. Isolation and characterization of protein from normal infant lenses and old lens peripheries. *Invest. Ophthal.* 15: *394-399* (1976).

Roy, D. & A. Spector. Human insoluble lens proteins. II. Isolation and characterization of a 9,600 dalton polypeptide. *Expl. Eye Res.*: in press (1978).

Shinohara, T. & J. Piatigorsky. Regulation of protein synthesis, intracellular electrolytes and cataract formation in vitro. *Nature* 270: *406-411* (1977).

van Heyningen, R. The lens: Metabolism and cataract, in *The Eye,* Vol. 1, 2nd Ed. (ed. Durson, H.) Academic Press, London, 1969, pp. *381-488.*

Wannemacher, C.F. & A. Spector. Protein synthesis in the core of calf lens. *Expl. Eye Res.* 7: *623-625* (1968).

Weber, K. & M. Osborn. The reliability of molecular weight determinations by dodecyl sulfate-polyacrylamide gel electrophoresis. *J. biol. Chem.* 244: *4406-4412* (1969).

Authors' address:
Biochemistry and Molecular Biology Laboratory
Department of Ophthalmology
College of Physicans and Surgeons
Columbia University
New York 10032, USA

Docum. Ophthal. Proc. Series, Vol. 18

POLYPEPTIDES IN THE VERTEBRATE LENS

RUTH VAN HEYNINGEN, JOY E. SHIRLEY &
SIMON VAN HEYNINGEN

(Oxford, Edinburgh, England)

ABSTRACT

Using polyacrylamide gel electrophoresis in sodium dodecyl sulphate and urea, we have detected a range of polypeptides of molecular weight between about 2,000 and 9,000 in the human lens, and also, at lower concentrations, in bovine, rabbit, rat and monkey lens. The most prominent polypeptide(s) in this range, in all the lenses examined by this method, had a molecular weight of about 7,500; preparations of α-crystallin also contain a polypeptide that separates in the same position after gel electrophoresis.

INTRODUCTION

The dry weight of the vertebrate lens is at least one-third of the wet weight and is almost entirely protein. The crystallins, α, β, and γ, account for more than 90% of this protein. The lens grows throughout life within a capsule, and sheds no cells. The youngest growing cells and fibres in the outer cortex are responsible for the synthesis of the crystallins. The central core of the lens contains the proteins synthesized in embryonic and infant life and any changes in their composition are believed to be post-synthetic.

In the animal lens the central core gradually becomes dehydrated and hard during ageing, as the overlying fibres are laid down, but in the human lens this does not occur, and the dry weight of about 35% of wet weight is maintained throughout life.

α-crystallin from the bovine lens, the most intensively studied of the crystallins, appears to be subject to at least three irreversible changes during the process of normal ageing: (i) the formation of high molecular weight aggregates (ii) progressive deamidation of primary polypeptide chains and (iii) defined degradation of polypeptides starting from the carboxyl terminal end (Bloemendal, 1977).

In the human lens these processes also occur but are far more complex and have been less fully investigated; the formation of high molecular aggregates involves all the crystallins and is highly complex (see Harding & Dilley, 1976).

The mechanisms underlying the post-synthetic changes are not understood, but as α-crystallin is a substrate of the neutral proteinase that is found in the lens, *in vivo* proteolysis may be involved in the degradation (Blow, Van Heyningen & Barrett, 1975).

101

It seemed possible that the neutral proteinase in the centre of the human lens might be responsible for the slow autolysis of some of the crystallins, with the formation of a variety of peptides. Since, in contrast to the bovine lens, the human lens contains barely detectable traces of leucine amino peptidase (Hanson, 1962; Trayhurn & Van Heyningen, 1976), an enzyme that in any case has little activity at neutral pH, these peptides might not be further degraded. Roy & Spector (1976) considered that the disappearance of low molecular weight α-crystallin from the human lens nucleus could possibly be due to a preferential modification or destruction of the A chain polypeptides, brought about by proteolysis.

We studied the total peptide composition of the centre and cortex of various types of lenses after destruction of non-covalent bonds by use of SDS*. Electrophoresis in polyacrylamide gels with 0.1% SDS containing 8M urea by the method of Swank & Munkres (1971) enables the separation of oligopeptides in the molecular range of about 1,200 to 10,000 and gives a first approximation of their molecular weight. The fact that the solution (Swank & Munkres, 1971) of 1% SDS, 8M urea, and 1% mercaptoethanol dissolves the whole lens leaving virtually no residue is important; by the usual methods of extraction well over half the protein in the nucleus of many cataractous lenses is insoluble in water and in 8M urea (Dilley & Pirie, 1974).

EXPERIMENTAL

Animal lenses were removed from the eye soon after death and stored deep-frozen. Human lenses (more than twenty cataractous and one normal) were from operation and used at once or stored deep-frozen. The foetal and 12 year lenses were from post mortem material and had remained in the eye for one or two days after death.

The lenses were divided into approximately equal weights of cortex and nucleus. These were weighed and dissolved in a solution containing 1% SDS, 8M urea and 1% mercaptoethanol according to the method of Swank & Munkres (1971). A volume containing the equivalent of 300 μg fresh tissue was taken for analysis by polyacrylamide gel electrophoresis. The method of Swank & Munkres was followed closely, using a concentration of urea of 8M, polyacrylamide 12.5% and a cross linkage ratio of 1:10 bis:acrylamide. A current of 1.8 mA per gel was applied for 16 hours along gels of 12 cm length. Bromphenol Blue was used as internal standard and marker gels of α-crystallin, and the four cyanogen bromide cleavage products of myoglobin were always included. Myoglobin and the three cyanogen bromide cleavage products of cytochrome c were also used. Alpha-crystallin was prepared from adult bovine lenses by gel chromatography on Sephadex G200 (see Bloemendal, 1977).

---

* Abbreviation: SDS, sodium dodecylsulphate

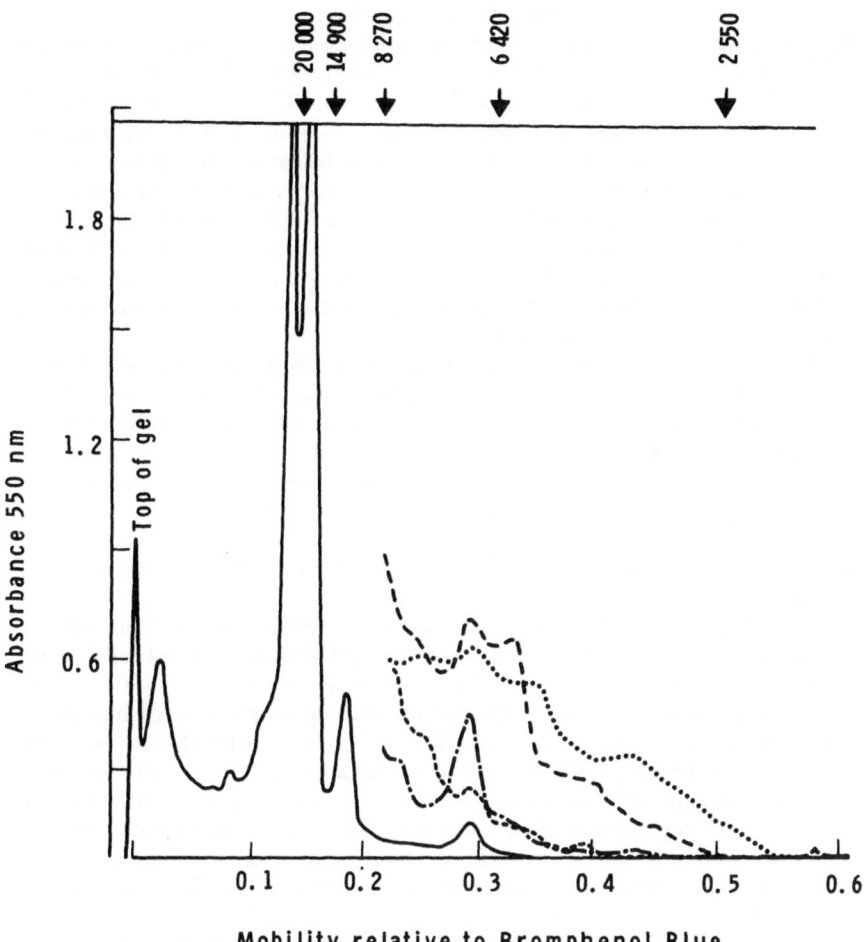

Fig. 1. Scans of the stained bands of polypeptides separated from lens tissue by polyacrylamide gel electrophoresis in sodium dodecyl sulphate and urea.

α-crystallin (10 μg) and the equivalent of about 300 μg fresh tissue (roughly 100 μg protein) were applied to the gels. The standards were α-crystallin molecular weight 20,000 and the cyanogen bromide peptides of myoglobin I plus II, I, II and III, molecular weights 14,900; 8,270; 6,420 and 2,550 (Swank & Munkres, 1971).

———— α-crystallin; —·—·—· nucleus of bovine lens; —— whole foetal human lens; ————— nucleus of normal human lens (aged 59); ..... brown nucleus of human cataractous lens (aged 68).

RESULTS AND DISCUSSION

Fig. 1 shows the scans of the polypeptides in the human and bovine lens nucleus, and in the whole foetal lens obtained after polyacrylamide gel electrophoresis in SDS and 8M urea; the cortex of the lens invariably contained fewer peptides, on a wet or dry weight basis, and those of the higher molecular weight range were less abundant or absent. For clarity only the scans of the polypeptides of molecular weight below about 9,000 are given, but the whole spectrum obtained from bovine α-crystallin is included, together with the position of the standards. The other scans are lined up so that the peaks of mobility of 0.29 (relative to the internal marker bromphenol Blue), coincide. This gives a fairly accurate overall picture of the results but as the distance from the top of the gel to the dye varied between 10 and 12 cm, the alignment of the traces is not precise.

The figure shows that the lens contains peptides of molecular weight less than about 9,000. Not shown are the findings from the lens nucleus of the rabbit, monkey and rat. All these contained peptides giving a profile similar to that of the bovine lens.

In all the old human lenses studied there was a range of peptides of molecular weight less than about 5,000; these were absent or scarce in the animal lenses. The brown degenerate lens nucleus tended to contain more low molecular weight peptides than the normal nucleus (coloured pale yellow but this was not always the case).

An unexpected finding was the presence in all the lenses from all the species examined of a band of relative mobility 0.29, running just behind the myoglobin cyanogen bromide peptide II of molecular weight 6,420. A band in the identical position was also found after electrophoresis of human or bovine α-crystallin (fig. 1). This position was confirmed by electrophoresing a mixture of the cyanogen bromide peptides and a sample of lens nucleus. The unknown appeared as a separate band just behind peptide II. A plot of linear rate of migration against the logarithm of molecular weight, gives a molecular weight of this peptide(s) of about 7,500; but according to Swank & Munkres (1971) the standard deviation from the correct value could be at least 18%.

Alpha-crystallin chains, degraded from the carboxyl end, have been found in the bovine lens, in increasing concentration towards the lens nucleus (Van Kleef, Willems-Thijssen & Hoenders, 1976). These chains called α A_2 1-101 have 101 amino acid residues compared with the 173 residues of α-crystallin itself. It is possible that this polypeptide(s) we have detected in all lenses constitutes the remaining 72 amino acid residues.

A fourth band occurs consistently after electrophoresis of human or bovine α-crystallin (fig. 1) corresponding to a molecular weight of 13,500 ± 18% (relative mobility 0.18). It is likely that this denotes the presence of α A_2 (1-101) itself.

We are currently attempting to isolate and analyse these polypeptides in α-crystallin and in the lens.

REFERENCES

Bloemendal, H. The vertebrate eye lens. *Science* 197: *127-138* (1977).

Blow, A.M.J., R. Van Heyningen & A.J. Barrett. Metal-dependent proteinase of the lens. *Biochem. J.* 145: *591-599* (1975).

Hanson, H. Proteolytic enzymes. *Expl. Eye Res.* 1: *468-479* (1962).

Harding, J.J. & K.J. Dilley. Structural proteins of the mammalian lens: A review with emphasis on changes in development, ageing and cataract. *Expl. Eye Res.* 22: *1-73* (1976).

Roy, D. & A. Spector. Absence of low-molecular weight α-crystallin in nuclear region of old human lenses. *Proc. Watl. Acad. Sci. USA* 73: *3484-3487* (1976).

Swank, R.T. & K.D. Munkres. Molecular weight analysis of oligopeptides by electrophoresis in polyacrylamide gel with sodium dodecyl sulfate. *Analyt. Biochem.* 39: *462-477* (1971).

Trayhurn, P. & R. Van Heyningen. Neutral proteinase activity in the human lens. *Expl. Eye Res.* 22: *251-257* (1976).

Van Kleef, F.S.M., W. Willems-Thijssen & H.J. Hoenders. Intracellular degradation and deamidation of α-crystallin subunits. *Eur. J. Biochem.* 66: *477-483* (1976).

Authors' addresses:
Ruth van Heyningen
Nuffield Laboratory of Ophthalmology
University of Oxford
Walton Street
Oxford, OX2 6AW
England

Simon van Heyningen
Department of Biochemistry
University of Edinburgh Medical School
Teviot Place
Edinburgh, EH8 9AG
Scotland, U.K.

Docum. Ophthal. Proc. Series, Vol. 18

UTILIZATION OF BENCYCLANE-HYDROGEN-FUMARATE AS A SUBSTRATE FOR THE CITRIC ACID CYCLE OF BOVINE LENSES

OTTO HOCKWIN, MECHTHILD GÜNTER & ELSE NOLL

(Bonn, West Germany)

ABSTRACT

Bovine lenses incubated in TC 199 in the presence of bencyclane-hydrogen-fumarate (BCHF) show, in contrast to controls incubated without addition of BCHF, an increased metabolite-level of malate and α-ketoglutarate which is due to metabolism of the fumarate portion of the BCHF. This effect is most obvious after pre-incubation under conditions of endogenous substrate deficiency. Addition of disodium fumarate does not show any effect which may be due to different permeation properties with respect to BCHF. – Results support former findings that an activation of the carbohydrate metabolism through bencyclane-hydrogen-fumarate is due to its utilization as a substrate of the citric acid cycle.

INTRODUCTION

Investigations on bovine lens homogenates (Korte et al., 1976; Hockwin et al., 1977) and on intact bovine lenses which, due to deficiency of endogenous substrates, had sustained a serious disturbance of their metabolic balance (Hockwin et al., 1978), showed that bencyclane-hydrogen-fumarate is able to reactivate the carbohydrate metabolism to a great extent. Bencyclane-hydrogen-fumarate (BCHF) is a N-[3-(1-bencyl-cycloheptyl-oxy)-propyl] -N, N-dimethyl-ammoniumhydrogen fumarate*. The molecule has certain salt-like properties; the bencyclane part is linked to the anionic fumarate portion as its cationic partner. The substance plays a vasoactive role (Denck, 1973). With some of the vasoactive clinical effects an improved metabolic condition is observed (Hapke, 1974; Gärtner et al., 1974; Kiss et al., 1977), which may in most cases be interpreted as an activation of the carbohydrate breakdown (Spaan & Hild, 1974).

The lens investigations gave rise to the question of whether the fumarate part of BCHF might be responsible for the observed alterations of biochemical parameters of the carbohydrate and energy metabolism. Korte et al. (1977) were able to prove that the enzyme fumarase (EC. 4.2.1.2) metabolizes the fumarate portion of the molecule. The substrate affinities of the

---

* Trade name: Fludilat®, Manufacturers Dr. Thiemann GmbH, Chem.-pharm. Fabrik, D-4670 Lünen, Westf., Fed. Rep. Germany, to whom we are indebted for the substance.

enzyme were about $K_m = 1.3 \times 10^{-3}M$, and did not show any dependence on the cationic component. These results supported the assumption that the fumarate portion of BCHF might be utilized as a substrate for the citric acid cycle (Hockwin, 1977, Hockwin et al., 1978).

For a long time the problem of whether the citric acid cycle is involved in the carbohydrate breakdown had been open to question (Leinfelder & Christiansen, 1952; Kinoshita & Wachtl, 1958; van Heyningen, 1962). The results of F.P. Fischer (1934), Kronfeld (1927, 1933), Huysman & Fischer (1941), Ely & Robbie (1950), Kinsey & Frohman (1951), Harris et al. (1953), Heinrichs & Harris (1956), and Hockwin (1956) gave first evidence of its presence. Its importance was pointed out by Hockwin et al. (1956) and Hockwin (1961), who finally succeeded in determining the possible role of this metabolic pathway in the energy metabolism of the lens (Hockwin & Korte, 1966; Blum, 1969; Murata & Hockwin, 1969; Hockwin et al., 1971; Radetzky, 1971; Korte & Hockwin, 1972). The results of Trayhurn (1972) and Trayhurn & van Heyningen (1971/1973) verify the activity of the citric acid cycle and its involvement in energy providing processes.

The model of the substrate deficient lens, the physiologic balance of which has been altered, now allowed investigations on the activation of lens metabolism with whole lenses (Hockwin et al., 1978) which had formerly only been possible with lens homogenates (Korte & Hockwin, 1978). In our investigations we tried to elucidate whether the increased metabolism of the fumarate part of the BCHF leads to changes in the content of metabolites of the citric acid cycle even in the presence of glucose. For this purpose we determined the content of malate and α-ketoglutarate in a pairwise test assay under various incubation conditions. One lens of each pair was subjected to bencyclane-hydrogen-fumarate. As a parameter for measurements malate was chosen, since it is formed from fumarate by the enzyme fumarase (Korte et al., 1977), and also α-ketoglutarate, which is formed from fumarate after several intermediate steps.

MATERIALS AND METHODS

Bovine eyes from the local slaughter house immediately after the death of the animals, were put pairwise into a cooled Dewar and brought to the laboratory. Preparation and medium for the substrate deficiency tests (Krebs-Ringer) and for the recovery phase (TC 199) have been described elsewhere (Hockwin et al., 1978).

In a first series BCHF (10 mM/l) was added to the medium. For comparison, another series, where BCHF was replaced by disodium fumarate, (10 mM/l) was performed. The periods of pre-incubation in Krebs-Ringer solution at 37°C varied; the phase of recovery was kept constant with 3 hrs at 37°C.

Following incubation the lenses were rinsed in ice-cold H_2O for 3 min., dried on filter paper, weighed again and homogenized in 0.6 N $HClO_4$ (1 g lens/7 ml). The protein was separated by centrifuging (17.000 x g) at 4°C for 20 min. From the supernatant 7 ml were diluted with 1.4 ml of 1.75 M

K_3PO_4 and kept in an icebath for 15 min. The precipitated $KClO_4$ was filtered off, and the filtrate showed an average of pH = 7.19.

α-Ketoglutaric-acid was determined after Wallenfels and Christian (1974), using 4 ml of the lens extract. Malate determination was performed with 0.2 ml of lens extract after Gutmann & Wahlefeld, (1974).

RESULTS

Table 1 shows the concentrations of α-ketoglutarate and malate found in bovine lenses under various conditions of incubation. If freshly obtained lenses were incubated for 3 hrs in TC 199 the content of α-ketoglutarate increased with addition of 10 mM/l BCHF by about 108 per cent (p $<$ 0.001) compared to controls. If, previous to the above procedure, the lenses were incubated in Krebs-Ringer solution for 4 hrs, the increase in α-ketoglutarate was about 187 per cent (p $<$ 0.001) compared to the fellow lens. A 20-hr pre-incubation in Krebs-Ringer solution creating substrate deficiency, effected an increase in α-ketoglutarate through BCHF of more than 850 per cent during the 3 hr-phase of recovery. This was mainly due to the fact that

Table 1. Contents of α-ketoglutarate and malate in bovine lenses after various periods of pre-incubation and with addition of 10 mM/l bencyclane-hydrogen-fumurate or disodiumfumarate respectively during the 3 hr-recovery-phase in TC 199. Means in μM/100 g lens wet weight with standard deviation.

Pre-incubation Krebs-Ringer	n =	3 hr incubation in TC 199		3 hr incubation in TC 199 with 10 mM/l bencyclane -hydrogen-fumorate	
hrs		α-Keto-gluta-rate	Malate	α-Keto-gluta-rate	Malate
		Concentrations in μM/100 g lens wet weight			
0	12	0.83 ±0.27	23.08 ±6.54	1.71 ±0.28	52.20 ±5.24
4	18	0.57 ±0.27	41.52 ±8.96	1.38 ±0.38	80.52 ±14.02
20	15	0.14 ±0.24	35.64 ±11.47	1.30 ±0.65	80.69 ±14.34
				TC 199 with 10 mM/l Na$_2$-fumarate	
0	27 (18)	1.02 ±0.34	28.6 ±7.58	1.15 ±0.34	32.2 ±10.9
4	16	0.73 ±0.46	26.3 ±8.13	0.95 ±0.38	29.6 ±7.6

the lenses incubated without BCHF did not regain their initial physiologic level of α-ketoglutarate during the 3 hr-incubation in TC 199, while the lenses subjected to BCHF could fully regain their initial level. In this context the time of pre-incubation and therefore the degree of substrate deficiency plays an important role. The longer the pre-incubation, the lower the α-keto-glutarate content which, in contrast to that in the BCHF-treated lenses, never reached initial values again during the 3 hr recovery-phase in TC 199.

Similar results were obtained for the malate concentrations of these lenses, where different pre-treatment, however, did not play such an important role. Lenses subjected to BCHF during the 3 hr-recovery-phase regained initial values and the differences between lens and fellow-lens were significant with $p < 0.001$ and lie between 100 and about 150 percent, since the lenses without BCHF-influence showed a decreased malate concentration.

Fig. 1 shows the results obtained for lenses and fellow-lenses with different kinds of preparation.

Fig. 1a represents the values for lenses without pre-incubation, 1b shows the values after 4 hrs, and 1c after 20 hrs of pre-incubation. Along the abscissa, the lenses are plotted according to their content of α-ketoglutarate or malate, respectively, after a 3 hr-incubation in TC 199. Values for the relative fellow-lenses, subjected to the additional influence of 10 mM/l BCHF during the 3 hr-recovery period are plotted on the ordinate. Values obtained for these lens pairs have been connected. If BCHF-treatment had not shown any effect, the values would lie on or about the straight line. In this figure absolute values are given instead of values percent.

Disodium-fumarate as a substrate added to the TC 199 medium for the 3 hr-incubation hardly influenced the content of α-ketoglutarate and malate of fresh lenses or of lenses pre-incubated for 4 hrs in Krebs-Ringer solution. The differences between lenses and fellow lenses for 28 lens pairs had a 13 percent higher content of α-ketoglutarate and of malate for the fresh lenses incubated in TC 199. 17 lens pairs were pre-incubated for 4 hrs in Krebs-Ringer solution, then left to recover in TC 199, (i.e. 1 lens of each pair in TC 199 + Na_2 — fumarate for 3 hrs.) Compared to controls, values for α-ketoglutarate were higher by 30 per cent, those for malate by 12 per cent in lenses treated with disodium-fumarate. This difference is not significant (p > 0.05), vis. Table 1.

DISCUSSION

Today, it is an accepted fact that the citric acid cycle is an important factor in lens metabolism. Investigations on its ability to metabolize substrates have repeatedly been undertaken. Trayhurn (1972) and Trayhurn & van Heyningen (1971 a, b, 1973) have performed such experiments with some of the aminoacids. Werner (1969) was able to verify its ability to metabolize endogenous lipids.

Kleifeld et al. (1956) and Kleifeld & Hockwin (1956) assayed lens homogenates to verify not only its metabolic ability but also its relevance to metabolic processes. It could, for instance, be shown that in the presence of

110

pyruvate considerable incorporation of $^{32}PO_4{}^{3-}$ into ATP ($AT^{32}P$) takes place. Using the model of the reversible cation shift (Harris et al., 1951, 1953, 1954 a, b) Heinrichs & Harris (1956) investigated the recovery of the physiologic Na^+/K^+-equilibrium and found that acetate, pyruvate or α-keto-glutarate were not able to replace glucose, although a partial recovery could be observed, giving proof of a certain influence of these substances.

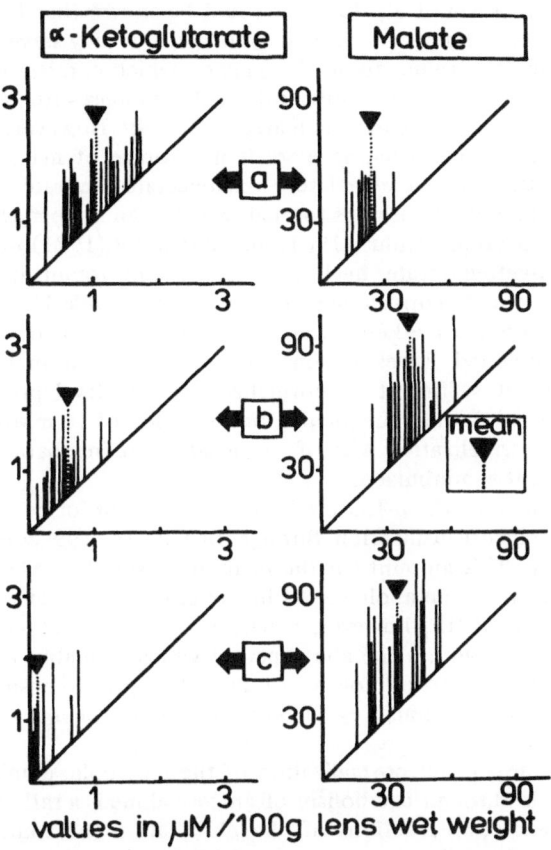

Fig. 1. Content of α-ketoglutarate and malate in bovine lenses. Comparison of results from pairwise test assays. Concentrations given in μM/100 g lens wet weight. Contents of α-ketoglutarate or malate respectively of lenses incubated in TC 199 without addition of bencyclane-hydrogen-fumarate are plotted along the abscissa.

Contents found in the relevant fellow-lens are plotted along the ordinate. The lenses of each pair are connected by a straight line. The values were measured after 3 hrs of incubation in TC 199 with and without addition of 10 mM/1 bencyclane

a) non-pre-incubated lenses
b) 4 hrs pre-incubation ⎱ in Krebs-Ringer solution to achieve
c) 20 hrs pre-incubation ⎰ substrate deficiency

Since investigations on the utilization of BCHF on lens homogenates (Hockwin et al., 1977) and on intact bovine lenses (Hockwin et al., 1978) indicated that the observed activation of the carbohydrate breakdown and the associated improvement of the energy equilibrium is due to metabolism of the fumarate portion of the BCHF (Korte et al., 1977), the problem as to whether this involves changes in the content of α-ketoglutarate and malate seemed interesting. Using lenses which, through their special incubation, showed substrate deficiency and therefore a disturbed physiologic metabolic equilibrium (Hockwin et al., 1978) it could be shown that BCHF as a substrate is metabolized in the citric-acid cycle where it may serve to restore the metabolic level. The values found for malate, which correspond to those of Krause & Stack (1939), are significantly higher in lenses treated with BCHF than in equally prepared lenses incubated in TC 199. However, values do not exceed the physiologic level, as there is no storage of malate. By further steps in the citric-acid cycle (malate → oxaloacetate → citrate → cis-aconitate → isocitrate →) α-ketoglutarate is formed, which is an important link towards amino-acid utilization. Paulus (1961) and Radetzky (1971) determined the content of α-ketoglutarate in bovine lenses and found it to be about 1-2 $\mu M/100$ g, which corresponds to our results (Table 1). In contrast to malate, the content of α-ketoglutarate is rather dependent on the kind of incubation employed. Investigations showed that a 3 hr-incubation in TC 199 alone is not sufficient to normalize the low level provoked by the substrate changes through pre-incubation. Addition of 10 mM/l BCHF, however, enables normalization even if, by a 20-hr pre-incubation, the α-ketoglutarate content is minimized.

This behaviour of the α-KG level may also explain former findings on an activation of glucose utilization through BCHF. TC 199 contains 1 g glucose/1 medium. This amount (or the medium as such) is evidently not able to restore the initial metabolite level in the citric-acid cycle within 3 hrs. In the presence of BCHF, however, malate as well as α-ketoglutarate regain their initial values within the above period which probably means that the requisite amount of carrier molecules is available again to ensure the smooth functioning of the citric-acid cycle, in which lies the energy supply through ATP.

It is well known that normalization of the metabolic equilibrium in the citric-acid cycle through catabolism of glucose alone is a rather slow process due to the restricting reactions of phosphorylation (hexokinase, phosphofructokinase) especially in case of the ATP-deficiency characteristic for a state of disturbed equilibria. Utilization of the fumarate portion of the BCHF enables regeneration of this energetically effective system, thus creating the basis for a ready supply of metabolic energy. This could be demonstrated by determining the ATP-content in bovine lenses after a 2 hr-recovery phase in TC 199 to which 0.1 mM/1 BCHF was added. Compared to that in lenses incubated without BCHF, it is significantly increased and concentrations of the glycolytic intermediates indicate increased glucosebreakdown (Hockwin et al., 1978).

We cannot as yet explain why the disodium-salt of fumarate does not or only to a slight degree show the effects observed with BCHF. However, differences in the permeation properties of the substances may be responsible.

Our investigations reinforce the importance of the citric-acid cycle for the energy balance of the lens, and indicate that utilization of bencyclane-hydrogen-fumarate and its breakdown may serve to compensate disturbances in the metabolite level of the tricarboxylic-acid cycle, as could be shown with α-ketoglutarate and malate, demonstrating that the disturbed metabolic equilibria can be restored to a physiologic steady state insuring the energy balance.

REFERENCES

Blum, G. Versuch einer Bilanzierung der Kohlenhydratabbauwege in Kälber- und Kaninchenlinsen. Dissertation Bonn (1969).

Denk, H. Behandlung peripherer Durchblutungsstörungen mit Bencyclan. *Wien. Med. Wschr.* 123: *174-178* (1973).

Ely, L.O., Robbie, W.A. The cyanide sensitivity and cytochrome-c content of the crystalline lens. *Am. J. Ophthal.* 33: *269-272* (1950).

Fischer, F.P. Wasserbindung, Durchsichtigkeit und Durchlässigkeit der Linse. *Arch. Augenheilk.* 108: *80-125* (1934).

Fischer, F.P. Die reduzierenden Substanzen der Linse. *Arch. Augenheilk.* 108: *527-543* (1934).

Gärtner, E., Enzenross, H.G., Vlahov, V., Schanzenbächer, P., Brandt, H., Betz, E. Durchblutung, pO_2 und pH des zerebralen Kortex unter Einwirkung van Fludilat[®]. *Therapiewoche* 23: *25:2824* (1974).

Gutmann, J., Wahlefeld, A.W. in Bergmeyer, H.-U.: Methoden der enzymatischen Analyse. 3. Aufl. Bd. II, S. *1632-1635*; Verlag Weinheim/Bergstr. 1974.

Hapke, H.J. Wirkung von Fludilat auf die Blut-Hirnschranke. *Therapiewoche* 24: 25: 2853 (1974).

Harris, J.E., Gehrsitz, L.B. Significance of changes in potassium and sodium content of the lens; mechanism for lenticular intumescence, *Am. J. Ophthal.* 34: (II), *131-138* (1951).

Harris, J.E., Gehrsitz, L.B., Nordquist, L.T. The in vitro reversal of the lenticular cation shift induced by cold or calcium deficiency. *Am. J. Ophthal.* 36: (II), *39-50* (1953).

Harris, J.E., Hauschildt, J.D., Nordquist, L.T. Lens metabolism as studied with the reversible cation shift. I. The role of glucose. *Am. J. Ophthal.* 38 (II), *141-147* (1954) a.

Harris, J.E., Hauschildt, J.D., Nordquist, L.T. Lens metabolism as studied with the reversible cation shift. II. The effect of oxygen and glutamic acid. *Am. J. Ophthal.* 38 (II), *148-152* (1954)b.

Heinrichs, D., Harris, J.E. Lens metabolism with the reversible cation shift. IV. The ability of various metabolites to replace glucose. *Am. J. Ophthal.* 42: *358-362* (1956).

Heyningen, van, R. The lens. II. General metabolism of the lens. 6. Citric acid cycle, in (ed. Davson, H.) The Eye, Vol. I, Academic Press New York and London, 1962. p. 228.

Hockwin, O. Untersuchungen von Stoffwechselvorgängen in der Linse unter Anwendung der polarographischen Analysenmethode. Dissertation Bonn 1956.

Hockwin, O. Experimenteller Beitrag zur Wirkung von Röntgenstrahlen auf Stoffwechselabläufe der Augenlinse in Abhängigkeit vom Lebensalter. Habilitationsschrift Bonn 1961; *Fortschr. Medizin* 80: *659-666* (1962).

Hockwin, O. Zur Wirkungsweise des Fludilat auf Vorgänge des Kohlenhydratstoffwechsels. Fortschr. Ther. in: *Fortschr. der Med.* 95: *1837-1840* (1977).

Hockwin, O., Korte, I. Biochemistry of the various catabolic pathways of the lens. Symp. Biochemistry of the Eye, Tutzing Castle 1966; Karger, Basel-New York 1968, pp. *216-225*.

Hockwin, O., Kleifeld, O., Arens, P.: Einfluß des Kaliumcyanid und der Monojodessigsäure auf den Stoffwechselablauf der Linse. *A. v. Graefes Arch. Ophthal.* 158: *47-53* (1956).

Hockwin, O., Korte, I., Breuer, R., Schmidt, G., Rast-Czyborra, F. In vitro Inkubation von Linsen. Modell zur Untersuchung der Substratverwertbarkeit von Substanzen für den Energiestoffwechsel am Beispiel des Bencyclanhydrogenfumarats. *A. v. Graefes Arch. klin. exp. Ophthal.* 1978, im Druck.

Hockwin, O., Blum, G., Korte, I., Murata, T., Radetzky, W., Rast, F. Studies on the citric acid cycle and its portion of glucose breakdown by calf and bovine lenses in vitro. *Ophthal. Res.* 2: *143-148* (1971).

Hockwin, O., Korte, I., Blum, G., Murata, T., Radetzky, W., Rast, F. Untersuchungen über den Anteil des Citronensäurezyklus am Kohlenhydratabbau der Linse. *Ber. dtsch. ophthal. Ges.* 70: *350-354* (1969).

Hockwin, O., Korte, I., Loth, C., Ohrloff, Ch., Fuss, R., Schmidt, G. Action of Bencyclane-hydrogen-fumarate on the Carbohydrate metabolism of Bovine Lens Homogenates. *Arzneim.-Forsch./Drug. Res.* 27: *1417-1420* (1977).

Huysmans, J.A., Fischer, F.P. Über den Gasstoffwechsel der Linse und des Glaskörpers. *Ophthalmologica (Basel)* 102: *275-286* (1941).

Kinoshita, J.H., Wachtl, C. A study of ^{14}C-glucose metabolism of the rabbit lens. *J. biol. Chem.* 233: *5-7* (1958).

Kinsey, E.V., Frohman, Ch.E. Studies on the crystalline lens. IV. Distribution of Cytochrome, Total Riboflavin, Lactate and Pyruvate and their Metabolic Significance. *Arch. Ophthal. (Chicago)* 46: *536-541* (1951).

Kiss, T., Smolenszky, T., Lelkes, J., Tekeres, M. Die Wirkung der Vasodilatoren Bencyclan und Tolazolin auf die Muskeldurchblutung im pharmakologischen und klinischen Experiment. *Therapiewoche* 22: *35:2791* (1972).

Kleifeld, O., Hockwin, O. Über den Kohlenhydratstoffwechsel der Linse in Abhängigkeit vom Lebensalter und bei experimentell erzeugten Stoffwechselstörungen. *Ber. dtsch. ophthal. Ges.* 60: *101-108* (1956).

Kleifeld, O., Ayberk, N., Hockwin, O. Über die Fähigkeit zur ATP-Bildung in Extrakten von Linsen junger und alter Tiere. *A. v. Graefes Arch. Ophthal.* 158: *34-38* (1956).

Korte, I., Hockwin, O. Studies on the citric acid cycle and its portion of glucose breakdown by calf and bovine lenses in vitro. lens symposium Utrecht, 1971; *Ophthal. Res.* 3: *13* (1972).

Korte, I., Hockwin, O. Content in adenosin-tri-, di- and monophosphate in bovine lens homogenate incubated in Ringer-solution and after addition of fructose-1,6-diphosphate. 3rd ISER-Congress, Osaka/Japan 1978.

Korte, I., Loth, C., Hockwin, O. The effect of bencyclane-hydrogen-fumarate (Fludilat [R]) on the gas exchange of lens homogenates. 17th Meeting AER, Guildford/England 1976; *Expl. Eye Res.* 24: *98* (1977).

Korte, I., Hockwin, O., Ohrloff, Ch., Schmidt, G., Fuss, R. Bestimmung des K_M-Wertes der Fumarase (EC 4.2.1.2) mit Bencyclanhydrogenfumarat als Substrat. *Arzneim.-Forsch./Drug Res.* 27: *1532-1534* (1977).

114

Krause, A.C., Stack, A.M. Citric and malic acid of the ocular tissues. *Arch. Ophthal. (Chicago)* 22: *66-72* (1939).

Kronfeld, P.C. Zur Frage der Linsenatmung. *Ber. dtsch. ophthal. Ges.* 46: *230-233* (1927).

Kronfeld, P.C. Metabolism of the normal and cataractous lens. *Am. J. Ophthal.* 16: *881-889* (1933).

Leinfelder, P.J., Christiansen, G.S. A critical study of lens metabolism. II. Glycolysis *Am. J. Ophthal.* 35: *33-38* (1952).

Murata, T., Hockwin, O. Der Gehalt an Zitronensäure in Linsen und einzelnen Linsenteilen unterschiedlich alter Rinder. *A. v. Graefes Arch. klin. exp. Ophthal.* 179: *32-40* (1969).

Paulus, W. Untersuchungen über den Gehalt von α-Ketoglutarsäure in Rinde und Kern verschieden alter Rinderlinsen. *A. v. Graefes Arch. Ophthal.* 163: *320-323* (1961).

Radetzky, W. Untersuchungen des Kohlenhydratstoffwechsels von Linsen nach Aufbewahrung in Nährlösung mit unterschiedlichem O_2-Partialdruck. Dissertation Bonn, 1971.

Spaan, G., Hild, R. Veränderungen einiger Stoffwechselparameter in der ischämischen Extremität durch Fludilat. *Therapiewoche* 24: 25:2833: *16-17* (1974).

Trayhurn, P. Metabolism of the citric acid cycle amino acids in the bovine lens. *Ophthal. Res.* 3: *13* (1972).

Trayhurn, P., van Heyningen, R. Aerobic metabolism in the bovine lens. *Exp. Eye Res.* bovine lens. *Biochem. J.* 124: *72 P* (1971a.).

Trayhurn, P., Van Heyningen, R. Aerobic metabolism in the bovine lens. *Exp. Eye Res.* 12: *315-327* (1971b.).

Trayhurn, P., van Heyningen, R. The Metabolism of Glutamine in the Bovine Lens: Glutamine as a source of glutamate. *Expl. Eye Res.* 17: *149-154* (1973).

Wallenfels, K., Christian, W. in Bergmeyer, H.-U.: Methoden der enzymatischen Analyse. 3. Aufl. Bd. II, S. 1624-1627, Verlag Chemie, Weinheim/Bergstr. 1974.

Werner, H. Oxidation of ^{14}C-labelled endogenous lipids by intact rabbit lenses. Ass. Res. Ophthal., Sarasota April 1969.

Authors' address:
Division Biochemistry of the Eye
Institute for Experimental Ophthalmology
University of Bonn, Fed. Rep. Germany
D-5300 Bonn-Venusberg.

DIFFERENCES IN THE SUSCEPTIBILITY OF VARIOUS ALDOSE REDUCTASES TO INHIBITION

PETER F. KADOR, LORENZO O. MEROLA &
JIN H. KINOSHITA

(Bethesda. USA)

ABSTRACT

The potency of the aldose reductase inhibitors 3,3-tetramethylene glutaric acid, *1*, Alrestatin, *2*, quercitrin, *3*, 7-hydroxy-4-oxo-4*H*-chromen-2-carboxylic acid, *4*, its ethyl ester, *5*, and 2-tetrazolyl-3-chloro-4-oxo-4*H*-chromen, *6*, was evaluated against human placental aldose reductase prepared via affinity column chromatography. The order of potencies obtained was *4 > 5 > 2 > 3 > 1 > 6*. This did not correlate with the order obtained against rat lens aldose reductase which was *3 > 2 > 4 = 5 = 1 = 6*. Except for 7-hydroxy-4-oxo-4*H*-chromen-2-carboxylic acid, *4*, all compounds displayed decreased inhibition against human placental aldose reductase as compared to rat lens aldose reductase. These findings indicate that the evaluation of aldose reductase inhibitors for potential clinical use may require the use of human aldose reductase.

INTRODUCTION

The sorbitol pathway of glucose metabolism contains two enzymes, aldose reductase (alditol: NADP oxidoreductase, EC 1.1.1.21) and sorbitol dehydrogenase (L-iditol: NAD oxidoreductase EC 1.1.1.14). Aldose reductase (AR) along with the coenzyme NADPH catalyzes the reduction of aldose to alditol (Collins & Corder, 1977, Hayman & Kinoshita, 1971). This enzyme has a broad substrate specificity, attacking many aldehyde containing compounds (Kinoshita, Varma & Fukui, 1976). Hexoses generally are poor substrates with high K_m's for AR; however, when their levels are elevated as in hyperglycemia or hypergalactosemia significant polyol formation can occur. In the lens the formation of excess sugar alcohol in the lens fibers followed by the osmotic accumulation of water has been implicated in the pathogenesis of diabetic and galactosemic cataracts (Kinoshita, 1974). Evidence also suggests AR to be involved in the major diabetic complications of neuropathy, nephropathy and retinopathy (Buzney et al., 1977, Gabbay, 1973).

Since AR appears to trigger the events that lead to sugar cataracts and possibly other diabetic complications, the development of potent and selective inhibitors of this enzyme is highly desirable. Currently an active search for AR inhibitors is being conducted and several compounds of diverse structure have been reported to show inhibitory activity. These include the Ayerst products 3,3-tetramethylene glutaric acid (TMG, *1*) and Alrestatin (AY-22,284, 1,2-dioxo-1*H*-benz[de]-isoquinoline-2-(3*H*) acetic acid, *2*), flavanoids such as quercitrin (2-3'4'-dihydroxyphenyl-3-0-rhamnosyl-5,7-dihy-droxy-4-oxo-4H-chromen, 3) and chromones such as 7-hydroxy-4-oxo-4H-chromen-2-carboxylic acid, 4, its ethyl ester, 5, and 2-tetrazolyl-3-chloro-4-oxo-4H-chromen, 6 (Jedziniak & Kinoshita, 1971, Kinoshita, 1974, Varma & Kinoshita, 1976 and Kador & Sharpless, 1978).

In evaluating the potency of these compounds, AR from animal lenses has been used. This source was assumed to be adequate due to the difficulty in obtaining human lenses and the amount of material required to obtain adequate amounts of the enzyme. The placenta, however, is a readily available source of human AR (Clemens & Winegrad, 1972). Here we report the evaluation of known AR inhibitors with human placental aldose reductase (HPAR) and compare these results with those obtained using rat lens aldose reductase (RLAR).

METHODS

Compounds 1 and 2 were obtained from the Ayerst Chemical Company, Montreal, Canada, compound 3 from K and K Laboratories, Inc., and compounds 4-6 from Dr. G.P. Ellis, Department of Chemistry, the University of Wales Institute of Science and Technology, Cardiff, U.K. NADPH (type I), NADP and DL-glyceraldehyde were obtained from Sigma Chemical Company and Boehringer Mannheim GmbH. AH-Sepharose 4B was obtained from Pharmacia Fine Chemicals, 4-carboxybenzaldehyde from Aldrich Chemical Company and 1-ethyl-3-(3-dimethylaminopropyl)-carbodiimide hydrochloride (EDC) from Pierce Chemical Company. Human placental homogenate solution was supplied by Drs. J. Barranger and J. Kusiak of NIH as the effluent from a Con A-Sepharose 4B column (Pharmacia). This solution was prepared by homogenizing 1 kg of placenta with 2 l of 25 mM phosphate buffer pH 6.4 and centrifuging at 17,000 g for 30 min.

Preparation of Affinity Column To a 100 ml solution of 1:1 dioxane-water containing 2.0 g of 4-carboxybenzaldehyde was added 15 g of AH-Sepharose 4B previously swollen in 200 ml of 0.5 M sodium chloride and washed on a sintered glass filter with 3 l of distilled water. To the slurry was added dropwise 1.88 g of EDC dissolved in 10 ml of water. The mixture rapidly became cloudy and an additional 30 ml of tetrahydrofuran was added. The mixture was placed on a shaker at room temperature while the pH was maintained below 5.0 for the first hr. After 72 hr the clear mixture was washed with 2 x 250 ml of 1:1 dioxane-water and 2 l of water. This was then followed by washing with 250 ml buffer containing .1 M borate and .5 M sodium chloride, pH 8 and .1 M acetate and .5 M sodium chloride, pH 4. Finally the coupled Sepharose was washed with buffer containing .1 M NaK phosphate and 0.01 M mercaptoethanol, pH 6.2 (standard buffer) and packed in a Pharmacia K 16/40 column.

Preparation of HPAR To 1500 ml of the placental solution was added 125 mg of NADP and 1000 ml of saturated ammonium sulfate solution. After standing for 30 min the solution was centrifuged at 45,000 g for 10 min and an additional 250 ml of saturated ammonium sulfate solution was added to the supernatant. After standing 30 min and centrifugation, 427 g of powdered ammonium sulfate was added with stirring. The precipitate recovered (*ca.* 50-70% saturation) upon standing and centrifugation was dissolved in a minimum amount of standard buffer and dialyzed against 2 changes of 6 l standard buffer. This solution was stored by freezing in liquid nitrogen. Aliquots of this solution were passed through the above column with the standard buffer. The enzyme could then be obtained by elution with standard buffer containing a 1 *M* sodium chloride gradient. Alternatively, crude placental solution was directly passed through the column and after washing with standard buffer, the HPAR could be obtained via a 1 *M* sodium chloride gradient in standard buffer.

Preparation of RLAR This enzyme was prepared as previously described (Kador & Sharpless, 1978).

AR activity was assayed spectrophotometrically by determining the decrease in the NADPH concentration at 340 nm in a Gilford 2400-2 automated compensating double beam spectrophotometer. The reaction mixture contained *ca.* 0.1 *M* phosphate buffer, pH 6.2; 0.104 *mM* NADPH; and 10 *mM* *DL*-glyceraldehyde in a total volume of 1.00 ml. The reference blank contained all of the above compounds except the glyceraldehyde substrate. Appropriate blanks to correct for the nonspecific reduction of NADPH and any absorbance of the inhibitor were used. The percent inhibition of each compound was calculated by comparing the reaction rate of the solution containing substrate and compound at a given concentration with that of the control solution containing only substrate. The average rate for the control solution was 1.72 ± .52 ng/ml/min. Protein concentrations were spectrophotometrically determined according to the method of Bradford (1976) and by using the equation $1.45A_{280} - .74A_{260} = $ mg/ml (Kalckar, 1947).

RESULTS AND DISCUSSION

In order to assess the inhibitory activity of compounds *1-6* a partial purification of HPAR was required since AR activity in the crude homogenate can not be accurately assessed due to competing reactions. Clemens & Winegard (1972) have reported a six step purification of HPAR involving treatment with calcium phosphate gel, ammonium sulfate fractionation, DEAE cellulose and Sephadex G-100 chromatography and repeated isoelectric focusing.

In this study affinity chromatography using a 4-carboxybenzaldehyde coupled AH-Sepharose 4B led to a preparation of HPAR of sufficient purity to permit evaluation of AR inhibitors. Upon elution with a sodium chloride gradient the enzyme can be obtained with some fractions of the gradient having up to 300 fold purification. Elution with the sodium chloride gradient was better than with 0.1 *M* glyceraldehyde, a substrate of AR, which only partially removed bound AR from the column or NADP which had no effect.

The crude placental homogenate rapidly loses AR activity upon standing for several days at 4°C. However, through ammonium sulfate fractionation and dialysis a more stable solution can be obtained. During this procedure the addition of NADP appears to stabilize the enzyme. No significant loss in activity was observed upon freezing in liquid nitrogen and storing at −78°C for 1 month. Chromatography with this preparation, which corresponds to the elution pattern of Figure 1, resulted in 86% recovery of enzyme activity. Upon extended use of the column, especially with the ammonium sulfate fractions, a build-up of proteins due to nonspecific binding occurred. This resulted in a decreased efficiency of the column.

The purified enzyme appeared to be quite unstable, rapidly losing activity upon standing overnight at 4°C. Moreover, it could not be concentrated with an Amicon PM-30 filter without significant loss of activity. We plan to continue the purification of HPAR; however, for evaluating the AR inhibitors the enzyme immediately recovered from affinity column chromatography was used.

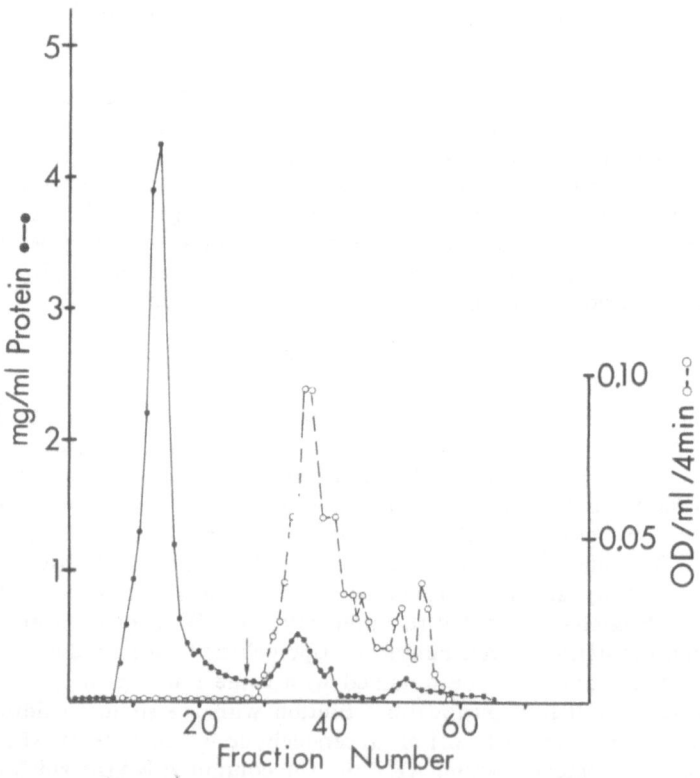

Fig. 1. Elution of dialyzed ammonium sulfate fraction on 4-carboxybenzaldehyde coupled AH-Sepharose 4B with .1 *M* phosphate buffer, pH 6.2, containing .01 *M* mercaptoethanol. Arrow represents start of a linear 1 *M* sodium chloride gradient (400 ml). Fractions were collected in 5 ml aliquots.

120

Enzyme kinetic studies with Alrestatin ($1 \times 10^{-6} M$), quercitrin ($1 \times 10^{-6} M$) and 7-hydroxy-4-oxo-4H-chromen-2-carboxylic acid ($5 \times 10^{-7} M$) indicated that all three noncompetitively inhibited HPAR. Similar inhibition has been observed with RLAR (Varma & Kinoshita, 1976) although quercitrin and 7-hydroxychromene-2-carboxylic acid have been shown to uncompetitively inhibit at $1 \times 10^{-6} M$ and to noncompetitively inhibit at higher concentrations (Kador & Sharpless, 1978).

The inhibitory activity of compounds *1-6* assessed in both HPAR and RLAR is summarized in Table *1*. From the percent inhibition obtained, semilogarithmic dose-response curves of the percent inhibition vs log concentration of inhibitor were constructed (Figure *2*). Although S-shaped curves are obtained straight lines can be approximated through regression analysis since the middle parts of the curve approximate straight lines. The activity of these inhibitors can, therefore, be estimated as the concentration needed to elicit 50% inhibition (IC_{50}). This value, which represents the affinity of the inhibitor for the enzyme is proportional to the K_I obtained by Michaelis-Menton kinetics (Wenke, 1971).

Against HPAR 7-hydroxy-4-oxo-4H-chromen-2-carboxylic acid, *4*, appeared to be the most potent inhibitor with an IC_{50} of $1.8 \times 10^{-6} M$. This was followed in decreasing order by 7-hydroxy-4-oxo-4H-chromen-2-carboxylic acid, ethyl ester, *5*, $IC_{50} = 5.0 \times 10^{-6} M$, Alrestatin, *2*, $IC_{50} = 6.5 \times 10^{-6} M$, TMG *1*, $IC_{50} = 2.5 \times 10^{-5} M$ and 2-tetrazolyl-3-chloro-4-oxo-4H-

Table 1. Summary of inhibitions obtained against HPAR and RLAR.

Inhibitor		% Inhibition $10^{-5}M$ $10^{-6}M$ $10^{-7}M$			IC_{50} $\times 10^{-6} M$	$\dfrac{IC_{50} \text{ HPAR}}{IC_{50} \text{ RLAR}}$
1	HPAR	50	trace	0	25.	11.4
	RLAR	87	34	trace*	2.2	
2	HPAR	65	30	0	6.5	4.3
	RLAR	86	50	7	1.5	
3	HPAR	57	20	0	7.1	11.6
	RLAR	91	65	20	.61	
4	HPAR	73	46	14	1.8	0.8
	RLAR	79	33	11	2.2	
5	HPAR	72	20	trace	5.0	2.2
	RLAR	77	31	13	2.3	
6	HPAR	47	21	trace	41.	16.4
	RLAR	77	34	7	2.5	

n=3-10, S.E.≤10 ; *trace ≤5

121

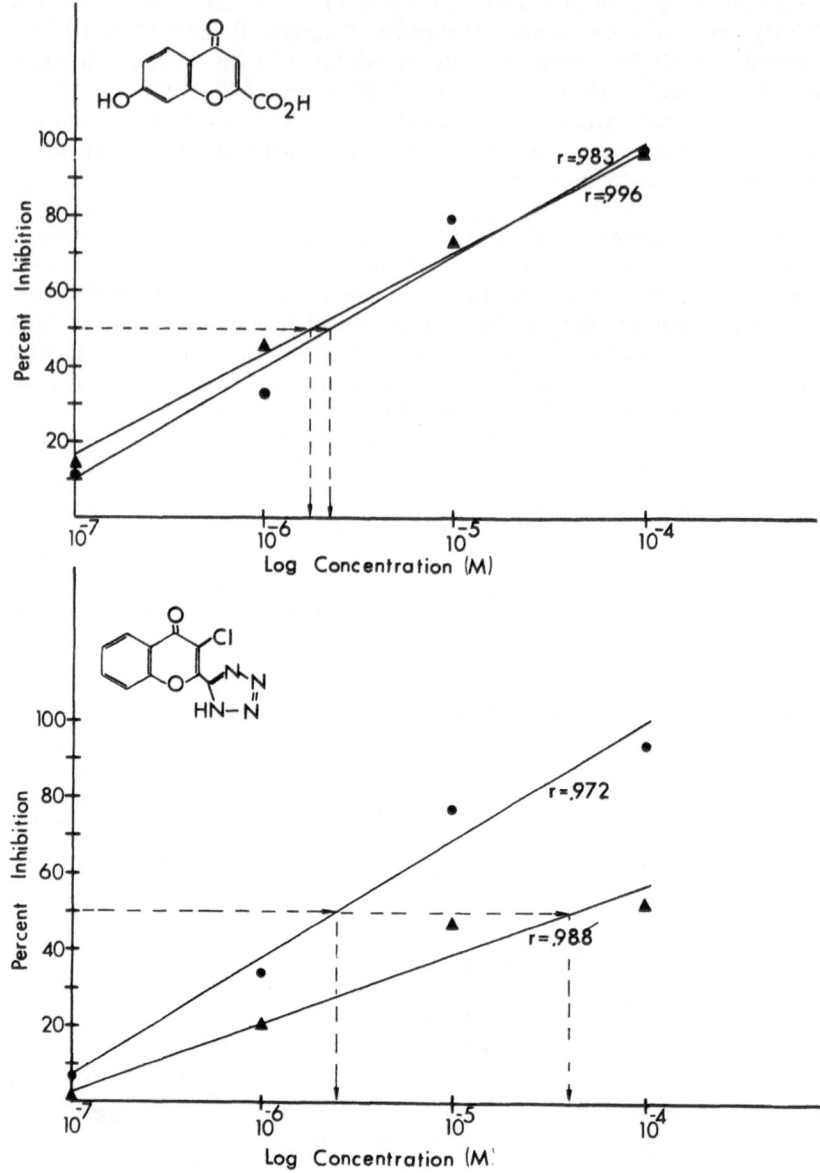

Fig. 2. Dose-response plots of the percent inhibition versus log concentration of 7-hydroxy-4-oxo-4*H*-chromen-2-carboxylic acid (top) and 2-tetrazolyl-3-chloro-4-oxo-4*H*-chromen (bottom) against HPAR (▲) and RLAR (●). Arrows indicate IC_{50} values.

122

chromen, 6, IC_{50} = 4.1 x $10^{-5} M$. Against RLAR quercitrin, 3, was the most potent inhibitor (IC_{50} = 6.1 x $10^{-7} M$) followed by Alrestatin, 2, IC_{50} = 1.5 x $10^{-6} M$. The remaining inhibitors were all equipotent, IC_{50} = 2.2-2.5 x $10^{-6} M$. With the exception of 7-hydroxy-4-oxo-4H-chromen-2-carboxylic acid, 4, which slightly increased in potency, all of the compounds displayed decreased inhibition against HPAR as compared to RLAR. This decreased potency, respectively, was 2-tetrazolyl-3-chloro- 4-oxo-4H-chromen, 6, 16x, Quercitrin, 3, 12x, TMG, 1, 11x, Alrestatin, 2, 4x, and 7-hydroxy-4-oxo-4H-chromen- 2-carboxylic acid, ethyl ester, 5, 2x.

As pointed out by Clemens & Winegrad (1971), HPAR resembles AR from animal sources in many ways including its ability to be stimulated by lithium sulfate and ammonium sulfate, and by its broad substrate specificity. Moreover, HPAR also has a broad pH optimum between 5.6-6.8. With respect to inhibition, however, although similar mechanisms of inhibition are observed against both HPAR and RLAR, the relative potency of inhibitors against RLAR does not correlate with their activity against HPAR. This may be due to different degrees of bulk tolerance exhibited by the two enzymes. These findings therefore indicate that the evaluation of aldose reductase inhibitors for potential clinical use may require the use of human aldose reductase.

REFERENCES

Bradford, M.M., A rapid and sensitive method for the quantitation of microgram quantities of protein utilizing the principle of protein-binding. *Analyt. Biochem.* 72: *248-254* (1976).

Buzney, S.M., Frank, R.N., Varma, S.D., Tanishima, T. & Gabbay, K.H. Aldose reductase in retinal mural cells. *Invest. Ophthal. Vis. Sci.* 16: *392-396* (1977).

Clemens, R.S. Jr. & Winegrad, A.I. Purification of alditol: NADP oxidoreductase from human placenta. *Biochem. Biophys. Res. Commun.* 47: *1473-1479* (1972).

Collins, J.G. & Corder, C.N. Aldose reductase and sorbitol dehydrogenase distribution in substructures of normal and diabetic rat lens. *Invest. Ophthal. Vis. Sci.* 16: *242-243* (1977).

Gabbay, K.H. The sorbitol pathway and the complications of diabetics. New Engl. *J. Med.* 288: *831-836* (1973).

Gabbay, K.H. & Kinoshita, J.H. in Methods of Enzymology vol XLI (ed. Wood W.A.) Academic Press, New York 1975.

Hayman, S. & Kinoshita, J.H. Isolation and properties of lens aldose reductase. *J. Biol. Chem.* 240: *877-882* (1971).

Jedziniak, J.A. & Kinoshita, J.H. Activators and inhibitors of aldose reductase. *Invest. Ophthal.* 10: *357-366* (1971).

Kador, P.F. & Sharpless, N.E. Structure-activity studies of aldose reductase inhibitors containing the 4-oxo-4H-chromen ring system. *Biophys. Chem.* 8: (1978) in press.

Kalckar, H. Differential spectrophotometry of purine compounds by means of specific enzymes. III. Studies of the enzymes of purine metabolism. *J. Biol. Chem.* 167: *461-475* (1947).

Kinoshita, J.H. Mechanisms initiating cataract formation. *Invest. Ophthal.* 13: *713-724* (1974).

Kinoshita, J.H., Varma, S.D. & Fukui, H.N. Aldose reductase in diabetes. *Jap. J. Ophthal.* 20: *399-410* (1976).

Varma, S.D. & Kinoshita, J.H. Inhibition of lens aldose reductase by flavanoids – their possible role in the prevention of diabetic cataracts. *Biochem. Pharmac.* 25: *2505-2513* (1976).

Wenke, M. in Fundamentals of Biochemical Pharmacology (ed. Bacg. Z.M.) Pergamon Press, New York 1971.

Authors' address:
Laboratory of Vision Research
National Eye Institute
National Institutes of Health
Bethesda, Md. 20014 USA

124

Docum. Ophthal. Proc. Series, Vol. 18

STUDIES ON THE CRYSTALLINE LENS. XXVIII.
THE INTERRELATIONSHIP OF HYDRATION, OSMOLARITY AND ELECTROLYTE CONTENT IN LENSES OF VARYING WEIGHTS FROM YOUNG RABBITS*

V. EVERETT KINSEY & KENNETH R. HIGHTOWER*

(Rochester, Michigan, U.S.A.)

ABSTRACT

The percentage of water in lenses decreases linearly with increasing lens weight as does the osmolarity of the intralenticular fluid. The latter change parallels a decrease in potassium concentration associated with a substantial increase in total water content in lenses of increasing weight. Values for osmolarity of lenses weighing between 250 and 500 mg are consistently lower than that of aqueous humor, 270 vs. 310 milliosmoles/ kg water, respectively. The value for the osmolarity of the intact lens, as measured by gain or loss of water of lenses bathed in media of various osmotic strengths, is approximately the same as that determined directly on the intralenticular fluid.

INTRODUCTION

Lens hydration is controlled by osmotic gradients between intralenticular fluid and the bathing media. Kinoshita et al. (1965) showed that lens hydration varies in a direct manner with osmolarity of the bathing media following incubation for 20 hours, swelling in hypotonic media and shrinking in hypertonic media, acting, therefore, as an osmometer. Cotlier et al. (1968) determined the osmolarity of intralenticular fluid of rabbit lenses and observed that changes in lens hydration occur as a result of water movement in response to osmotic gradients established between this fluid and the bathing media. They showed that within a range of 238-368 milliosmoles/kg water the lens behaves as a 'perfect osmometer.' From measurements of osmolarity of intralenticular fluid they concluded that the rabbit lens is isosmotic with aqueous humor at approximately 302 milliosmoles/kg water, which is intermediate between values found earlier by Nordmann (1935) in lenses from rabbits and human beings, viz. 285 and 312 milliosmoles/kg water, respectively. Duncan (1970) found a value for osmolarity of rabbit lenses (301 milliosmoles/kg water) similar to that of Cotlier et al. He also showed that in

* This work was presented at the national meeting of the Association for Research in Vision and Ophthalmology, Sarasota, Florida U.S.A. May, 1978. Supported in part by Research Grant Nos. EY 00483 and EY 05092 from the National Eye Institute of the National Institutes of Health, United States Energy Research and Development Administration, Contract No. E(11-1)-2012-36
* Recipient of United States Public Health Service National Research Service Award.

125

amphibians and rats the osmolarities of intralenticular fluid and aqueous humor were in excellent agreement. All these results suggest that there is no water pump in the lens, although Fowlks (1973a) has shown that a hypotonic fluid accumulates on the anterior surface of lenses bathed in silicone oil.

Patterson (1976) and Patterson & Fournier (1976) observed that hydration of rat lenses is affected not only by changes in osmolar concentrations of the media, but is also influenced by changes in permeability to potassium which they interpret as evidence for volume regulation.

The osmolarity of intralenticular fluid, according to Harris & Gruber (1962), depends upon metabolic activity of the lens which controls cation transport. The degree of hydration can be accounted for by the increase in total base (Na + K) and attendant shifts in anions under varying conditions that affect ion pumps. They found that when exchange of sodium and potassium is equivalent, the water content in the lens remains essentially constant, but when the transport mechanisms responsible for excretion of sodium and concentration of potassium are blocked sufficiently, more sodium is gained than potassium lost and, predictably, the lenses hydrate. Other studies by Kinoshita et al. (1961) show that the lens fails to maintain its normal hydration and cation relationship in the absence of glucose and oxygen as well as in the presence of rather low concentrations of iodoacetate. This observation was confirmed by Becker (1962) who noted that this poison blocks the uptake of rubidium.

The present study is designed to determine the interrelationship of lens hydration, osmolarity of intralenticular fluid in the intact lens, and the electrolyte concentrations under conditions associated with weight changes of lenses from young rabbits, undisturbed by exposure to widely varying solute concentrations in the bathing media or to such factors as chilling or exposure to metabolic poisons.

METHODS

Intralenticular osmolarities were determined by measuring the depression of the freezing point using an Advanced Instruments precision osmometer (Osmette). Lenses were blotted, weighed and homogenized in 1 ml of distilled water. The homogenate was centrifuged for 30 minutes at 16,000 g and aliquots of 0.2 ml of the supernatant were assayed for osmolarity immediately following standardization of the Osmette using solutions of 100 and 500 milliosmoles/kg water obtained from Advanced Instruments Inc. Readings of the supernatant were multiplied by the appropriate dilution factors assuming an average water concentration to be 65% of the fresh weight of the lens. Corrections were made to take into account the decrease in the osmotic coefficient of KCl due to dilution of the potassium salts in the intralenticular fluid of the lens. The correction factor (0.96) was based on values for KCl reported by Robinson & Stokes (1959).

Intralenticular osmolarity in intact lenses was estimated by establishing the tonicity of a bathing fluid which caused neither gain nor loss of water

126

when lenses were immersed for time periods of less than one minute, i.e., short enough to minimize movement of solutes. This technique was adapted from one employed by Goldstein & Solomon (1960) for the red blood cell and is thought to provide a measure of what they refer to as the 'operative' osmotic pressure, i.e., $\pi_0 = \sigma\pi$ where π is the measured osmotic pressure and σ the reflection coefficient (Staverman, 1951, 1952).

Lenses were carefully dissected free from the globe and gently rolled on filter paper moistened with saline to remove excessive vitreous or zonular fibers prior to weighing on a precision torsion balance in which the weighing pan was replaced with a wire loop. After placing the lens on the loop it was dipped into the test media for one second to offset possible dehydration of the capsule in case of excessive blotting. A reference, or zero time, weight was obtained by again gently blotting the lens on its posterior side and reweighing. Lenses supported by the loop were subsequently immersed in different warmed (37°C) test solutions of various strengths, blotted and reweighed at 5, 15 and 30 second intervals. Weighings were reproducible to within 0.1 mg. Test solutions consisted of NaCl, KCl, sucrose, glucose or urea made up in stock solutions of 1M strength and diluted to the desired concentrations prior to the experiment. The osmolarities were determined several times.

Sodium and potassium analyses were performed on the same aqueous extracts employed for determining osmolarity of the intralenticular fluid after removing protein by adding 4 ml of 2.5.% trichloroacetic acid (TCA) to 0.25 ml of the extract. The pipette used in transferring the extract was rinsed with water which was then added to the TCA solution. Protein in the TCA homogenate was removed by centrifugation and the cations in the supernatant were analyzed using an Hitachi-Perkin Elmer flame photometer.

Chloride was also determined on aqueous extracts employed for measurements of osmolarity. One half ml of the extract, along with an additional 0.5 ml of distilled water used to rinse the pipette, was added to 0.5 ml of 7.5 mM solution of diamide. The mixture was kept at 37°C for 2 hours to oxidize all the glutathione in the extract because reduced glutathione titrates electrometrically like chloride on a one-to-one basis. Protein in this mixture was removed by precipitation with 0.5 ml of 40% TCA. After centrifugation, 2 ml of water were added to 1 ml of supernatant and 1 ml aliquots were titrated electrometrically using a Cotlove Chloridometer. Standard solutions of chloride were prepared by adding diamide and TCA in the same concentration as employed with lens extracts.

No correction was made in calculating the ionic concentration to take into account the volume of protein in the original water extract of the lens.

Linear regression analyses were employed in fitting most of the data, and standard deviation of the error of estimate, when used, were employed to establish confidence limits for the regression lines using the relation: $S_e = S_y (1 - r^2)^{1/2}$ where S_y is the standard deviation of the dependent variable and r is the correlation coefficient of linearity between dependent and independent variables.

RESULTS

Figure 1 shows that water content of the lens decreases linearly from about 67% for lenses weighing 250 mg to 62% for those weighing 500 mg. The linear relation between percentage of water in the lens and lens weight was established by regression analysis, the correlation coefficient, r, being 0.9 for the group of 25 lenses.

While the percentage of water decreases with lens weight, Figure 2 shows that the absolute amount of water in the lens increases in direct proportion tolens weight, approximately doubling, for a two-fold increase in weight. The figure also shows that dry weight, as determined by drying under high va-

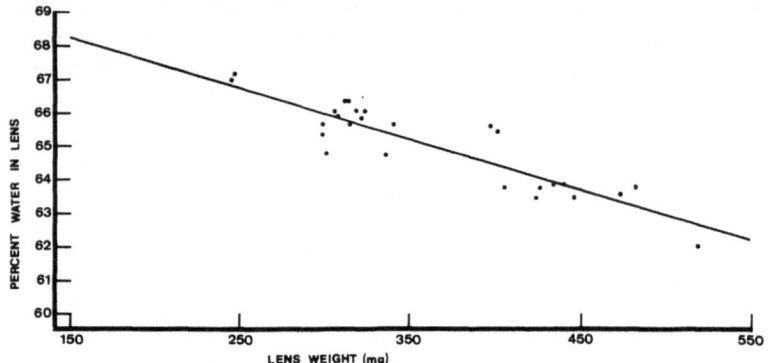

Fig. 1. Lens water calculated as percentage wet weight.

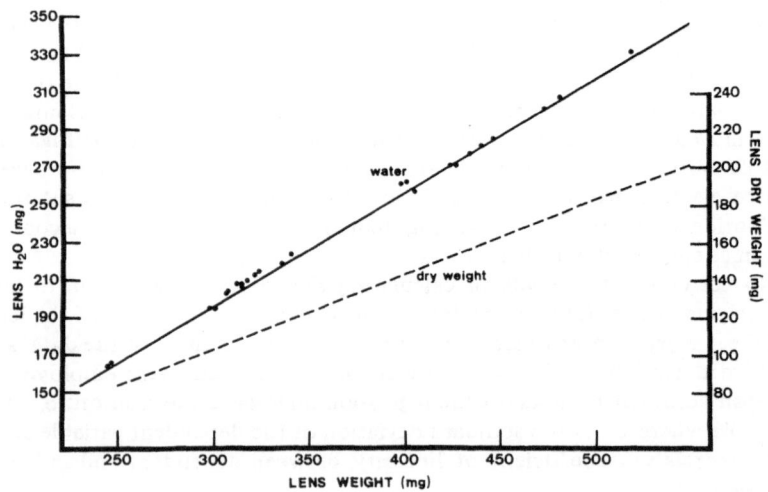

Fig. 2. Water and dry weight of lenses varying in weight from 250 to 500 mg.

128

cuum to constant weight, also increases linearly maintaining approximately a 1-to-3 ratio to that of lens. The correlation coefficient between lens water and lens weight, as well as dry weight and lens weight, was 0.95.

While both lens water and dry weight increase together with weight of the lenses, osmolarity decreased linearly with lens weight, from approximately 280 for the smallest lenses to 240 milliosmoles/kg lens water for lenses weighing 500 mg (Figure 3). The correlation between osmolarity and

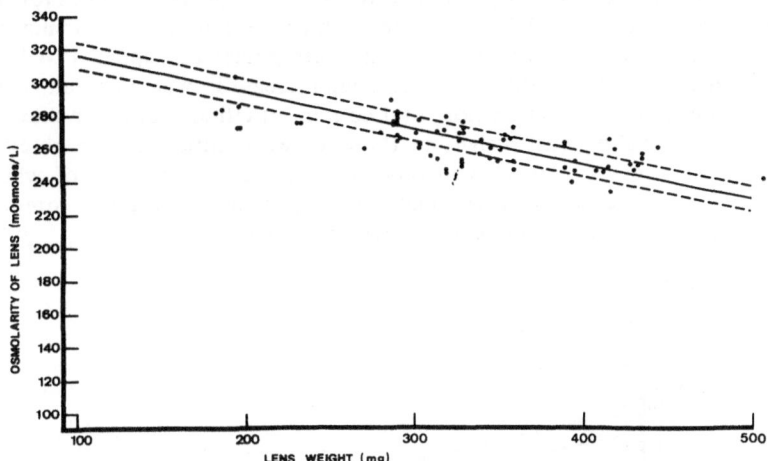

Fig. 3. Osmolarity of intralenticular fluid of lenses of differing weights. Broken lines represent one standard deviation of the error of estimate.

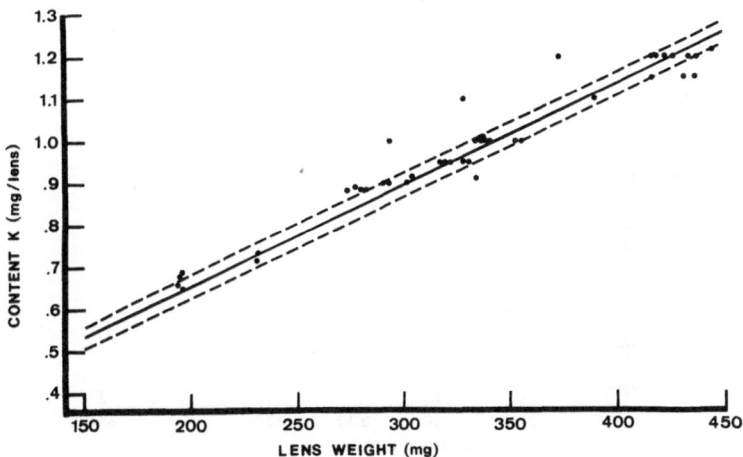

Fig. 4. Concentration of potassium in water of lenses of varying weights. Broken lines represent one standard deviation of the error of estimate.

129

weight was 0.79 for the 70 lenses employed and the standard deviation of the error of estimate was 8.6 milliosmoles/kg water as indicated by the broken lines.

The concentration and total content of sodium, potassium and chloride were determined in the intralenticular fluid in an effort to determine how they correlate with intralenticular osmolarity. Figure 4 shows that concentration of the electrolyte present in highest concentration, viz. potassium, decreases linearly with increase in lens weight while the total content of this ion increases linearly with weight (Figure 5). The respective r values for the correlations are 0.5 and 0.7. The decrease in concentration of potassium by approximately 20%, despite increase in total potassium, appears to be a consequence of dilution due to the striking increase in water content (Figure 2). Neither concentration nor total content of either sodium or chloride changed appreciably with weight in these lenses, contrary to the observations of Rink et al. (1977) who reported that sodium content of whole bovine lenses increased with age and lens weight, an increase not compensated by an equivalent decrease in potassium content.

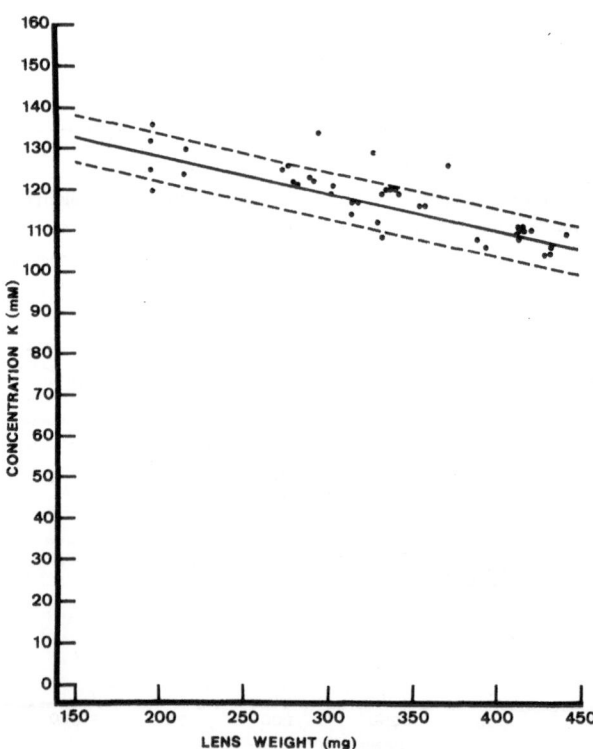

Fig. 5. Potassium content of lenses as a function of weight (solid line). Broken lines represent one standard deviation of the error of estimate.

The relation between changes in concentration of electrolytes in intralenticular fluid and its osmolarity is presented in Figure 6. Potassium concentration is obviously higher in lenses having greater osmolarity, which is the situation in smaller lenses, because of the inverse relation between osmolarity and lens weight (Figure 3). The apparent lack of dependence of the concentration of sodium and chloride on lens osmolarity, at least in the range of 230 to 300 milliosmoles/kg water, is consistent with the observation that concentration of these ions did not vary with lens weight. The sum of the concentrations of all three ions, likewise, was higher in lenses with high osmolarities, again in the lighter lenses.

The probable contribution of electrolytes to the observed osmolarity for lenses of varying weights is shown by the broken line of Figure 7 and was calculated by doubling the sum of values shown for concentration of potassium (Figure 4) and sodium (Figure 6) to take into account the contribution of the anions which must be associated with these cations (Figure 3). The solid line shows that actual osmolarity agrees well with that estimated for concentration of electrolytes.

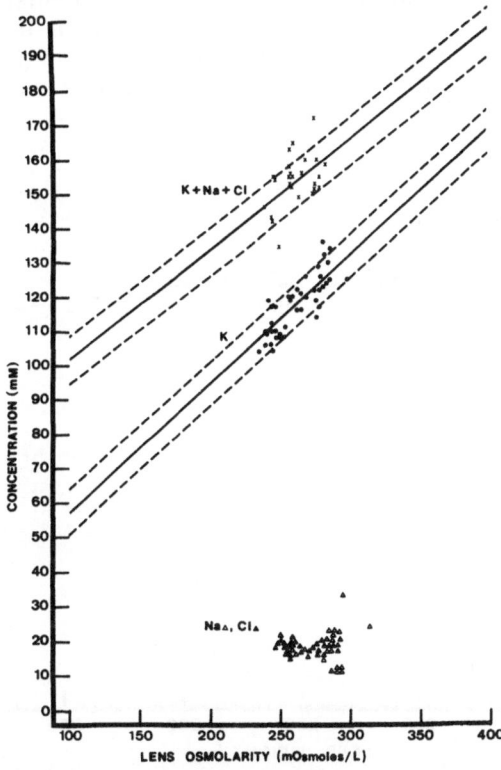

Fig. 6. Concentration of Na, Cl and K separately, and the total in the intralenticular fluid of lenses having different osmolarities depending upon their weight. Broken lines represent one standard deviation of the error of estimate.

DISCUSSION

The results of these studies show that the physical-chemical properties of the lens that affect hydration are highly dependent upon lens weight. Thus, lenses become decreasingly hydrated with increasing weight between 250 and 500 mg while osmolarity of intralenticular fluid decreases in parallel with an increase in total water content resulting in a concomitant decrease in concentration of potassium.

These observations suggest that decrease in concentration of intralenticular potassium may be largely responsible for osmolarity of the intralenticular fluid. For the entire range of weights studied, the values for osmolarity of intralenticular fluid were consistently lower than for that of aqueous humor (310 milliosmoles/kg water) (Kinsey, 1951). To determine whether the same difference exists between aqueous humor and the intact lens, gain or loss of water from lenses bathed for short periods in fluids of varying tonicity was determined and used as a measure of isotonicity.

The gain or loss in water resulting from immersion of lenses (average weight for 26 lenses of 304 mg) in solutions of NaCl of different concentrations for intervals up to 30 seconds is shown in Figure 8. It is evident that within this time span change in water content is linear with time. The rate of change in water content of the lenses was calculated from data in Figure 8

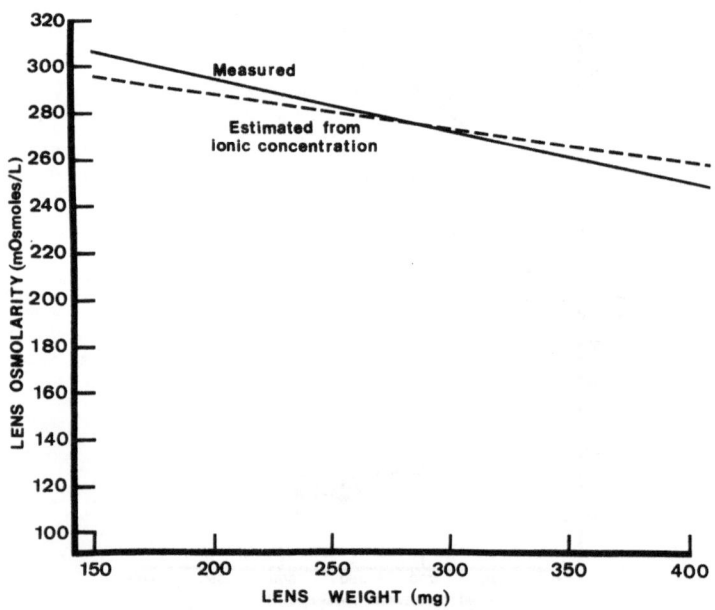

Fig. 7. Osmolarity of the intralenticular fluid as determined experimentally in lenses of varying weight (solid line) and as estimated from the ionic concentration (broken lines).

132

and the results are plotted in Figure 9 (solid line) as a function of the osmolarity of the media employed. Analogous experiments were performed using sucrose to vary the tonicity of the media and the resulting rates of change in water content of the lenses employed are also plotted (broken line) in Figure 9. The points for the experimental data for sodium chloride fall in a straight line and intercept the zero slope axis at 265 milliosmoles/kg water. The two points for data obtained for sucrose, when connected, intercept the zero slope axis at 260 milliosmoles/kg water. This intercept is the isosmotic concentration, assuming that the solute restricting membranes in the lens are sufficiently impermeable that sodium chloride and sucrose exert their full osmotic pressure and $\sigma = 1$.

Sodium propionate gave an isosmotic value indistinguishable from that of NaCl, but the data obtained while using urea and glycine intercepted the zero slope axis at 400 and 700 milliosmoles/kg water, respectively, suggesting that lens membranes are sufficiently more permeable to these substances such that they do not exert their full osmotic pressure, i.e., they have values of $\sigma < 1$.

The data from experiments of this kind are thought to provide a reasonably accurate measure of the initial rate of swelling or shrinking under conditions in which the lens remains in essentially the steady state condition prevailing in vivo with respect to water and solute distribution. It is note-

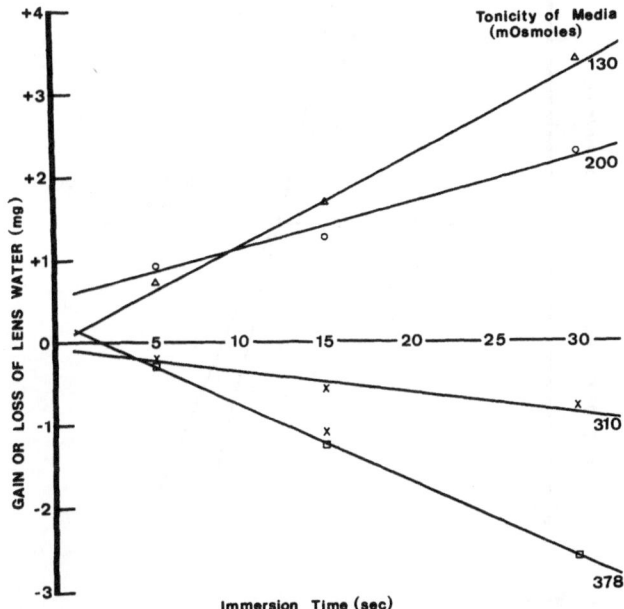

Fig. 8. Changes in water content of lenses immersed in solutions of NaCl of different tonicities for periods up to 30 seconds. Each line is a visual fit to data involving 6 to 8 lenses.

worthy that values obtained for isosmotic concentrations for the intact lens are also considerably lower than that of aqueous humor, and with respect to the saline solution they are in good agreement with the value, 274 milliosmoles/kg water, for lenses having a comparable weight, viz. 304 mg (Figure 3). Thus, an average value for osmolarity of lenses weighing approximately 300 mg in the present investigation would appear to be about 270 milliosmoles/kg water.

In the absence of knowledge of the weights used by others, it is not meaningful to compare this result with those reported previously, but only Nordmann's value of 285 milliosmoles/kg water appears to be significantly below the osmolarity of aqueous humor.

In an effort to strengthen evidence that the lens is, in fact, hyposmotic to aqueous humor, the possibility that some electrolytes are bound to insoluble protein in the aqueous extract, hence not included in the osmotic pressure, was investigated. Analyses of the pellet obtained from lens homogenates

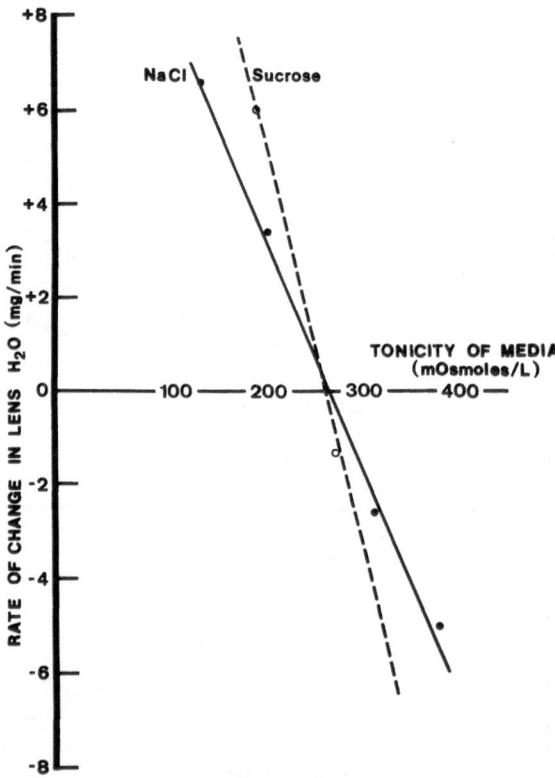

Fig. 9. Rate of change of water content of lenses immersed in solutions of NaCl or sucrose of different tonicities. The rates shown for the line for NaCl (solid) were obtained from the data plotted in Figure 8.

used in the preparation of aqueous extracts of the lens were extracted repeatedly in 10% TCA and then analyzed by flame photometry for the presence of sodium or potassium. No appreciable quantity was found, suggesting that the aqueous extracts employed for measurements of osmolarity include all the cations present and, therefore, the value of 270 milliosmoles/kg water is correct. In this regard, it is interesting to note that in results to be reported elsewhere the total concentration of those substances that would be expected to be osmotically active, i.e., calcium, magnesium, sodium, potassium, chloride, bicarbonate, amino acids, lactate and phosphate obtained by extracting lenses with TCA, add to a total of less than 270 milliosmoles/kg water.

If osmolarity of the lens is indeed as low as the results of these studies suggest, there would appear to be a substantial osmotic gradient between the fluid in the lens and the aqueous and vitreous humors. The mechanism needed to maintain the differences in water concentration, presumably active, between lens and bathing fluids is unknown, but it might be associated with the net movement of water through the lens as reported by Fowlks (1973b).

The authors acknowledge with greatful appreciation the skillful technical assistance of Mr. Victor Leverenz.

REFERENCES

Becker, B. Accumulation of ^{86}Rb by the rabbit lens. *Invest. Ophthal.* 1: *502-506* (1962).

Cotlier, E., Kwan, B. & Beaty, C. The lens as an osmometer and the effects of medium osmolarity on water transport, ^{86}Rb efflux and ^{86}Rb transport by the lens. *Biochim. biophys. Acta* 150: *705-722* (1968).

Duncan, G. Permeability of amphibian lens membranes to water. *Expl. Eye Res.* 9: *188-198* (1970).

Fowlks, W.L. Osmotic relations between the fluids of the rabbit eye. *Proc. Soc. exp. Biol. Med.* 143: *1176-1179* (1973a).

Fowlks, W.L. Demonstration of a net movement of water through the lens. *Experientia* 29: *548-549* (1973b).

Goldstein, D.A. & Solomon, A.K. Determination of equivalent pore radius for human red cells by osmotic pressure measurement. *J. gen. Physiol.* 44: *1-17* (1960).

Harris, J.E. & Gruber, L. The electrolyte and water balance of the lens. *Expl. Eye Res.* 1: *372-384* (1962).

Kinoshita, J.H., Kern, H.L. & Merola, L.O. Factors affecting the cation transport of calf lens. *Biochim. biophys. Acta* 47: *458-466* (1961).

Kinoshita, J., Merola, L. & Hayman, S. Osmotic effects on the amino acid-concentrating mechanism in the rabbit lens. *J. biol. Chem.* 240: *310-315* (1965).

Kinsey, V.E. The chemical composition and the osmotic pressure of the aqueous humor and plasma of the rabbit. *J. gen. Physiol.* 34: *389-402* (1951).

Nordmann, J. Etudes physio-chemiques sur le cristallin normal et pathologique. *Archs. Ophthal., Paris* 52: *78-114, 170-209* (1935).

Patterson, J.W. Cell volume regulation in the lens. *Docum. Ophthal. Proc. Ser.* 8: *219-227* (1976).

Patterson, J.W. & Fournier, D.J. The effect of tonicity on lens volume. *Invest. Ophthal.* 15: *866-869* (1976).

Rink, H., Münnighoff, J. & Hockwin, O.. Sodium, potassium and calcium contents of bovine lenses in dependence on age. *Ophthal. Res.* 9: *129-135* (1977).

Robinson, R.A. & Stokes, R.H. Electrolyte solutions. Academic Press, Inc., New York. Butterworths Scientific Publications London 1959, p. 559.

Staverman, A,J. The theory of measurement of osmotic pressure. Recl. Trar. chim Pays-Bas Blg. 70: *344-352* (1951).

Staverman, A.J. Apparent osmotic pressure of solutions of heterodisperse polymers. Recl. Trav. Chim. Pays – Bas Blg. 71: *623-633* (1952).

Authors' address:
Institute of Biological Sciences
Oakland University
Rochester, Michigan 48063, U.S.A.

Docum. Ophthal. Proc. Series, Vol. 18

CALCIUM AND TRANSPORT IN THE BOVINE LENS*

H.L. KERN

(Bronx, New York U.S.A.)

ABSTRACT

Selective changes in permeability and transport occur in the calf's lens on removal of Ca^{++} from the bathing solution. Our results suggest that the primary effect is a several-fold increase in passive permeability to Na^+ and K^+ across the cellular plasma membranes. This shift in cations is thought to be responsible for a progressive inhibition in uptake of solutes which undergo Na^+-dependent transport, including the systems for *myo*-inositol and the Gly-, β- and ASC-systems for amino acids. Efflux of amino acids which utilize Na^+-dependent systems is increased on removal of external Ca^{++}. Although inhibitory effects were also noted on uptake of amino acids which are transported by the Na^+-independent Ly^+- and L-systems, they were less drastic than those which are Na^+-dependent. Systems which were not significantly altered on removal of Ca^{++} included the Na^+-pump, and those for pyranoses and for nucleosides. Simple passive diffusion also appeared to be unchanged.

Ca^{++} was found to undergo comparable mediated uptake at both the anterior and posterior faces of the lens. The process was significantly increased at $0°C$.

INTRODUCTION

Calcium is an important factor in many cellular activities (Rasmussen, 1970; Robertson, 1976), and is essential for maintenance of structural integrity of biological membranes (Gitler, 1976; Montal, 1976). It has a regulated and complex transport, which apparently is designed to maintain a micromolar level of free cation in the cytosol of most animal cells (Wasserman, 1972). This is accomplished by extensive binding of the ion to cellular constituents, a low permeability of the plasma membrane to Ca^{++}, a (Ca^{++}, Mg^{++})-activated ATPase, which actively transports Ca^{++} out of the cell, and systems of transport in mitochondria and endoplasmic reticulum which are responsible for accumulating Ca^{++} in these organelles. There are several observations indicating the importance of calcium in lenticular metabolism and that its level must be regulated to preserve clarity: Ca^{++} was associated with increased opacity in freeze-fractured bovine lenses (Duncan & Bushell, 1976); it was increased in galactose cataract in the rat (Salit et al., 1942), and in human senile cortical cataract (Jedziniak et al., 1976; Duncan & Bushell, 1975); and

---

* This work was supported by Grant No. EY 00268 from the National Institutes of Health.

it caused aggregation of bovine and human α-crystallin (Spector & Roth-schild, 1973; Jedziniak et al., 1972; Jedziniak et al., 1973). There is evidence that Ca^{++} is necessary for normal membrane-permeability and transport with respect to a variety of substances in the lens, including entry of myo-inositol (Cotlier, 1970) and exit of Rb^+ (Becker & Cotlier, 1965) in the rabbit, maintenance of levels of Na^+ and K^+ in the calf (Merola et al., 1960), uptake of 2-aminoisobutyric acid, and retention of physiological passive permeabili-ty to Na^+ and K^+ in the rat (Thoft & Kinoshita, 1965). Thoft and Kinoshita noted that the extracellular space was increased in the absence of Ca^{++}. However, removal of Ca^{++} did not alter transport of D-glucose in the rat's lens (Elbrink & Bihler, 1972). We wish to present data regarding uptake of Ca^{++} by the calf's lens, and effects of omission of this ion from the medium on transport of various solutes.

MATERIALS AND METHODS

Paired calves' eyes were brought to the laboratory on ice, and the lenses removed and placed in balanced salt within 3 hr of the death of the animal. Incubation was at 37° with continual shaking (60 cycles/min) in 10-12 ml of a solution containing 140 mM Na^+, 5 mM K^+, 1.5 mM Ca^{++}, 1.0 mM Mg^{++}, 5.0 mM glucose, 27 mM HCO_3^-, 0.6 mM phosphate and 123 mM Cl^- (Kern, 1970). Prior to incubation, the media were gassed with a mixture of 95% air + 5% Co_2, and transferred to wide-mouth 25 ml Erlenmeyer flasks which were then stoppered. An equivalent amount of NaCl was substituted for Ca^{++} and/or Mg^{++} in experiments designed to investigate the effect of removal of these ions. Unless noted otherwise, the lenses were preincubated ½ hr or 1 hr in the presence or absence of Ca^{++}, then transferred on a loop and incubated an additional hour in fresh media which contained radioactive substrate with or without Ca^{++}. NaCl and KCl were replaced with tetraethylammonium chloride (TEAC) when a Na^+-free medium was employed. The non-saturable component of uptake of amino acids was determined as the residual uptake, linear with concentration, in the presence of at least a fiftyfold molar excess of appropriate competing amino acid. In these experiments, tonicity was maintained by isosmotic replacement of NaCl or TEAC.

Uptake of amino acids was characterized as shown in Table I (Kern et al., 1977). A fiftyfold or greater molar excess of amino acid was used where presence of competitor(s) is indicated in the last column of the Table. Exit of Rb^+ or Na^+ was estimated by loading the lenses for 2 hr or 3 hr respective-ly in ordinary balanced salt. This was followed by a ½ hr rinse in balanced salt ± Ca^{++}, and efflux was subsequently allowed to proceed for 1 hr into the 'rinse' media, with 0.1 mM ouabain present in the medium used to evaluate efflux of Rb^+.

After incubation, the lenses were rinsed briefly with 0.15 M NaCl, blot-ted, dispersed in 9.3 ml of 7.5% 5-sulfosalicylic acid, allowed to stand over-night with occasional agitation, and filtered through Whatman 42 paper. Equal volumes (1 ml) of the acid-extract and the medium in 7.5% sul-fosalicylic acid were counted in 12 ml of a scintillating solvent containing: toluene (10 ml), 2-(4-*tert*-butylphenyl)-5-(4-biphenylyl)-1,3,4-oxadiazole (40 mg), and BBS-3 (2 ml Beckman Instruments). Beckman Ready-Solv GP (12 ml) was also used as a pre-mixed liquid scintillation cocktail. In double label experiments, 1 mM (^{3}H)D-mannitol or (^{14}C)D-mannitol were taken as indicator of extracellular space. The correction amounted to 2-4% of the water-content of the lens under physiological conditions.

1-Aminocyclopentane-1-(^{14}C)carboxylic acid (ACPC), 2-amino(1-^{14}C)-isobutyric acid, D-glucose-U-^{14}C and *myo*-inositol-2-^{3}H were obtained from Amersham Corp.; sarcosine-1-^{14}C, L-serine-U-^{14}C and inulin(carboxyl-^{14}C), from California Bionuclear Corp.; L-arginine-U-^{14}C and adenosine-8-^{3}H, from Schwarz/Mann; taurine-1,2-^{14}C, b-2-aminobicyclo-(2,2,1)heptane-2-(^{14}C)-carboxylic acid, D-mannitol-1-^{3}H, D-mannitol-1-^{14}C, thiourea-^{14}C, sucrose-U-^{14}C, ^{22}NaCl, ^{86}RbCl, ^{45}CaCl$_2$, H$_2$^{35}SO$_4$ and ^{3}H$_2$O, from New England Nuclear. Stock tracers in alcoholic solution were evaporated to dryness prior to use. ^{3}H-compounds were diluted in the media to 0.5-1.0 uCi/ml, ^{14}C-compounds, to 0.07-0.40 uCi/ml, ^{35}SO$_4$$^=$, to 0.2 uCi/ml, and the radioactive inorganic cations, to 0.1-1.0 uCi/ml. All kinetic studies and analyses of efflux were done as double label with ^{3}H-mannitol in order to correct for the extracellular space of individual lenses. In the few experiments which were not double label, correction was made for 3% extracellular space after incubation for 1 hr.

The data are given as the mean of 3-6 observations ± the standard error of the mean.

Table I. Characterization of Systems of Transport in the Bovine Lens.

System	Symbol	Dependence on Na$^+$	Characterization
Alanine-preferring	A	+	Transport inhibitable by N-MeAIB*
Leucine-preferring	L	−	Transport inhibitable by L-methionine in Na$^+$-free medium
Alanine-serine-cysteine	ASC	+	Na$^+$-dependent transport in presence of sarcosine or glycine$^+$
Dibasic	Ly$^+$	−	Transport inhibitable by dibasic amino acid in Na$^+$-free medium
Glycine	Gly	+	Transport inhibitable by sarcosine or glycine in presence of L-methionine‡
Beta	β	+	Transport inhibitable by taurine

* N-MeAIB is N-methyl-2-aminoisobutyric acid.
$^+$ Sarcosine or glycine block A-system and Gly-system.
‡ L-Methionine blocks A-system and L-system.

RESULTS

A survey was made of the effect of omitting alkaline earth cations from the medium on transport of a variety of solutes by the calf's lens, and the data are summarized in Table II. Conditions for determination of efflux of Na^+ and Rb^+ are given in the Methods section. It is apparent that removal of Ca^{++}

Table II. Effect of Ca^{++} Absence on Transport of Various Substances by the Calf's Lens.

Substance (mM)	Uptake by Control nMoles/gm. Hr	Uptake Minus Ca^{++} % of Control
ACPC (0.1)	58.9 ± 3.6*	51*
Sarcosine (0.1)	36.0 ± 1.7*	44*
L-Arginine (0.1)	22.9 ± 0.4*	73*
L-Serine (0.1)	79.3 ± 4.0*	41*
Taurine (0.1)	3.2 ± 0.3*	83*
myo-Inositol (0.1)	9.1 ± 0.7*	31*
Na^+ entry (140)	2430 ± 160*; 1650 ± 260*	633*; 672*
Rb^+ exit	–	493-567
Na^+ exit	–	92-106
Rb^+ entry (1.0)	1020 ± 50[+]; 720 ± 16*	85[+]; 100*
Adenosine (0.1)	34.2 ± 0.9[+]; 29.3 ± 2.2*	88[+]; 92*
D-Glucose (1.0)	345 ± 9[+]	83[+]
HTO	23.1 ± 0.2 mMoles/gm.Hr[+]	101[+]
Thiourea (0.132)	26.0 ± 0.6*	109*

* Preincubated $\frac{1}{2}$ hr in balanced salt ± Ca^{++}; reincubated 1 hr ± Ca^{++}.
[+] No preincubation.

Table III. Effect of Ca^{++} Absence on Systems of Transport for Amino Acids in Calf's Lens*.

		Uptake, nMoles/gm.Hr					
		Saturable Component			Non-saturable Component		
0.1 mM Amino Acid	Transport System[+]	$+Ca^{++}$	$-Ca^{++}$	Percent of Control	$+Ca^{++}$	$-Ca^{++}$	Percent of Control
ACPC	L	54.3 ± 3.6	26.8 ± 1.8	49	4.65 ± 0.33	3.34 ± 0.24	72
Sarcosine	A	14.5 ± 0.6	4.92 ± 0.28	34	–	–	–
Sarcosine	Gly	22.0 ± 1.0	4.65 ± 0.84	21	3.47 ± 0.27	5.19 ± 0.57	150
L-Arginine	Ly[+]	21.2 ± 0.3	8.75 ± 0.21	41	1.70 ± 0.11	7.97 ± 0.48	468
L-Serine	ASC	61.3 ± 4.8	23.3 ± 1.4	38	–	–	–
Taurine	β	2.4[‡]	0.38[‡]	16	0.41[‡]	2.49[‡]	607

* Incubated 1 hr following preincubation for $\frac{1}{2}$ hr in Ca^{++}-containing (control) or in Ca^{++}-free TEAC- or Na^+-balanced salt.
[+] Component of uptake determined as described in Table I.
[‡] Determined from kinetic plot.
From Kern, 1978, with permission.

140

resulted in inhibition of uptake of all the amino acids examined and of
myo-inositol, and a marked increase in the passive fluxes of the alkali metal
cations. Little change was noted in the active cationic fluxes, and the rate of
entry of adenosine, D-glucose, tritiated water and thiourea. Formation of
lactate was not inhibited under the experimental conditions (Kern, unpublished observations). Removal of Mg^{++} had little effect on transport of the
substances listed in the Table, but absence of both Ca^{++} and Mg^{++} caused
more marked change in the passive cationic fluxes and in the non-saturable
component of taurine (see Table III) than absence of Ca^{++} only. A hypotoni-
city of 96 mOsmoles/L had effects similar to deletion of Ca^{++} except that
entry of Na^+ was increased only about 20% (Kern, unpublished observations).

A more detailed study was made of the effect of omission of Ca^{++} on
uptake of the amino acids, and the results are presented in Table III. The
components of uptake by the systems of transport listed in column 2 of the
Table were determined as described in the Methods section (Table I). It is
apparent that all the systems of transport were significantly inhibited, and
that the β-system was especially sensitive. The non-saturable component for
uptake of 4 of the 5 amino acids was also determined as the residual uptake

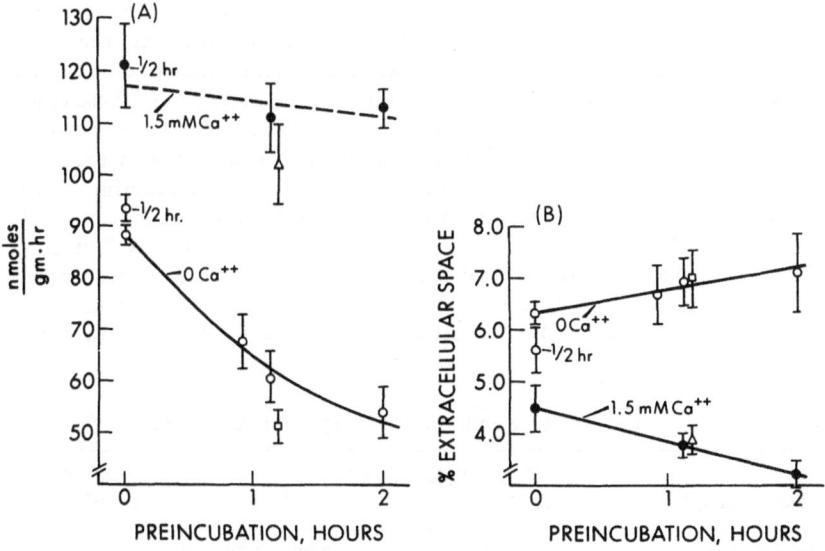

Fig. 1A. Effect of incubation time at 37° on uptake of 0.1 mM L-serine by the calf's
lens. Incubation time in the presence of L-serine was 1 hr (following pre-incubation for
0-2 hr) except as indicated. The medium was changed only for the points, Δ, □. Figure
1B. Effect of time of incubation with or without Ca^{++} on the extracellular space
expressed as a percentage of the total lenticular water. Conditions of incubation as in
Fig. 1A. The medium was changed only for the points, Δ, □. From Kern, 1978, with
permission.

in the presence of the competing amino acid(s). Selective effects were found with large increases occurring for L-arginine and taurine (last 3 columns in Table III). Therefore, the seemingly small effects on uptake of these two amino acids (Table II) actually reflect a large decrease in saturable uptake and a partially compensating increase in non-saturable uptake.

The deleterious effects of Ca^{++} omission increased with time of incubation as illustrated for uptake of 0.1 mM L-serine in Figure 1A. After exposure for ½ hr or 1 hr, the rate was about 77% of the control, whereas, after a total exposure of 3 hr, the rate was 48% of the control. The extracellular space measured with D-mannitol was increased in media having no added Ca^{++} as shown in Fig. 1B, but it did not increase significantly as the exposure to the deficient medium was increased from 1 hr to 3 hr. Table IV lists values measured with several indicators for extracellular space, as a percentage of the total lenticular water, in the presence and in the absence of Ca^{++}. The results indicate that removal of Ca^{++} caused a 50-100% increase in extracellular space, which could be correlated with increased hydration (Kern, unpublished observations).

Attempts were made to determine whether the effect of external Ca^{++} removal on transport of appropriate organic solutes was reversible. Table V gives data for the β-component of 0.1 mM taurine, and it may be seen that uptake in zero Ca^{++} after preincubation in 1.5 mM Ca^{++}, nMoles/gm. hr, was not significantly different from uptake in 1.5 mM Ca^{++} following pre-incubation in zero Ca^{++}, 1.40 nMoles/gm. hr. The results indicate, therefore, that the damage originating from removal of Ca^{++} is not readily reversed. The non-saturable component of taurine was about the same under these conditions, 0.31 ± 0.09 nMoles/gm. hr and 0.24 ± 0.10 nMoles/gm. hr respectively, whereas no significant non-saturable component was detected in the lenses incubated in 1.5 mM Ca^{++} throughout. A similarly designed experiment with 0.1 mM *myo*-inositol also showed little tendency for reversal in 1 hr of the damage done by omission of Ca^{++}. On the other hand, Thoft & Kinoshita, 1965, found that the extracellular space of the rat's lens, as measured with sucrose, returned to nearly normal 3 hr after restoring Ca^{++} to 0.75 mM. This effect was not apparent in our studies using D-mannitol as indicator of extracellular space.

Table IV. Effect of Ca^{++} Absence on Extracellular Space of Calf's Lens.

Indicator (mM)*	% Extracellular Space[+] $+Ca^{++}$	$-Ca^{++}$	$-Ca^{++}$ divided by $+Ca^{++}$
D-Mannitol (1)	4.03 ± 0.43	7.97 ± 0.78	1.98
Sucrose (1)	2.28 ± 0.20	4.47 ± 0.27	1.96
Inulin (0.12mg/ml)	1.92 ± 0.08	2.91 ± 0.46	1.52
Sulfate (1)	3.02 ± 0.28	4.48 ± 0.24	1.49

* Preincubated lenses in D-mannitol for $\frac{1}{2}$ hr in same medium as used for reincubation. Lenses in sucrose, inulin and sulfate were not preincubated.
[+] Determined after incubation for 1 hr.

It was also of interest to investigate the effect of removal of Ca^{++} on efflux of amino acids which utilize various systems of transport, selecting representatives which are not rapidly metabolized by the lens. Efflux of amino acids utilizing the A- and possibly the Gly-systems (2-aminoisobutyrate and sarcosine) was enhanced in a Ca^{++}-free medium, Table VI. There was also indication that efflux of taurine was increased, though no significant cellular efflux of this amino acid was detected in normal balanced salt. Efflux of amino acids utilizing the L- and Ly^+-systems was not dependent on the presence of external Ca^{++}. During the 3½ hr period of incubation, no metabolism of taurine or sarcosine was detected, but approximately 25% of the L-arginine was metabolized.

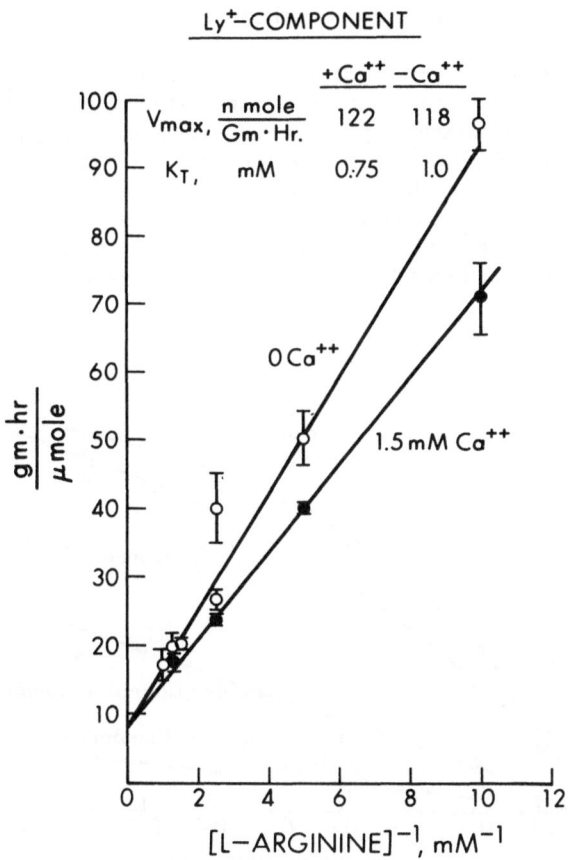

Fig. 2. Effect of Ca^{++} removal on kinetics of Ly^+-component of L-arginine, measured as uptake inhibitable by fiftyfold molar excess of L-lysine in Na^+-free medium. The lenses were preincubated ½ hr in the presence or in the absence of Ca^{++}, the medium was changed, and incubation was continued for 1 hr after adding the amino acids.

Kinetic studies were conducted to ascertain the effect of Ca^{++} on uptake by the Ly^+ and β-systems, since it appeared to depend on the presence of this cation (Table III). The parameters, K_T and v_{max}, for L-arginine were little changed (Fig. 2), as only a 33% increase in the coefficient for half saturation was obtained and v_{max} was unaltered. However, the non-saturable component of this amino acid increased about 3.5-fold in Ca^{++}-free medium (Fig. 3). More drastic effects occurred in the characteristics of uptake of taurine as illustrated in Figs. 4 and 5. The β-component was markedly reduced in the absence of Ca^{++} and saturability could not be demonstrated (Fig. 4). The decrease in saturable uptake was accompanied by an approximately equivalent increase in the non-saturable component (Fig. 5), and, therefore, total uptake was not much changed (Table II). Similar effects were observed on the Gly-component of sarcosine; saturability could not be demonstrated, and uptake via the Gly-system was markedly reduced when Ca^{++} was absent from the medium.

Preliminary studies of influx of Ca^{++} (^{45}Ca) at the anterior and posterior surfaces provided evidence of saturable system(s) for this ion, and indicate the existence of comparable high affinity (K_T, 0.05, 0.10 mM), low capacity (v_{max}, 7.9 nMoles/Cm^2.Hr) systems of transport, with the higher apparent affinity at the posterior surface. Reduction in temperature to 0°C. or the presence of 5 uM divalent ionophore, A23187 (Eli Lilly and Co.), increased the rate of entry 240% and 350% respectively. A twentyfold excess of Mg^{++}, Ba^{++} and Sr^{++} inhibited uptake of 0.05 mM Ca^{++} increasingly in the order given.

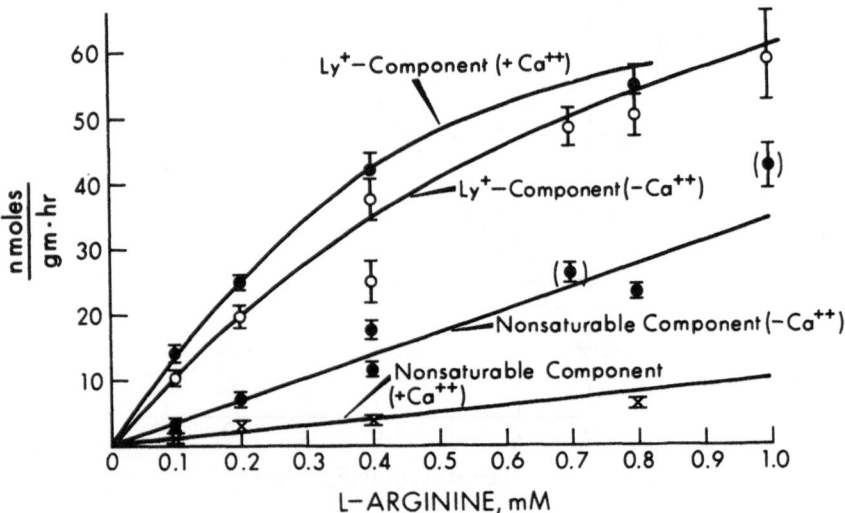

Fig. 3. Effect of Ca^{++} removal on Ly^+- and non-saturable-components of uptake of L-arginine. The non-saturable component was determined as the uptake remaining in the presence of a fiftyfold molar excess of L-lysine. Conditions of incubation as for Figure 2.

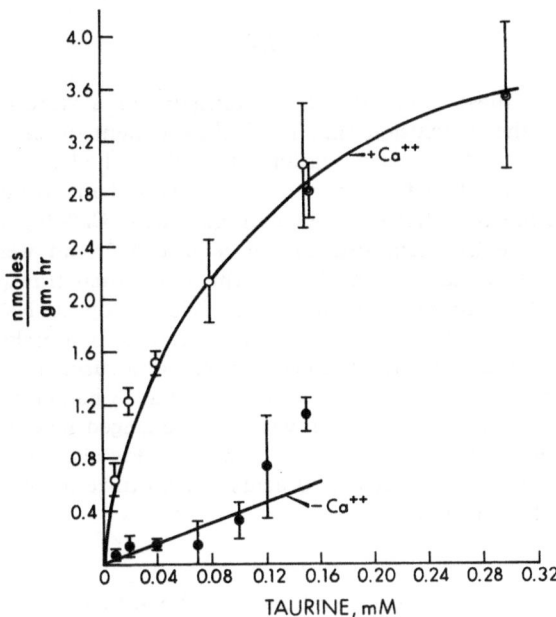

Fig. 4. Effect of Ca⁺⁺ removal on the β-component of taurine determined as uptake inhibitable by a fiftyfold molar excess of β-alanine. Clonditions of incubation as for Figure 2.

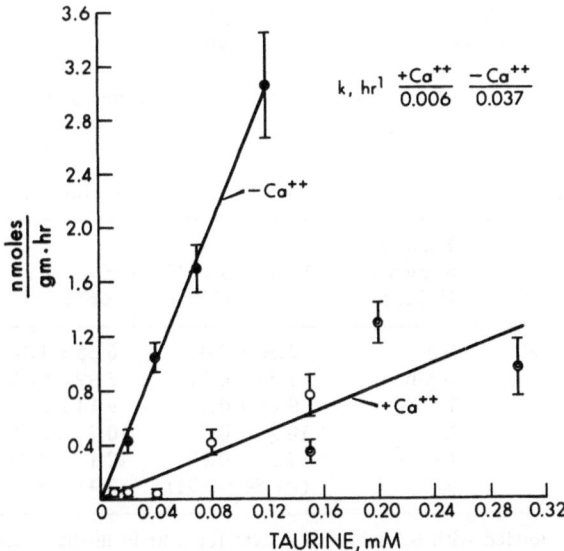

Fig. 5. Effect of Ca⁺⁺ removal on the non-saturable component of taurine determined as the uptake remaining in the presence of a fiftyfold molar excess of β-alanine. Conditions of incubation as for Fig. 2.

DISCUSSION

Consideration of these experiments on transport of a variety of organic solutes leads to the conclusion that the Na^+-dependent processes are most dependent on Ca^{++} in the solution bathing the cells of the lens. In support of this contention is the fact that entry of D-glucose and adenosine, processes that do not require Na^+ (Kern, 1978), exhibited little Ca^{++}-dependence. The Ly^+-system and the L-system also do not require Na^+, and were found to depend less on external Ca^{++} in the present study than transport by the Na^+-dependent Gly- and β-systems for amino acids, or by the Na^+-dependent system for *myo*-inositol. Comparison of the kinetics for uptake of taurine and of L-arginine illustrates the marked difference in susceptibility of these transport-systems to damage in the absence of Ca^{++}. Characteristics of uptake of L-arginine by the Ly^+-system were little changed whereas the β-system was markedly inhibited. Efflux of amino acids also appeared to be significantly increased only for amino acids which utilize the Na^+-dependent A-, Gly- or β-systems (Table VI).

Table V. Reversibility of Ca^{++}-Effect on Uptake of 0.1 mM Taurine.

| Condition of Incubation* | | Saturable Uptake | |
First Hour	Second Hour	nMoles/gm.Hr	% of Control
1.5 mM Ca	1.5 mM Ca	2.42 ± 0.31	–
0.0 Ca	0.0 Ca	0.71 ± 0.28	29
1.5 mM Ca	0.0 Ca	1.45 ± 0.13	60
0.0 Ca	1.5 mM Ca	1.40 ± 0.14	58

* The medium was changed after the first hour and taurine added at start of the second hour.

Table VI. Effect of External Ca^{++} on Amino Acid Efflux from the Calf's Lens.

| Amino Acid | Transport System Utilized | Efflux, % of Uptake* | | % of Control |
		1.5 mM Ca^{++}	0 Ca^{++}	
2-Aminoisobutyrate	A,L	2.30 ± 0.07	6.65 ± 1.10	289
Sarcosine	A,Gly	1.53 ± 0.11	5.99 ± 0.78	410
ACPC	L	9.09 ± 0.50	9.14 ± 0.34	101
BCH[+]	L	10.2 ± 0.27	10.7 ± 0.98	105
L-Arginine	Ly^+	9.5 ± 0.97	12.1 ± 0.94	129
Taurine	β	(−1.54 ± 0.31)	3.41 ± 0.56	–

* Lenses were loaded with 0.1 mM amino acid for 2 hr in media containing 1.5 mM Ca^{++}, washed for $\frac{1}{2}$ hr in media ± Ca^{++}, and efflux measured after 1 hr in 10 ml balanced salt ± Ca^{++}.

[+] b-D,L-2-Aminobicyclo-(2,2,1)-heptane-2-carboxylate.

146

It is possible that the selective damage to Na^+-dependent systems of transport may be secondary effects of the loss of selective permeability to the alkali metal cations in the absence of external Ca^{++} (Table II). This could produce a rapid elevation of Na^+ in the critical superficial cellular elements of the lens (epithelium and peripheral processes of fiber cells). The Na^+-gradient across these cellular membranes would be decreased or eliminated, with resultant inhibition of the Na^+-dependent processes for amino acids and inositol.

The slow development of the inhibition of uptake of 0.1 mM L-serine (increasing from ½ to 3 hr, Fig. 1), is also suggestive of a secondary effect of removal of Ca^{++} on transport of amino acids. In other words, the level of Na^+ in the peripheral areas of the lens may be increasing over this period, and the diminishing Na^+-gradient leads to a retardation of influx of the amino acid, which mainly utilizes the Na^+-dependent ASC-system at 0.1 mM.

It is more difficult to explain the smaller inhibitory effects noted on transport of amino acids which have affinity for the Na^+-independent L- and Ly^+-systems. However, these systems function by exchange of internal for external amino acid, and it is conceivable that the decreased influx noted at 0.1 mM ACPC or L-arginine results from a depressed level of intracellular amino acids.

REFERENCES

Becker, B. & E. Cotlier, The efflux of [86]rubidium from the rabbit lens. *Invest. Ophthal.* 4: *117-121* (1965).

Cotlier, E. Myo-inositol: active transport by the crystalline lens. *Invest. Ophthal.* 9: *681-691* (1970).

Duncan, G. & A.R. Bushell. Ion analysis of human cataractous lenses. *Expl. Eye Res.* 20: *223-230* (1975).

Duncan, G. & A.R. Bushell. The bovine lens as an ion exchanger: a comparison with ion levels in human cataractous lenses. *Expl. Eye Res.* 23: *341-353* (1976).

Elbrink, J. & I. Bihler. Characteristics of the membrane transport of sugars in the lens of the eye. *Biochim. biophys. Acta* 282: *337-351* (1972).

Gitler, G. On the nature of the lipid-protein interactions in biological membranes. In: The Enzymes of Biological Membranes; vol. V. 1. Physical and Chemical Techniques. (ed. Martonosi, A.) Plenum Press, New York pp. (1976), pp. 229-244.

Jedziniak, J.A., J.H. Kinoshita, E.M. Yates, L.O. Hocker & G.B. Benedek. Calcium-induced aggregation of bovine lens alpha crystallin. *Invest. Ophthals* 11: *905-915* (1972).

Jedziniak, J.A., J.H. Kinoshita, E.M. Yates, L.O. Hocker & G.B. Benedek. On the presence and mechanism of formation of heavy molecular weight aggregates in human normal and cataractous lenses. *Expl. Eye Res.* 15: *185-192* (1973).

Jedziniak, J.A., D.F. Nicoli, E.M. Yates & G.B. Benedek. On the calcium concentration of cataractous and normal human lenses and protein fractions of cataractous lenses. *Expl. Eye Res.* 23: *325-332* (1976).

Kern, H.L. Efflux of amino acids from the lens. *Invest. Ophthal.* 9: *692-702* (1970).

Kern, H.L. Transport of organic solutes in the lens. *Curr. Topics Eye* Res. 1: in press (1978).

Kern, H.L., C.-K. Ho & S.A. Ostrove. Comparison of transport at the anterior and posterior surfaces of the calf lens. *Expl. Eye Res.* 24: *559-570* (1977).

Merola, L.O., H.L. Kern & J.H. Kinoshita. The effect of calcium on the cations of calf lens. *Arch. Ophthal.* 63: *830-835* (1960).

Montal, M. Experimental membranes and mechanisms of bioenergy transductions. *Ann. Rev. Biophys. Bioeng.* 5: *119-175* (1976).

Rasmussen, H. Cell communication, calcium ion, and cyclic adenosine monophosphate. *Science* 170: *404-412* (1970).

Robertson, W.G. Cellular Ca^{++} and Ca^{++} transport. in: Calcium, Phosphate and Magnesium Metabolism. (ed. Nordin, B.E.C.) Churchill Livingstone, Edinburgh/New York, 1976, pp. *230-256*.

Salit, P.W., K.C. Swan & W.D. Paul. Changes in mineral composition of rat lenses with galactose cataract. *Am. J. Ophthal.* 25: *1482-1486* (1942).

Spector, A. & C. Rothschild. The effect of calcium upon the reaggregation of bovine α-crystallin. *Invest. Ophthal.* 12: *225-231* (1973).

Thoft, R.A. & J.H. Kinoshita. The effect of calcium on rat lens permeability. *Invest. Ophthal.* 4: *122-128* (1965).

Wasserman, R.H. Calcium transport by selected animal cells and tissues. In: Metabolic Pathways; vol. 6, 3rd Ed. (ed. Hokin, L.E.) Academic Press, New York, 1972. pp. *351-384*.

Author's address:
Department of Ophthalmology
Albert Einstein College of Medicine
of Yeshiva University
1300 Morris Park Avenue
Bronx, New York 10461, USA

Docum. Ophthal. Proc. Series, Vol. 18

STIMULATION OF AMINO ACIDS INCORPORATION INTO HUMAN LENS PROTEINS

JEAN KLETHI AND JEAN NORDMANN

(Strasbourg, France)

ABSTRACT

The amino acid incorporation into the soluble proteins of normal old human lenses was studied. In the presence of cyclic AMP and a phosphodiesterase inhibitor this incorporation could be stimulated.

INTRODUCTION

Observations made post mortem and in vivo show that the growth rate of the human lens slows down with age, but there is not a complete stop (Nordmann, Fink & Hockwin, 1974; Nordmann, 1977). On the other hand it was simultaneously published in New York and in Strasbourg, that the same diminution can be found concerning the incorporation of amino acids into human lens proteins. Spector, Stauffer, Roy, Li & Adams (1976) compared lenses obtained from newborns at maximum 5 days old to children of 1 to 20 months, Klethi (1976) investigated lenses of between 42 and 74 years of age. These results led us to study the possibility of stimulating the failing amino acids incorporation of old human lenses.

Preliminary experiments made with different substances on bovine lenses did not produce clear cut effects and no definite conclusion could be drawn (Klethi & Nordmann, 1978). This was also the case with human lenses except when cyclic AMP or prostaglandin were used as presumed stimulators.

MATERIAL AND METHODS

Human eyes more than 60 years old were enucleated at maximum 5 hours post mortem and rapidly brought to the eye department for a slit lamp examination of the lenses and then to the laboratory.

There, the lenses were extracted and the pair from the same donor was cultured in their intact capsule, each lens in a separate tube, for 12 hours in 3 ml TC 199 medium with 50 μCi equally distributed on ^{14}C-labeled leucine, lysine and tyrosine. The media of both lenses were gassed with air and

Institute of Biochemistry (Prof. P. Mandel) and the Eye Clinic (Prof. A. Bronner), Louis Pasteur University, Medical School.

CO_2 (95 : 5) and standard antibiotics were added. One of the tubes also contained the solution whose effect had to be tested.

After culture the lenses were rinsed with cold saline, homogenized in 0.002 M phosphate buffer at pH 6.8 and centrifuged for 30 minutes at 80.000 g. Samples were taken to determine the entrance into the capsular sac, the remainder of the soluble extract was dialyzed against a 100 fold excess of the same buffer with three changes during a 36 hours period.

The dialysate from each of the 2 human lenses was applied to a DEAE cellulose column (Whatman DE 52) previously equilibrated with 0.002 M phosphate buffer. Column dimensions were 1.0 x 15 cm and 4 ml fractions were collected.

The eluted proteins were monitored by measuring the absorption at 280 and 260 nm. Aliquots were taken for the determination of radioactivity by an Intertechnique scintillation counter using monophase 40 (Packard Instrument) as scintillation liquid.

RESULTS

In a first step we studied the amino acid incorporation into soluble proteins of cultured old transparent human lenses in a TC 199 medium which contained the radioactive amino acids as the sole addition. Table I shows the low variation rate obtained when lenses of the same pair are compared; the observed differences, concerning the specific activities, ranged from 5 to 13%.

This instigated us to study, in a second step, the effect of presumed 'protein synthesis stimulators' on a intraindividual basis. Preliminary experiments led us to conditions where the dibutyryl derivative of cyclic adenosine monophosphate (c AMP) was used in the presence of a protector, a diesterase inhibitor in the form of 3-isobutyl-1-methylxanthin.

Table 1. Amino acid incorporation into human soluble lens proteins, TC 199 contained only labeled amino acids. Lens a and b represent either the right or the left eye of the same donor.

	Age	76 years		61 years		62 years	
	Lens	a	b	a	b	a	b
	Before Dialysis						
1	Total c/m/lens	1.290.124	1.426.417	1.191.678	1.102.770	1.035.249	1.059.542
2	Specific Activity c/m/mg protein	23.941	22.966	19.759	20.088	15.286	16.211
	After Dialysis						
3	Total c/m/lens	40.409	45.687	14.560	13.248	20.576	18.426
4	Specific Activity c/m/mg protein	750	736	241	225	304	282
5	Ratio (4 : 2) in %	3.13	3.20	1.22	1.12	1.99	1.74
6	Relat. Spec. Activity $\dfrac{4}{1-3} \times 1000$	0.60	0.53	0.20	0.19	0.30	0.27

As relatively high levels are required for protection and as these inhibitors harm the incorporation process by itself, we tested the inhibitor used for a mean level which we found to be 0.5 mM.

Table II gives a scope of 3 typical experiments where human lenses were cultured in the same conditions, one lens of the pair with, the other without c AMP. Each time that c AMP was present in the medium, the total counts per lens, after dialysis of the lens extract, were higher than those of the controls. This was also the case for the other data registered after dialysis.

Table II. Amino acid incorporation into human soluble lens proteins from the same donor. a = TC 199 contained labeled amino acids and 0.5 mM phosphodiesterase inhibitor. b = TC 199 contained labeled amino acids, 0.5 mM phosphodiesterase inhibitor and 5 mM cyclic AMP.

	Age	64 years		73 years		64 years	
	Lens	a	b	a	b	a	b
	Before Dialysis						
1	Total c/m/lens	1.575.446	1.633.133	1.129.500	752.308	720.554	918.694
2	Specific Activity c/m/mg protein	25.720	25.100	16.300	10.400	13.300	16.120
	After Dialysis						
3	Total c/m/protein	27.821	38.573	12.751	14.629	11.642	23.629
4	Specific Activity c/m/mg protein	452	593	180	203	216	415
5	Ratio (4 : 2) in %	1.77	2.36	1.13	1.94	1.62	2.57
6	Rel. Spec. Activity $\frac{4}{1-3} \times 1000$	0.29	0.37	0.16	0.27	0.30	0.46

Table. III. Amino acid incorporation into human soluble lens proteins from the same 60 year old donor. a = TC 199 contained labeled amino acids, 5mM cAMP, and 0.5 mM phosphodiesterase inhibitor. b = TC 199 contained labeled amino acids, 5mM cAMP, 0.5 mM phosphodiesterase inhibitor and 0.20 mM cycloheximide.

	Lens	a	b
	Before Dialysis		
1	Total c/m/lens	997.702	1.032.471
2	Specific Activity c/m/mg protein	17.390	19.650
	After Dialysis		
3	Total c/m/lens	34.594	7.460
4	Specific Activity c/m/mg protein	603	144
5	Ratio (4 : 2) in %	3.47	0.74
6	Rel. Spec. Activity $\frac{4}{1-3} \times 1000$	0.62	0.14

151

Nevertheless, each experiment had a different development. Looking at the eventual effect on the uptake by c AMP all three possibilities are represented; but we cannot yet explain this inconsistency. In any case, the best expression which takes into account the mentioned irregularities is the relative specific activity. Judged on this basis, we obtained a stimulation of amino acid incorporation ranging from 27 to 71%.

We do think that c AMP can act in this way, as in other organs and tissue cultures, because in similar experiments where we replaced c AMP by a 1 μM Prostaglandin E_1 we had a similar stimulation. Unfortunately, as is well known, topical applications of prostaglandin produce a transient ocular hypertension. Such reactions are especially dangerous for old people and for that reason we have not continued, as yet, our observations on prostaglandins.

Table III summarizes one of our experiments where we added to c AMP and its protector 0.2 mM cycloheximide, which is known as a protein synthesis inhibitor. We observed a decrease in the amino acid incorporation by nearly 80%. It is to be noted that the amino acid uptake which is represented by the total counts per minute per lens remains constant under these conditions.

Finally, we were interested to know whether the stimulation by c AMP is a universal one or if it acts only on specific chromatographic peaks of human soluble lens proteins. In Table IV it is shown that the increase of specific activity due to the effect of c AMP is not uniform and this leads us to think that there are preferential actions of the stimulation. But this was not always true, since in other experiments in nearly all peaks a 60% increase was noted. So we can answer our question: the increase is general, but not always homogeneous.

DISCUSSION

The first question which arises, is: Do we really stimulate the incorporation into the lens proteins by the addition of c AMP? Our answer is affirmative for the following reasons: 1) the extraction of the incorporated amino acids

Table IV. Chromatographic DEAE cellulose peaks of human soluble lens proteins from the same 64 year old donor. a = TC 199 contained labeled amino acids and 0.5 mM phosphodiesterase inhibitor. b = TC 199 contained labeled amino acids, 0.5 mM phosphodiesterase inhibitor and 5 mM cyclic AMP.

Phosphate Eluant	a		b		Increase in %	
	Spec. Activity	Rel. Spec. Activity (see Table I)	Spec. Activity	Rel. Spec. Activity	Spec. Activity	Rel. Spec. Activity
0.03 M a	287	0.185	470	0.295	64	60
0.03 M b	386	0.249	504	0.316	41	27
0.05 M	467	0.302	699	0.438	68	45
0.08 M	219	0.142	273	0.171	25	20
0.4 M	280	0.181	336	0.211	20	17

by 10% hot TCA resulted in a loss of only 8-10% of the radioactive material; 2) parallel experiments in the presence of 0.1 mM puromycine greatly reduce the incorporation and this change reached 80%; 3) another potent inhibitor of proteosynthesis, the 0.2 mM cycloheximide, gave the same result (Table III).

A second question we have to discuss, is the reproducibility of our experiments. As can be seen in our tables, this reproducibility exists in an intraindividual manner, but not in an interindividual one, i.e. that for the two lenses of the same donor the difference in specific activity after dialysis did not exceed 7, 8%, when the TC 199 contained only the labeled amino acids. Lenses from different donors had a very important spread, as often observed in human lenses.

One of the factors explaining this spread of the interindividual results, could be the post mortem extraction of the lenses, although we discarded all the lenses removed from eyes enucleated more than 5 hours after death. In fact our experiments on bovines have shown that there is no difference between the incorporation into lenses brought rapidly on ice from the slaughterhouse, extracted and immediately cultured and lenses transported without refrigeration, extracted and cultured only 5 hours later.

The last question concerns the age of the lenses. We were especially interested in old lenses, because in this life period the lens may, in certain circumstances, need stimulation of its protein synthesis. A study of Young lenses which are much more difficult to obtain a few hours after death, will follow later.

ACKNOWLEDGEMENTS

The authors are very grateful to Mrs. Margaret Bakish for her excellent technical assistance.

REFERENCES

Klethi, J. Incorporation of glutamic acid into soluble protein as a function of age. *Invest. Ophthal.* 15: *430-433* (1976).

Klethi, J. & Nordmann, J. Problems concerning aging of the lens – bovine and human – and senile cataract. *Interdiscipl. Topics Geront.* 13: in press. (Karger, Basel 1978).

Nordmann, J. Au sujet du vieillissement du cristallin humain et de la pathogénie de la cataracte sénile. *Adv. Ophthal.* vol. 34, pp. *1-73* (Karger, Basel 1977).

Nordmann, J., Fink, H. & Hockwin, O. Die Wachstumskurve der menschlichen Linse. *Albrech v. Graefes Arch. klin. exp. Ophthal.* 191: *165-175* (1974).

Spector, A., Stauffer, J., Roy, D., Li, L.-K. & Adams, D. Human alpha-crystallin. I. The isolation and characterization of newly synthesized alpha-crystallin. *Invest. Ophthal.* 15: *288-296* (1976).

Authors' address:
Louis Pasteur University
Medical School
Strasbourg
France

Docum. Ophthal. Proc. Series, Vol. 18

ANTERIOR FUSIFORM CATARACT (*CAT-B*): A NEW TYPE OF RECESSIVELY INHERITED LENS OPACITY IN THE SPRAGUE DAWLEY RAT

HANS-REINHARD KOCH, HORST BAUMGARTEN &
JANA KRATOCHVILOVA

(Bonn and Neuherberg, Fed. Rep. Germany)

ABSTRACT

A new mutant Sprague Dawley rat is described, in which the occurrence of bilateral nuclear lens opacities with a fusiform or pyramidal connection to the anterior lens pole (*cat-b*) is a recessively inherited trait. The gene has about 99% penetrance and a slight variation in expression. During lens development the opaque nucleus-pole connection eventually becomes disrupted so that all animals have mere nuclear cataracts, when they reach the age of 100 days. Lens fresh weights are reduced in affected animals under the age of 16 days.

INTRODUCTION

While there are numerous papers on inherited congenital cataracts in the mouse, information on such opacities in rats is scarce. In recent years we have had the opportunity to detect several different types of hereditary lens opacities in laboratory rats. Amongst these two were briefly documented in the literature: a sutural opacity of the *posterior* embryonic nucleus (Koch et al., 1976) and a spherical opacity of the *anterior* embryonic nucleus (Koch et al., 1977).

The present paper presents the mode of inherintance and the morphological features of a third type of congenital opacity. It was first observed in some Sprague Dawley rats, when we were screening animals for a different study (Baumgarten, 1977). The trait was called *cat-b* (provisional name).

MATERIAL AND METHODS

The source of our animals is the outbred Sprague Dawley strain of Zentralinstitut für Versuchstiere (Hannover, BRD). Controls are from the same source. Animals were first mated when 8-12 weeks old and permanent monogamous breeding was continued for 4-5 generations.

The animals were kept in Macrolon cages. They were given Altromin[R] standard diet and water was given ad libitum. Body weights were checked regularly. The eyes were examined at a Zeiss photo slit lamp in mydriasis (atropine eye drops, 1%). Findings were documented by drawings and by photos on Agfa CT 21.

To determine lens fresh weights, animals were killed in ether anesthesia, and the eyes were enucleated. The lenses were removed by posterior approach and weighed on a Mettler microbalance. They were then freeze-dried or deep-frozen for later biochemical investigations (to be published).

RESULTS

INHERITANCE

The mutant condition was first noted in a litter of commercially-obtained Sprague Dawley rats. From 12 offspring, 4 displayed a lens opacity. The mother was then confirmed to have the same type of opacity, while the father was not available at the time of investigation.

The breeding tests showed that 71 offspring from crosses between affected and normal unrelated animals were phenotypically normal. Offspring from crosses between the phenotypically normal F_1 heterozygotes segregated 8 : 35, which is close to the expected 1 : 3 ratio for recessive genes. Of 116 offspring from crosses between affected animals only, 110 were affected by pronounced nuclear or anterior fusiform cataracts on at least one eye. Five animals showed reduced expression of the lens opacity in that both lenses exhibited only minor nuclear changes and 1 animal was normal (Table I).

It could be concluded that the cataract is a recessively-inherited trait. The penetrance of the recessive gene is about 99%. There is slight variation in expression of the gene observed in about 5% of the affected animals.

Apart from the cataracts the animals appeared normal in all other respects. Reproductive capacity was not reduced. Mean litter sizes are incorporated into Table 1; they did not differ significantly between the groups in an analysis of variance. No associated deformations or disorders were observed and mortality was not increased. The development of the body weights was the same in controls and mutants.

Table I. Segregation of *cat-b* and mean litter sizes

Cross:			Phenotype:			Litter size:		
♂	x	♀	cat-b	cat-b$_{red}$	+	$\bar{x}$	±	s
cat-b/cat-b x +/+			0	0	45	9.0	±	1.4
	+/+ x cat-b/cat-b		0	0	26	8.7	±	2.5
	cat-b/+ x cat-b/+		7	1	35	7.7	±	3.0
cat-b/cat-b x cat-b/cat-b			110	5	1	7.8	±	2.5
	controls (+/+ x +/+)		–	–	158	8,8	±	3,1

cat-b = cataract Baumgarten (provisional name)
cat-b$_{red}$ = *cat-b* with reduced expression
+ = normal phenotype

A litter of 10 *cat-b* homozygotes was followed up at the slit lamp for 6 months. The first examination was carried out at the age of 14 days, shortly after opening of the eyes. All animals had congenital lens opacities, which varied somewhat in severity (Fig. 1-3).

A clear inner portion of the lens nucleus was surrounded by an opaque layer with a larger, markedly opaque area in the anterior nucleus. In six animals, there was an opaque protrusion of fusiform or pyramidal appearance (Fig. 1) from this area touching the anterior surface of the lens. A small circular anterior polar opacity was present where this protrusion reached the anterior lens capsule. The 4 remaining animals have somewhat less pronounced opacities, lacking the fusiform interconnection between nucleus and anterior pole, and in 2 of them one eye was affected even less so that there was only a discrete opaque layer in the outer nuclear portion. This latter finding was termed 'reduced expression' in the breeding series, when it occurred bilaterally.

An interesting finding was observed in 3 animals of the breeding series although not in the follow-up group. It was the occurrence of filamentous remnants of the pupillary membrane, inserting at the anterior lens pole at the apex of the fusiform opacity.

During the follow-up period the opacities did not progress. Newly formed fibres were clear and while the lenses grew the nuclear opacity became relatively smaller and receded into the inner nuclear region (Fig. 2). During this process the interconnection between nucleus and anterior pole became slimmer in the 6 animals affected in this way. At 41 days the nuclear opacities had pyramidal extrusions, from the apex of which there was a filamentous connection with a discrete anterior sub-capsular opacity. At 81 days, the connection was completely disrupted in three of the 6 rats and at

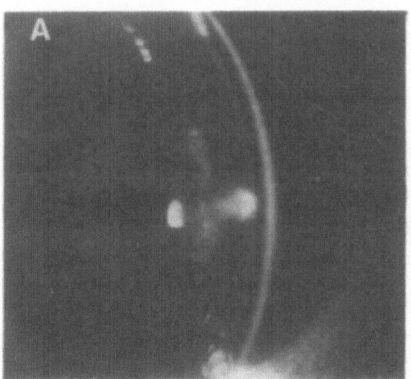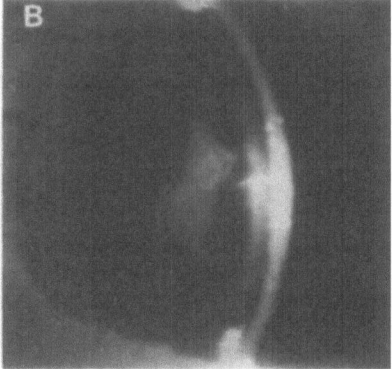

Fig 1. Slit lamp photography of two examples of *cat-b* mutants at 14 days of age with fusiform (A) or pyramidal (B) protrusion from a nuclear opaque layer to the anterior lens pole.

157

109 days in all animals. Thus, a small nuclear opacity remained, with an apex pointing the anterior lens pole (Fig. 3).

LENS FRESH WEIGHTS

The larger part of the homozygous offspring from breeding tests as well as unaffected Sprague Dawley rats were sacrificed at different dates after birth, to obtain lenses for biochemical investigations. At this stage we are only able to present preliminary results of the lens fresh weights (Fig. 4). It can be seen that there was an initial retardation of lens growth in *cat-b* rats, which became compensated by the time the animals opened their eyes.

DISCUSSION

After reviewing the pertinent literature on inherited lens opacities in laboratory animals we found this opacity to be quite unique. None of the rat mutants with hereditary cataracts described so far (Jess, 1925; Lambert & Sciuchetti, 1935; Bourne & Grüneberg, 1939; Smith & Barrentine, 1943; Léonard & Maisin, 1965; Smith et al., 1969; Kern & Schärer, 1970) had comparable opacities.

The peculiar feature of the new recessive cataract mutant is that 60% of the animals have a pathological fusiform or pyramidal opaque connection between lens nucleus and anterior pole. This connection becomes disrupted in the course of lens growth by layers of newly formed fibre cells. Thus, we may assume that a similar interconnection may originally have existed in *all* animals but has been disrupted before the opening of the eyes.

The opacities observed in our mutant rats have a strong resemblance to a human type of congenital cataract, in which an opaque nucleus is connected of an anterior polar opacity. Such cases have been published by Vogt (1931)

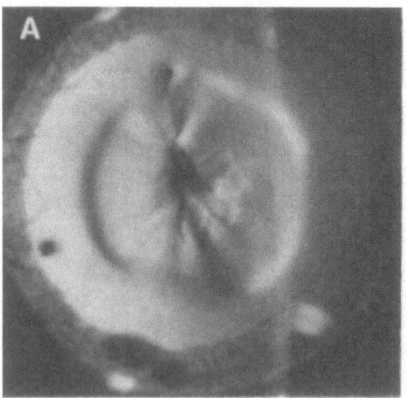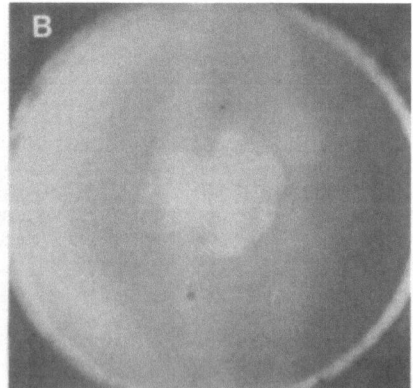

Fig. 2. Slit lamp photos in retroillumination of *cat-b*. Relative decrease in size of the opaque nuclear portion from age of 14 days (A) to the age of 189 days (B).

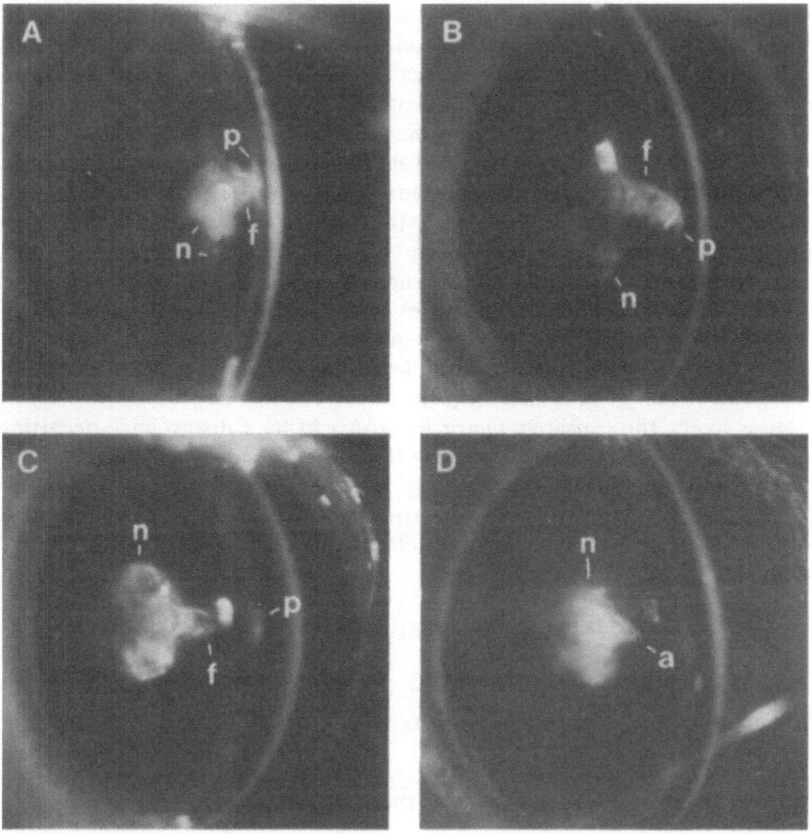

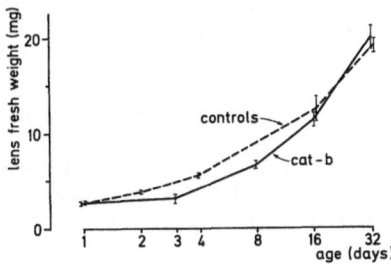

Fig. 3. Regression of anterior fusiform opacity during lens development: A: broad connection (f) between nuclear opacity (n) and anterior polar opacity (p) at 14 days; B: stalklike connection at 21 days; C: disruption of fusiform protrusion from anterior polar opacity at 109 days; D: nuclear opacity with apex pointed to the anterior lens pole at 189 days.

Fig. 4. Mean lens fresh weights and standard deviations in normal controls and *cat-b* mutants. Each mean is based on 20-40 values.

159

and by Lisch (1943). The association with remnants of the pupillary membrane observed in a few of our animals had also been observed in humans (cf. Waardenburg, 1961). The absence of the fusiform interconnection in part of our animals suggests that some of the more common nuclear congenital cataracts in man may belong into the same group.

The mechanism of development of such opacities is up-to-date unknown. Early papers (cf. von Hess, 1893; Mann, 1937) have discussed a disturbed segregation of the lens anlage from the surface ectoderm resulting in a pathological adherence of the primary lens fibres to the anterior lens pole. This hypothesis may be applicable to the cataracts observed in the rat line of Léonard & Maisin (1965), which we ourselves had the opportunity to study in detail (unpublished; cf. Gorthy & Abdelbaki, 1974). It is probably not applicable to our new mutant, as the inner centre of the lens nucleus, containing the primary fibres, is not opaque.

More likely the causative factor in *cat-b* will be a disturbance occurring later in lens development and affecting the early secondary lens fibres.

Further biochemical and embryological experiments with *cat-b* rats are in progress and we hope that the new mutant will prove a suitable animal model to clarify some of the problems related to anterior fusiform and nuclear cataract development.

ACKNOWLEDGEMENT

We are grateful to Professor Dr. Otto Hockwin for helpful discussions.
This investigation was supported by Deutsche Forschungsgemeinschaft (grout Ko 594/2).

REFERENCES

Baumgarten, H. Versuche zur experimentellen Rötelnembryopathie bei der Ratte. Diplomarbeit: Bonn (1977).

Bourne, M.C. & Grüneberg, H. Degeneration of the retina and cataract. A new recessive gene in the rat (rattus norvegicus). *J. Heredity* 30: *131-136* (1939).

Gorthy, W.C. & Abdelbaki, Y.Z. Morphology of a hereditary cataract in the rat. *Expl. Eye Res.* 19: *147-156* (1974).

Hess, v. Zur Pathologie und pathologischen Anatomie verschiedener Starformen. Cataracta centralis, Cataracta perinuclearis. – Zur Erklärung der angeborenen Cataractformen. – Cataracta punctata. *Albrecht v. Graefes Arch. Ophthal.* 39, I: *183-220* (1893).

Jess, A. Über kongenitale und vererbbare Staarformen der weißen Ratte nebst Bemerkungen über die Frage des Verhaltens der Linsen bei vitaminfreier Ernährung. *Klin. Mbl. Augenheilk.* 74: *49-56* (1925).

Kern, R. & Schäfer, K. Über eine angeborene Katarakt der Ratte. I: Linsenveränderungen während der ersten 14 Tage. *Ophthalmologica* 161: *255-263* (1970).

Koch, H.-R., Fischer, A. & Kaufmann, H. Occurrence of cataracts in spontaneously *ophthal.* 1: *55-62* (1976).

Koch, H.-R., Fischer, A. & Kaufmann, H. Occurrence of cataracts in spontaneously hypertensive rats. *Ophthal. Res.* 9: *189-193* (1977).

Lambert, W.V. & Sciuchetti, A. A dwarf mutation in the rat. *Science* 81: *278* (1935).

Léonard, A. & Maisin, J.R. Hereditary cataract induced by X-irradiation of young rats. *Nature* 205: *615-616* (1965).

Lisch, K. Zur Genese des vorderen Polstars. *Graefes Arch. Ophthal.* 145: *393-396* (1943).

Mann, I. Developmental abnormalities of the eye. University Press: Cambridge (1937).

Smith, S.E. & Barrentine, B.F. Hereditary cataract. A new dominant gene in the rat. *J. Hered.* 34: *8-16* (1943).

Smith, R., Hoffman, H. & Cisar, C. Congenital cataract in the rat. *Arch. Ophthal., Chicago* 81: *259-263* (1969).

Vogt, A. Vorderer Polstar bei Schichtstar. In: Lehrbuch und Atlas der Spaltlampenmikroskopie des lebenden Auges. Vol. 2, p. *407*. Springer: Berlin (1931) p. *407*.

Waardenburg, P.J. The lens, in, Genetics and Ophthalmology. Vol. 1, p. *847-951*. Van Gorkum: Assen (1961).

Authors' address:
Priv. Doz. Dr. H.-R. Koch
Dipl. Biol. H. Baumgarten
Institute of experimental Ophthalmology
Division Biochemistry of the Eye
University of Bonn, D-5300 Bonn Fed. Rep. Germany

Dr. J. Kratochvilova
Abteilung für Genetik
Gesellschaft für Strahlen- und Umweltforschung
D-8042 Neuherberg, Fed. Rep. Germany

Docum. Ophthal. Proc. Series, Vol. 18

UTILIZATION OF FRUCTOSE-1,6-DIPHOSPHATE AS GLYCOLYTIC SUBSTRATE IN BOVINE LENS HOMOGENATES

INGE KORTE, OTTO HOCKWIN & DIETER KASKEL

(Bonn, Fed. Rep. Germany)

ABSTRACT

Cortex and nucleus of bovine lenses of different ages were homogenized and incubated in the presence of glucose at 37°C for different periods. A balance of the free adenine nucleotides is produced, which is nearly independent of the amount of glucose added (12.5; 25; 37 mM) and shows certain deviations from the physiologic values. These might be interpreted as due to a decreased rate of glycolytic catabolization. Possibly the phosphorylation of the glucose, which is present in sufficient amounts, is inhibited. If, for instance, fructose-1,6-diphosphate in a concentration of 10^{-4}M is added to homogenates with such a disturbed nucleotide balance, a normalization takes place within 30 min, and the values of the initial physiologic equilibrium are restored. Due to the difference in the metabolic condition, there are differences between the behaviour of the cortex homogenate and that of the nucleus. The original equilibrium of the free nucleotides present in homogenates of lens nuclei is more stable during incubation in the presence of glucose. Most obvious is the improvement of the equilibrium in the presence of fructose-1,6-diphosphate. Besides the analytical evaluation of the free nucleotides the values of the concentrations of di-hydroxyacetone-phosphate, pyruvic acid and lactate clearly show that fructose-1,6-diphosphate may be utilized as a substrate for the glycolysis of lens homogenates.

In a pilot study we investigated the *in vitro* penetration of FDP from a Krebs-Ringer solution into the bovine lens. At a concentration of 10^{-2}M FDP in the medium, the lenses showed a considerably increased FDP – content after 3 hrs. *In vivo* investigations with rabbits showed that the content of FDP in the aqueous was significantly increased after a subconjuctival injection of a 10^{-1} M FDP solution as well as after topical application with a 20 percent eye ointment. These findings may be of importance in view to a possible activation of the carbohydrate metabolism of the lens *in vitro* and probably also *in vivo*.

INTRODUCTION

The rate of glycolysis of the eye lens is considerably affected by the ageing process, for which the impaired activities of the phosphorylating enzymes, phosphofructokinase and hexokinase, are in part responsible. Without having been able to determine the enzyme itself, Müller et al. as early as 1958 assumed phosphofructokinase formed a bottleneck in glycolysis; Hockwin (1972), and most recently Cheng & Chylack (1977) have confirmed its existence. The reasons for this bottleneck in glucose catabolism at the step from F6P to F-1,6-DP are posttranslational alterations of the enzyme phosphofructokinase with the age-related occurrence of a metazyme which has a considerably lower substrate affinity than the original enzyme (Ohrloff et al., 1977, Ohrloff, 1978; Bous et al., 1977). The lens nucleus is always much more affected by the ageing process than the lens cortex.

Kleifeld et al. (1956, a, b) showed with rabbit lenses that the rate of AT ^{32}P-formation (i.e. the incorporation of inorganic $^{32}PO_4^{3-}$ into ATP which can be electrophoretically isolated and determined by β-radioactivity scanning of the electropherogram) can be stimulated by adding fructose-1,6-diphosphate instead of glucose to the fresh homogenates. This was a first indication of a possible activation of the glycolytic processes in lens homogenates by replacing glucose in the medium with phosphorylated intermediates.

Investigating the stability of the adenine nucleotide equilibrium in the homogenates of bovine lenses incubated in glucose-containing medium we observed (Hockwin et al., 1977) that the ATP/ADP/AMP equilibrium existing at the beginning of the test reaches values characteristic of disturbances in the carbohydrate breakdown within 1 hr of incubation at 37°C (pO$_2$ = 20 percent in the presence of 25mM or or 37mM glucose respectively (Korte et al., 1968): the content of ATP is decreased, that of AMP increased accordingly. In these homogenates of whole bovine lenses glucose was not able to maintain the original steady state of the adenine nucleotide distribution. Only by adding a compound containing an anionic fumarate portion (bencyclane-hydrogen-fumarate) could the original equilibrium be stabilized, or within an already disturbed system could reactions be initiated which lead to normalization (Hockwin et al., 1977, 1978a, 1978b). The present investigations, based on the findings of Kleifeld et al. (1956a, 1956b) with fructose-1,6-diphosphate aimed at elucidating the question as to whether this substance may be utilized instead of glucose to normalize a disturbed physiologic balance of ATP/ADP/AMP in the homogenates of cortex and nucleus of bovine lenses of different age. To verify the utilization of F-1,6 DP as a substrate, the content of dihydroxyacetone-phosphate, pyruvate and lactate were determined besides the content of free nucleotides.

In a preliminary series we examined whether or not the test procedure is also feasible for intact lenses, and whether their incubation in a F-1,6-DP containing medium leads to an increase of this substrate in the lens. Further, *in vivo* investigations with rabbits were performed to show whether the content of F-1,6-DP in the aqueous is increased after application of an appropriate eye ointment and after subconjunctival injection.

MATERIALS AND METHODS

Studies with homogenates

Calf and bovine eyes from the local slaughterhouse were used for the investigations. Following preparation the lenses were separated into cortex and nucleus and each part homogenized (lg lens wet weight/10 ml) using a Krebs-

Ringer salt solution (96 ml 0.154 M NaCl; 2 ml 0.154 M KCl; 2 ml 0.110 M CaCl$_2$, and 20 ml 0.155 M NaHCO$_3$).

The homogenates from cortex and nucleus respectively were each divided into four parts. One part was deproteinized using perchloric acid to determine the initial values. To the other three test assays glucose was added in amounts relative to the intended time of incubation (Korte et al., 1976), so that the following initial glucose concentrations were present in the homogenates:

a)   30 min. incubation = 12.5 mM
b)   60 min. incubation = 25   mM
c)   90 min. incubation = 37   mM

After the incubation time of 30 or 60 min. respectively, the homogenates a) and b) were each divided into two parts. One part was deproteinized by perchloric acid, the other incubated in the presence of fructose-1,6-diphosphate (sodium salt) in a concentration of 10^{-4} M for another 30 min., then the reactions were stopped by deproteinizing. Homogenate c was deproteinized after 90 min. All homogenates were incubated in a gently shaking Warburg apparatus at 37°C and a pO$_2$ of 20%. In the deproteinized extracts the following substances were determined enzymatically after Bergmeyer (1974) using chemicals from Biochemica Boehringer: adenosine-triphosphate, adenosine-diphosphate, adenosine-monophosphate, dihydroxy-acetonephosphate, pyruvate and lactate.

In-vitro incubation of intact lenses

Intact bovine lens pairs were incubated in Krebs-Ringer solution at 37°C for 3 hrs, in such a way that one lens of each pair was incubated in a solution with added inulin, the other in solution with added F-1,6-diphosphate. After 3 hrs the lenses were rinsed in a 0.9 percent NaCl-solution, then deproteinized. The same metabolic parameters as in the homogenates were then determined. Additionally, their content in F-1,6-DP was determined according to Bergmeyer (1974).

In-vivo experiments with rabbits

Rabbits with a mean body weight of about 2-2.5 kg were given 2 subconjunctival injections of 0.5 ml each at 2 opposite places of a 10^{-1} M FDP-solution (aqua bidest.) in one eye. Both eyes were punctured after 30, 60 and 120 min. (5 animals each time), and the content of F-1,6-DP determined in the collected aqueous (Kaskel et al., 1975). Further, by means of an ophthalmic ointment base a 20 percent fructose-1,6-diphosphate ointment was prepared, and about 0.2 to 0.25 g was applied to one eye of each rabbit, using the other one as control. 30 and 60 min. after application, aqueous from both eyes was collected (6 animals for each period) and the content of F-1,6-DP measured.

RESULTS AND DISCUSSION

Tables 1-6 show the values obtained for all substances investigated in the homogenates of lens cortex and nucleus of bovine lenses of different age. Data of concentrations are means, number of cases and standard deviation of means are given. Significant differences have been checked by t-test in a pairwise assay.

All tables show that the equilibria of the free adenine nucleotides as well as the concentrations of the glycolytic intermediates existing in the fresh homogenates are altered when incubated in the presence of glucose. Under the above conditions of incubation, the changed equilibrium of the free adenine nucleotides in the homogenates with a strong decrease in ATP and an increase in AMP indicates characteristic disturbances in energy metabolism (Korte et al., 1968).

If, after the 30 or 60 min. incubation period in the presence of glucose which had caused the reported changes, the incubation is continued with addition of 10^{-4} M F-1,6-DP, nearly all investigated parameters are restored to the approximate initial values found in the fresh homogenates. With F-1,6-DP, the metabolic equilibrium disturbed by glucose was again nearly balanced. There are, however, certain differences in the influence of the F-1,6-DP which depend on the kind of homogenate as well as on the age of animal. Table 1 shows that the decrease in ATP of the cortex homogenates occurs mostly in the first half hour, and is stronger in the bovine lens than in the calf lens. Addition of F-1,6-DP to the medium of calf cortex homogenates after 30 or 60 min. resulted in an approximation of the lowered ATP

Table 1. ATP content in μM/100 g 1ww in incubated 10 percent homogenates of cortex and nucleus from calf and bovine lenses after different durations and with various amounts of glucose and after additional supplement of F-1,6-DP.

| Incubation: with glucose | | Continuation with further addition of F-1,6-DP 10^{-4} M | *ATP* | | | | |
| | | | *Calf* n = 8 μM/100 g | | Bovine n = 12 μM/100 g | | |
10^{-2} M	min.	min.	lww	s	lww	s	
0	0	0	209.54 *	23.58	165.67 *	21.80	
1.25	30	0	160.47 *	26.69	76.31 *	12.80	
1.25	30	30	218.63	21.30	112.62	15.01	
2.5	60	0	151.48 *	20.35	56.75 *	5.69	*Cortex*
2.5	60	30	221.54	32.82	101.16	23.89	
3.75	90	0	137.73	26.38	39.99	12.06	
0	0	0	53.40	7.39	29.26	7.80	
1.25	30	0	49.17 *	8.96	41.42 *	13.84	
1.25	30	30	69.26	9.77	73.49	25.15	
2.5	60	0	44.94 *	5.27	35.95 *	13.22	*Nucleus*
2.5	60	30	69.26	5.96	64.68	17.43	
3.75	90	0	39.92	8.11	32.78	10.08	
					* $p < 0.05$		

Table 2. ADP content in $\mu M/100$ g 1ww in incubated 10 percent homogenates of cortex and nucleus from calf and bovine lenses after different durations and with various amounts of glucose and after additional supplement of F-1,6-DP.

Incubation with glucose 10^{-2} M	min.	continuation with further addition of F-1,6-DP 10^{-4} M min.	ADP Calf n = 8 $\mu M/100$ g lww	s	Bovine n = 12 $\mu M/100$ g lww	s	
0	0	0	51.66 *	6.87	51.12	7.33	
1.25	30	0	79.76 *	8.80	64.99	16.12	
1.25	30	30	45.69	4.75	60.54	4.94	
2.5	60	0	88.50 *	6.33	61.69 *	7.80	Cortex
2.5	60	30	47.77	7.99	64.37	16.80	
3.75	90	0	92.19	9.42	47.29	12.23	
0	0	0	24.88	4.42	16.65	5.57	
1.25	30	0	25.09	1.37	20.79	17.73	
1.25	30	30	22.91	7.57	10.90	7.63	
2.5	60	0	26.24	3.65	14.81	5.57	Nucleus
2.5	60	30	23.71	3.43	12.89	7.74	
3.75	90	0	27.39	14.84	18.41	6.39	

* $p < 0.05$

Table 3. AMP content in $\mu M/100$ g lww in incubated 10 percent homogenates of cortex and nucleus from calf and bovine lenses after different durations and with various amounts of glucose and after additional supplement of F-1,6-DP.

Incubation: with glucose 10^{-2} M	min.	continuation with further addition of F-1,6-DP 10^{-4} M min.	AMP Calf n = 8 $\mu M/100$ g lww	s	Bovine n = 12 $\mu M/100$ g lww	s	
0	0	0	6.27 *	1.86	10.44 *	1.63	
1.25	30	0	26.01 *	3.5	40.70 *	6.92	
1.25	30	30	5.87	1.87	22.40	5.26	
2.5	60	0	20.43 *	5.37	43.35 *	11.12	Cortex
2.5	60	30	6.27	1.62	31.46	12.11	
3.75	90	0	18.70	8.79	51.48	9.43	
0	0	0	15.94	7.71	9.02	2.07	
1.25	30	0	16.86 *	2.13	10.96 *	5.06	
1.25	30	30	5.51	2.41	5.79	3.21	
2.5	60	0	21.81 *	3.57	10.32 *	4.80	Nucleus
2.5	60	30	6.85	2.13	4.68	1.59	
3.75	90	0	23.88	5.04	13.12	5.77	

* $p < 0.05$

content to the values of the fresh homogenates, which also was true for the cortex homogenates of bovine lenses. The values of the fresh controls, however, were not fully reached. In the homogenate of calf nuclei, the ATP content showed only a slight, non-significant decrease. In both age groups the increase in the ATP content through addition of F-1,6-DP after 30 or 60 min. respectively was significant, and the values measured were higher than those of the fresh nucleus homogenates. This means that application of F-1,6-DP stimulates ATP-formation in all homogenates. Table 2 shows the values for ADP. A significant increase of the content of ADP by incubation in a glucose-containing salt solution was only found with the cortex homogenates of calf lenses, and took place mostly within the first half hour. In the homogenate of bovine lens cortex the increase of the ADP content found was not significant. Addition of F-1,6-DP effected a normalization of the ADP-content. A similar behaviour was found with the homogenates of nuclei.

The AMP content (Table 3) in the homogenate of calf and bovine cortex increased significantly during incubation in the presence of glucose. It happened mainly in the first half hour and was more apparent in the bovine than in the calf lens. In all cases, addition of F-1,6-DP effected a decrease in AMP. In the cortex homogenates of calves the initial values were regained, in those of bovines only a partial recovery, as in the case of ATP, took place.

In the nucleus homogenate of both age groups the increase of AMP in the presence of glucose could be lowered to below that of the fresh homogenates.

The concentrations of dihydroxyacetone-phosphate, pyruvate, and lactate show in part changes dependent on kind of incubation and homogenate.

The values demonstrated in Table 4 show that the content of DAP in the homogenates is rather stable, and even an addition of F-1,6-DP hardly changes its concentration. Only in the nucleus homogenates of bovine lenses was a remarkable increase of DAP-concentrations observed, by far exceeding that of the fresh homogenates. This phenomenon might be due to the considerable changes of the enzymes glyceraldehyde-phosphate-dehydrogenase and enolase through posttranslational influences (Ohrloff, 1978; Berdjis, in prep.).

The pyruvate concentrations (Table 5) increased in the presence of glucose in all homogenates except in that of the bovine cortex. This increase was even higher and in part significant when F-1,6-DP was added.

The content of lactate (Table 6) increased significantly in the cortex homogenates of calf lenses in the presence of glucose, where addition of F-1,6-DP was of little effect. A similar behaviour could be observed in the nucleus homogenates of calf and bovine, although less distinct, here the differences were not significant. The cortex homogenates of the bovine lenses showed a different behaviour, and indicate that here the catabolization of glucose to lactate did not take place within the test time. Addition of F-1,6-DP, however, effected a certain but non-significant increase in lactate.

It is not possible to apply the results obtained with homogenates to the whole lens (Hockwin et al., 1978a). Previous to our current studies on the utilization of F-1,6-DP in the case of substrate-deficient lenses, we examined the question of whether the substance was able to permeate from the medium into the lens. Table 7 shows results obtained after a 3 hr incubation of bovine lenses in a medium with added 10^{-2} M F-1,6-DP and inulin respectively. The content of F-1,6-DP in lens equator was remarkably increased compared to that under inulin.

The lactate content was also increased. All other parameters of this *in vitro* test did not show any changes. This is certainly due to the fact that in the lenses of this test assay the physiologic balance was intact. Since the ATP-concentration was in accordance with the physiologic level, the lens need not necessarily utilize an alternative substrate, even if F-1,6-DP offered more favorable conditions.

In a further pilot study we tried to find out whether it was possible to increase *in vivo* the F-1,6-DP content in the aqueous as the natural medium of the lens. Table 8 demonstrates that this holds true. In the aqueous of rabbits the content of F-1,6-DP is considerably increased after a subconjunctival injection as well as after application of the substrate in a special ointment, compared to the untreated eye.

At present we do not intend to draw conclusions from the results of this study on the mechanisms of permeation, or to discuss the importance of certain tissue properties with respect to the permeation of F-1,6-DP. We only wanted to look into the question of whether it would be worth while to attempt an increase of F-1,6-DP in the aqueous with a view to its availability in the lens as an alternative substrate, which would be of great impor-

Table 4. DAP content in $\mu M/100$ g 1ww in incubated 10 percent homogenates of cortex and nucleus from calf and bovine lenses after different durations and with various amounts of glucose and after additional supplement of F-1,6-DP.

Incubation: with glucose 10^{-2} M	min.	continuation with further addition of F-1,6-DP 10^{-4} M min.	*Calf* n = 8 $\mu M/100$ g lww	s	*Bovine* n = 12 $\mu M/100$ g lww	s	
0	0	0	12.26	4.03	13.12	3.81	
1.25	30	0	12.61	4.83	8.89	1.78	
1.25	30	30	16.61	3.42	8.88	2.17	
2.5	60	0	15.10	3.01	10.60	1.95	*Cortex*
2.5	60	30	17.33	2.94	9.69	2.14	
3.75	90	0	16.08	4.59	11.31	2.14	
0	0	0	14.66	7.24	8.92	3.10	
1.25	30	0	13.91	6.54	5.45 *	2.54	
1.25	30	30	13.77	3.74	47.86	26.26	*Nucleus*
2.5	60	0	12.53	4.48	12.26 *	11.58	
2.5	60	30	13.77	3.68	55.10	21.70	
3.75	90	0	15.10	6.44	12.67	14.70	

$* \quad p < 0.05$

Table 5. Pyruvate content in $\mu M/100$ g lww in incubated 10 percent homogenates of cortex and nucleus from calf and bovine lenses after different durations and with various amounts of glucose and after additional supplement of F-1,6-DP.

Incubation: with glucose 10^{-2} M	min.	continuation with further addition of F-1,6-DP 10^{-4} M min.	Pyruvate Calf n = 8 $\mu M/100$ g lww	s	Bovine n = 12 $\mu M/100$ g lww	s	
0	0	0	26.39 *	4.50	18.89	4.95	
1.25	30	0	34.03 *	6.56	20.48 *	5.79	
1.25	30	30	57.75	6.75	39.62	7.73	
2.5	60	0	42.56	6.71	18.60 *	4.18	Cortex
2.5	60	30	52.15	11.29	33.99	9.69	
3.75	90	0	39.80	15.19	16.22	3.48	
0	0	0	17.59	1.96	8.98	4.20	
1.25	30	0	21.94	12.08	16.17	4.68	
1.25	30	30	25.59	3.31	12.97	6.02	
2.5	60	0	19.55 *	4.85	12.20	4.06	Nucleus
2.5	60	30	26.92	5.07	13.33	5.13	
3.75	90	0	17.32	6.02	17.38	11.32	

$*\ p < 0.05$

Table 6. Lactate content in $\mu M/100$ g lww in incubated 10 percent homogenates of cortex and nucleus from calf and bovine lenses after different durations and with various amounts of glucose and after additional supplement of F-1,6-DP.

Incubation with glucose 10^{-2}	min.	continuation with further addition of F-1,6-DP 10^{-4} M min.	Lactate Calf n = 8 $\mu M/100$ g lww	s	Bovine n = 12 $\mu M/100$ g lww	s	
0	0	0	666.74 *	112.32	546.71	84.06	
1.25	30	0	977.62	211.61	574.90	210.10	
1.25	30	30	856.14	130.45	611.21	193.45	
2.5	60	0	1041.07	175.50	535.78	136.12	Cortex
2.5	60	30	1034.26	215.74	623.20	143.31	
3.75	90	0	1078.08	199.26	532.19	160.79	
0	0	0	552.00	172.91	270.71	61.04	
1.25	30	0	568.39	212.67	326.05	154.86	
1.25	30	30	501.24	198.65	431.09	189.27	
2.5	60	0	592.18	158.67	299.90	299.90	Nucleus
2.5	60	30	572.09	129.20	435.68	216.91	
3.75	90	0	583.19	121.49	495.28	365.79	

$*\ p < 0.05$

tance in case of disturbances in the carbohydrate and energy metabolism of the lens.

CONCLUSION

Some years ago Nordmann (1954) and Müller (1956) suggested that a disturbed energy metabolism is one of the main causes of cataract formation. A decrease of the energy-rich compounds increases the susceptibility of the lens to the formation of opacities and makes the lens more sensitive to additional risk factors.

Table 7. Content of free adenine nucleotides and intermediates of glycolysis in $\mu M/100$ g lww in bovine lensequators after 3 hrs. incubation in a Krebs-Ringer solution with 10^{-2} M F-1,6-DP or inulin resp. w = 5-12.

addition of 10^{-2} M	ATP	s	ADP	s	AMP	s
Inulin	133.87	42.03	66.26	4.67	16.92	2.98
F-1,6-DP	116.04	28.46	58.34	17.00	17.90	3.16
	DAP	s	lactate	s	Pyruvate	s
Inulin	2.69	1.55	464.77	71.57	10.17	5.17
F-1,6-DP	3.39	1.16	560.63 *	82.63	10.14	8.10
			F-1 6-DP	s		
Inulin			1.31	0.57		
F-1,6-DP			55.74 *	35.38	* p < 0.05	

Table 8. F-1,6-DP content in $\mu M/100$ ml in the aqueous of rabbit eyes after subconjunctival injection of 1.0 ml 10^{-1} M F-1.6-DP (a) or topical application of about 50 mg F-1,6-DP by eye ointment (b).

		a) injection			b) ointment		
		$\bar{x}$	s	n	$\bar{x}$	s	n
30'	Control	4.73	1.41	5	3.21	0.85	6
	F-1,6-DP	19.50 *	9.83	5	8.17 *	3.58	6
60'	Control	6.90	0.80	5	3.12	0.56	6
	F-1,6-DP	25.43 *	10.11	5	13.55 *	5.39	6
120'	Control	5.06	0.44	5	* p < 0.05		
	F-1,6-DP	8.36	2.65	5			

171

Without any visible influence, the energy balance undergoes changes during the ageing process (Hockwin et al., 1978). Investigations on the behaviour of enzyme activities of the carbohydrate metabolism as the main source of energy showed that particularly the enzymes hexokinase and phosphofructokinase are subject to age-related alterations which may well be responsible for the impaired energy condition (Müller et al., 1958; Hockwin et al., 1977; Cheng & Chylack, 1977; Ohrloff, 1978).

A decrease in total and specific activities of these enzymes and also lowered substrate affinities through metazyme forms occurring with age (Ohrloff et al., 1977; Bous et al., 1977; Ohrloff, 1978) are obvious causes for the age-induced lowered rate of glycolysis and its consequences.

There have been several attempts to replace glucose in its role as energy source. Kleifeld et al. (1956a, b) have used F-1,6-DP besides other intermediates of the carbohydrate metabolism. Their results with the homogenate of rabbit-lenses indicated that a stimulation of the ATP-formation is possible.

In previous investigations we learned that glucose in the homogenate of whole bovine lenses is not able to maintain the physiologic equilibrium of the free adenine nucleotides. We therefore tried to improve the balance conditions disturbed by glucose through utilizing fructose-1,6-diphosphate. Our results show that the observed alterations in the homogenates of nucleus and cortex of calf and bovine lenses, which indicated a disturbed carbohydrate and energy metabolism, may for the better part, be repaired.

As could be demonstrated by *in vitro* tests, F-1,6-DP is also able to permeate into the lens, if present in the medium in sufficient amounts. By subconjunctival injection and also by local application by means of an eye ointment, the F-1,6-DP content in the aqueous of rabbits could be increased.

Considering these results, we feel justified in continuing our attempts to improve conditions of the energy metabolism in the ageing lens by utilizing alternative substrates.

Thus the ageing lens may be provided with a potential that might help to delay or even avoid cataract formation.

REFERENCES

Berdjis, H. Altersbedingte Veränderungen des kinetischen und physiko-chemischen Verhaltens der Glycerinaldehyd-3-phosphat-Dehydrogenase (EC 1.2.1.12), 3-Phosphoglycerat-Kinase (EC 2.7.2.3), Phosphoglycerat-Mutase (EC 2.7.5.3) und Enolase (EC 4.2.1.11) in Rinderlinsen. Thesis, in preparation.

Bergmeyer, H.U. Methoden der enzymatischen Analyse, 3. Aufl. Bd.ll. Verlag Chemie, Weinheim, Bergstrasse, 1974.

Bous, F., Hockwin, O., Ohrloff, C. & Bours, J. Investigations on phosphofructokinase (PFK, EC 2.7.1.11) in bovine lenses in dependence on age, topographic distribution and water-soluble proteins. *Expl. Eye Res* 24: *383-389* (1977).

Cheng, H.M. & Chylack, L.T.jr. Factors affecting the rate of lactate production in rat lens. *Ophthal. Res.* 9: *381-387* (1977).

Hockwin, O. Biochemie des Linsenstoffwechsels und die Möglichkeit der medikamentösen Beeinflussung. *Vers. Rhein.-Westf. Augenärzte* 125: *24-33* (1972).

Hockwin, O., Korte, I., Breuer, R., Schmidt, G. & Rast, F. In vitro Inkubation von Linsen. Modell zur Untersuchung der Substratverwertbarkeit von Substanzen für den Energiestoffwechsel am Beispiel des Bencyclanhydrogenfumarats. Albrecht *v. Graefes Arch. klin. exp. Ophthal.* in press, 207: *169-180* (1978a).

Hockwin, O., Fink, H. & Ohrloff, C. Carbohydrate metabolism of the lens depending on age. Evaluation of factor analysis. 5th Europ. Symp. Basic Res. in Gerontology, 632-645, 1977, Weimar, GDR, Verlag Dr. med. Straube, Erlangen.

Hockwin, O., Günther, M. & Noll, E. Utilization of bencyclanehydrogen fumarate as a substrate for the critic acid cycle of bovine lenses. *Doc. Ophthal. Proc. Ser.* 18: *107-115.* (1978b).

Hockwin, O., Korte, I., Breuer, R., Schmidt, G. & Rast, F. In vitro Inkubation von clanehydrogen fumarate on the carbohydrate metabolism of bovine lens homogenates. *Drug. Res.* 27: *1141-1142* (1977).

Kaskel, D., Scholz, R., Hockwin, O. & Ziesmer, W. Composition of aqueous humour and lens after carotid ligation. *Ophthal. Res.* 7: *409-415* (1957).

Kleifeld, O., Ayberk, N., Hockwin, O. Über die Fähigkeit zur ATP-Bildung in Extrakten von Linsen junger und alter Tiere. *Albrecht von Graefes Arch. klin. exp. Ophthal.* 158: *34-38* (1956a).

Kleifeld, O. & Hockwin, O. Über den Kohlenhydratstoffwechsel der Linse in Abhängigkeit vom Lebensalter und bei experimentell erzeugten Stoffwechselstörungen. *Ber. dtsch. Ophthal. Ges. Heidelberg* 60: *101-108* (1956b).

Korte, I., Hockwin, O., Schmack, W. & Cremer-Bartels, G. Weitere Untersuchungen zur in vitro-Aufbewahrung von Augenlinsen. *Albrecht v. Graefes Arch. klin. exp. Ophthal.* 175: *235-241* (1968).

Korte, I., Hockwin, O., Winkler, F. & Rabe, P. Studies on the mode of action of 1-hydroxy-pyrido-(3,2α)-5-phenoxazone-3-carboxylic acid in bovine lenses. *Doc. Ophthal. Proc. Ser.* 8: *205-211* (1976).

Müller, H.K., Dardenne, U., Hockwin, O., Kleifeld, O. & Schafhausen, G. Altersbedingte Veränderungen im Stoffwechsel der Linse. XVIII Conc. Ophthalm. Belgica, *750-763* (1958).

Müller, H.K., Kleifeld, O., Arens, H.P., Dardenne, U., Fuchs, R. & Hockwin, O. The phosphorus metabolism of the lens. *Am. J. Ophthal.* 42: *431-473* (1956).

Nordmann, J. Biologie du Cristallin, Masson et Cie, Paris, 1954.

Ohrloff, C. Age changes of Enzyme Properties in Crystallin Lens. *Interdiscipl. Topics Geront.* 12: *158-179* (1978).

Ohrloff, C., Hockwin, O., Bous, F. & Bours, J. Investigations on the phosphofructokinase (EC 2.7.1.11) in bovine lenses depending on age. 5th Europ. Symp. Basic Res. in Gerontology, 646-656, 1977, Weimar, GDR, Verlag Dr. med. Straube, Erlangen.

Schmack, W., Hockwin, O. & Adusa-Amankwa, K.K. Der Einfluss cytostatischer Substanzen [Cyclophosphamid und 2,3,5-Tris-aethylenimino-benzochinon-(1,4)] auf den Energiestoffwechsel junger und alter Rinderlinsen. *Ber. dtsch. ophthal. Ges.* 70: *376-380* (1969).

Authors' address:
Division Biochemistry of the Eye
Institute of experimental Ophthalmology
University of Bonn, Fed. Rep. Germany

Docum. Ophthal. Proc. Series, Vol. 18

EFFECT OF LONG-WAVE ULTRAVIOLET LIGHT ON THE LENS
III. A STUDY OF FACTORS INFLUENCING UV-INDUCED INJURY TO THE LENS IN VITRO

JOHN F.R. KUCK, Jr.

(Atlanta, Georgia U.S.A.)

ABSTRACT

Long-wave ultraviolet light affects the lens in vitro by depressing amino acid uptake and partly destroying glutathione. Later and more serious injury is manifested by lens swelling. The injury is enhanced in the presence of oxygen and is not reversed by a subsequent period of incubation in the dark. Toxic material released from irradiated lenses may affect shielded lenses bathed in the same medium. Evidence points to the injury as a catastrophe which is characterized as a rather sudden, overpowering and irreversible change. This effect has been demonstrated for the first time with human lenses whose rate of leucine incorporation is reduced to 5% of the level found in the non irradiated contralateral mate.

INTRODUCTION

Long-wave ultraviolet light (here called UV) affects cells by two mechanisms: (1) injury to DNA resulting in subsequent defective protein synthesis; the effective dose is relatively small and there is a time lag before an obvious defect occurs; a photosensitizer is usually required. (2) Injury produced directly on more sensitive parts of the cell such as the membranes; the effect may appear within hours if the intensity and duration of radiation are enough to overcome the considerable capacity of the cell to resist and repair damage; a photosensitizer is not usually required but may enhance the effect.

The direct effect, the subject of this paper, appears to be mediated by activated molecules which are not the small highly energetic free radicals produced by ionizing radiation. Instead they are species of organic molecules which have become activated by absorbing energy (McCormick & Thomason, 1978), which may be re-radiated at longer wave lengths (fluorescence) or consumed in altering the molecule (photoactivation or photodecomposition). A related phenomenon is the photodynamic effect which was first studied in the lens by Harris et al. (1959). Here the toxicity of oxygen was induced by interaction with methylene blue. In this case the effective wavelength of light is that absorbed by the dye, which behaves in somewhat the same way as light-activated molecules. We are concerned here chiefly with the action of such altered molecules whose effects are not easy to detect or quantitate, especially early in the process.

175

Experimental methods of assessing early damage to the lens include: determination of depressed glutathione levels, measurement of depressed amino acid uptake or incorporation, and swelling of the lens due to water imbibition. In earlier reports we have shown the utility of these methods (Kuck, 1976, 1977). Now we present a study of some of the factors involved in the mechanism of damage.

MATERIALS AND METHODS

Lenses were removed from eyes of rats, chicks or human eyebank material and incubated in a bicarbonate-buffered balanced salt solution in 50 ml round bottom centrifuge tubes with the bottoms in contact with a UV lamp (G.E. F-15T8 BLB) submerged in the water bath. The lenses were about 2-3 mm away from the lamp surface which had a flux intensity of about 2.5 mwatts per cm^2. The medium was gassed with 5% CO_2 in O_2 through a tube positioned just above the pool of lenses; this served to maintain the pH and to produce thermal and compositional equilibrium in the medium. Pre-incubations in 10-30 ml of medium were carried out for as long as 24 hours, then the lenses were transferred to 2 ml of medium containing tracer amino acid and incubation continued for 2 hours for rat lenses, 6 hours for human lenses. After the tracer incubation the lenses were removed, rinsed, blotted dry, weighed and homogenized in a solution containing 0.1% each of NaF, NaN_3 and EDTA. Whenever possible an experimental lens pool consisted of one lens from each of the required number of rats while the other lens went into the control pool.

In some experiments a special twin-tube was employed, constructed from two 50 ml centrifuge tubes joined about 1.5 cm from the bottom by a connecting tube which allowed medium to pass but not the lenses. One compartment was exposed to UV, the other compartment and the connecting tube were shielded. By means of a tube extending to the bottom of the UV-compartment medium was pumped into the shielded compartment at about 15 ml per minute. Liquid levels in the compartments were equalized by flow through the connecting tube. With this apparatus it was possible to submit a pool of shielded lenses to medium from the exposed lenses or to medium exposed to UV in the absence of lenses.

The tracer amino acids were from Amersham/Searle: 2-amino-^{14}C (αAIB) and DL-1-^{14}C leucine, used at concentrations of 1 and 2 μCi/ml, respectively.

Glutathione was analyzed by Ellman's procedure as modified by Sedlak & Lindsay (1968). Incorporation of leucine into lens proteins was measured by the method of Spector & Kinoshita (1964).

RESULTS

Duration of Irradiation

The effect of duration of incubation on the swelling and glutathione (GSH)

Table 1. The effect of duration of UV irradiation on swelling and glutathione level of chick lenses.

	Lens Weight (mg)		Glutathione, mg%	
HOURS	DK	UV	DK	UV
6	38.48 ± 1.65	41.73 ± 1.51	82.8 ± 6.1	72.7 ± 9.0
8	41.88 ± 3.61	42.80 ± 3.84	69.1 ± 9.3	71.2 ± 5.2
12	40.60 ± 2.53	41.58 ± 1.17	76.6 ± 16.6	63.8 ± 17.0
18	38.48 ± 0.43	47.80 ± 1.10	68.9 ± 3.5	35.0 ± 15.0

DK = shielded lenses, UV = irradiated lenses.
Each pool had 4 lenses pre-incubated in a solution containing 10 mM aminotriazole for the indicated time, then analyzed individually for glutathione.

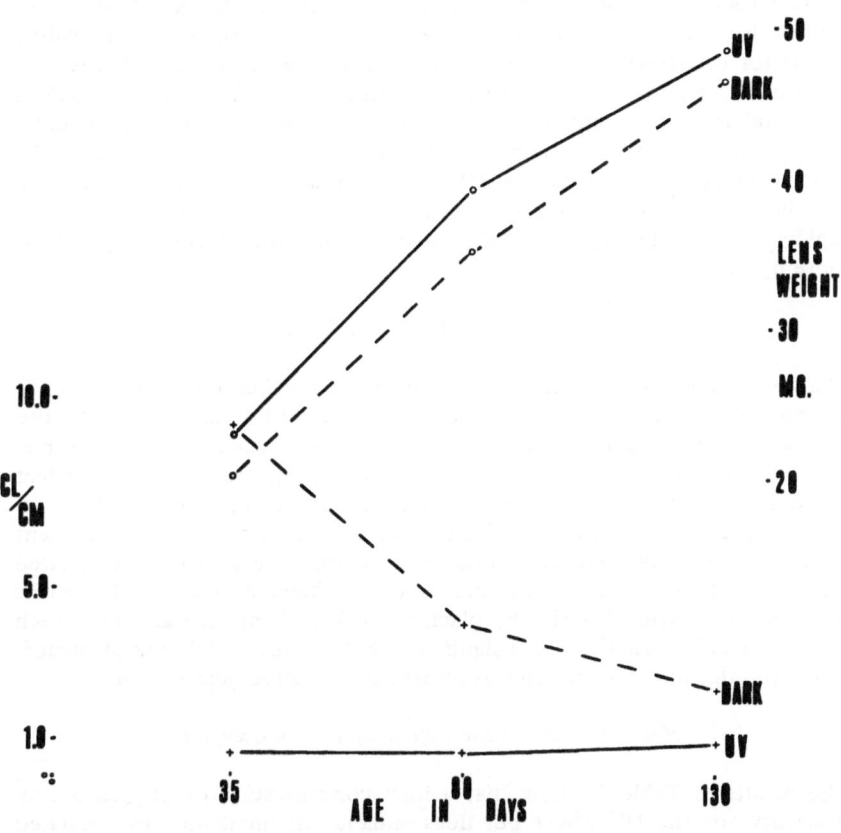

Fig. 1. The effect of rat lens age on the severity of UV-induced injury to the lens as measured by depression of amino acid uptake. CL/CM is the concentration of α-AIB in the lens water divided by that in the incubation medium. A value of CL/CM < 1.0 indicates transport in by diffusion only.

level in chick lenses is shown in Table 1. There was no significant water imbition or loss of GSH until after 12 hours of UV. By 18 hours the changes in both parameters were marked. This result was confirmed by several rat lens experiments showing that maintenance of GSH levels failed after 12 hours of UV.

Effect of Age of Lens

The effect of lens age on resistance to UV is shown in Fig. 1. The upper curves rising to the right are for lens weight; the vertical distance between points for the same age represents mg swelling in UV; thus none of these lenses underwent much swelling although the two younger groups exposed to UV were significantly larger (12-13%) than their shielded mates. On the other hand, when CL/CM (Lens concentration/Medium concentration) for αAIB is used as an index of lens integrity, all three groups exhibited depression of the amino acid pump, ranging from 61 to 94%. Analysis of individual results for the largest lenses show that for three the CL/CM is 1.24 while for the remaining three the value is 0.67; the weights are all very close together. This emphasizes the points that have become apparent in many experiments: (1) the amino acid pump is more sensitive to UV than is maintenance of water balance. (2) The effect of UV on CL/CM is catastrophic; once a single lens begins to lose its pump, the capacity to accumulate amino acid is rapidly and completely lost and what amino acid is transported in appears to move by diffusion.

Indirect Effect of Products of Irradiation

That lenses may be affected by some means other than direct irradiation is shown in Table 2. Here the lens pool designated DKirr was incubated in the shielded compartment of the twin-tube but was continually bathed in medium which was circulating through the UV compartment. Thus the effect could have been mediated only by substances released from the lens, including extraneous tissue not cleaned off in dissection, which underwent conversion to toxic materials during irradiation. The lens pool designated DK was incubated in a separate tube and was shielded from UV. These lens pools were matched for size by placing one lens from each animal in each tube. The effect on CL/CM is significant but required 21 hours of incubation; even this long incubation was insufficient to affect lens weight.

Enhancement of the Effect of UV by Oxygen

The results in Table 3. show that a high concentration of oxygen is not necessary for the UV effect but does enhance it. Incubation of irradiated lenses in medium gassed with 95% N_2-5% CO_2 for 24 hours produced a significant reduction in CL/CM as compared with shielded lenses. For older lenses there was no effect on CL/CM. There was no effect on lens weight for either size lens. In similar experiments using lenses of comparable age and even

178

shorter incubation times, gassing with oxygen during UV irradiation caused a complete loss of amino acid pump activity (i.e., CL/CM $<$ 1.0); an example appears in Fig. 1 where the two smaller sizes of lenses after incubation in medium gassed with 95% O_2-5% CO_2 during 8 hours of UV had only 6-15% of the normal CL/CM.

Failure of Recovery from UV-induced Damage

The results of Fig. 1 suggested that the effect of UV is catastrophic; additional evidence on this point is provided by experiments where a barely detectable level of damage was produced by 6 hours of UV, then the lenses were incubated further in the dark for 4 hours to see if any recovery was evident. The first two columns (Control) of Table 4. are for lenses which were incubated in tracer after the 6 hour irradiation period to show the effect before a possible recovery period; the depression in CL/CM by UV is 54%. The last two columns (Recovery) show the results for comparable lenses which were allowed to preincubate an additional 4 hours in the dark before the tracer incubation. In this case the UV-injured lenses showed no evidence of recovery; the apparent further degradation is not statistically significant.

Table 2. The effect of irradiated medium on shielded rat lenses. Lens swelling and uptake of α-AIB.

	DK Control	DKirrad.
Lens Weight, mg	30.86 ± 0.88	30.97 ± 1.18
CL/CM	7.08 ± 1.37	2.70 ± 0.68

The DKirrad lenses were shielded but were bathed in medium exposed to UV in another compartment. The DK control lenses were incubated in a separate, shielded vessel.

Table 3. The effect of UV on rat lenses in a medium gassed with a mixture containing nitrogen instead of oxygen.

	DK	UV
Lens Weight, mg		
Small	16.63 ± 0.05	16.35 ± 0.57
Large	43.90 ± 1.20	43.77 ± 1.12
CL/CM		
Small	9.24 ± 0.90	5.59 ± 1.23
Large	1.75 ± 0.19	1.70 ± 0.16

179

Table 5 shows the results for 8 pairs of human lenses in pilot experiments designed to elicit without fail a significant response to UV as measured by the effect on leucine incorporation and lens swelling. The small amount of swelling is significant only in the sense that the irradiated lens always weighed more than its shielded mate. However UV produced a tremendous reduction of leucine incorporation, to about 5% of the value for the shielded mates. Because of the heterogeneous nature of this small groups of lenses, no other correlations (e.g., with age) could be found.

DISCUSSION

It is clear from the results given above that the effect of UV on the lens is a complex process depending on several variables. Important parameters are the age of the lens and the duration of UV-exposure. Not unexpectedly, younger lenses are significantly more sensitive than older lenses, perhaps only because the young lens presents relatively more cortex to the environment than older, larger lenses. For younger lenses the UV effect was ap-

Table 4. Failure of rat lenses to recover from UV during a subsequent incubation in the dark.

	Control		Recovery	
	DK	UV	DK	UV
Lens Weight, mg	33.11 ± 0.73	37.59 ± 1.16	33.00 ± 1.30	40.41 ± 2.83
CL/CM	3.92 ± 0.51	0.68 ± 0.12	4.11 ± 0.62	0.58 ± 0.12

Table 5. The effect of UV on leucine incorporation into human lens proteins in vitro.

No.	Age	% Swelling	Leucine Incorporation		% Depression
			UV	Dark	
81	75	13.	55.2	3997.	98.6
82	67	16.	71.2	3069.	97.7
83	67	3.5	285.2	4055.	93.0
84	59	2.7	107.2	1979.	94.6
92	63	1.0	75.2	2654.	97.2
93	82	6.6	108.6	1126.	90.4
98	45	0.7	171.1	1800.	90.5
99	77	11.	54.6	1409.	96.1

The leucine incorporation, as cpm/mg protein, was calculated on the assumption that protein was 30% (Klethi, 1976) of the nominal fresh weight of the lens using the ages given here and the table in Weekers et al. (1975). Only lenses No. 92 and 98 were badly swollen on this basis.

parent in the virtual absence of oxygen but only after a relatively long pre-incubation with UV. Older lenses showed no difference for this same incubation time. It is significant that lenses subjected to an irradiation period just long enough to affect CL/CM but not lens swelling showed no recovery during a subsequent incubation in the dark.

It is important to prove that UV can affect the human lens as well as colorless animal lenses. The data presented here concerning the nearly complete blockade of leucine incorporation by UV are new information. This effect lends credence to the idea that a sufficient insult of this kind to the human lens may initiate or be a contributing factor to senile cortical cataract, the type which includes the vast majority of human senile cataracts.

ACKNOWLEDGEMENTS

This work was supported by NIH Grant EY 00260. The Georgia Lions Eye Bank — Atlanta was the source of human lenses employed in this investigation.

REFERENCES

Harris, J.E., Gruber, L., Talman, E. & Hoskinson, G. The influence of oxygen on the photodynamic action of methylene blue on cation transport in the rabbit lens. *Am. J. Ophthal.* 48: *528-535* (1959).

Klethi, J. Sodium and potassium in the normal human lens in relation with age. *Doc. Ophthalmol.* 8: *213-217* (1976).

Kuck, J.F.R. Effect of long-wave ultraviolet light on the lens. I. Model system for detecting and measuring effect on the lens in vitro. *Invest. Ophthal.* 15: *405-407* (1976).

Kuck, J.F.R. Effect of long-wave ultraviolet light on the lens. II. Metabolic inhibitors synergistic with UV in vitro. *Doc. Ophthalmol.* 8: *261-265* (1976).

McCormick, J.P. & T. Thomason. Near-ultraviolet photooxidation of tryptophan. Proof of formation of superoxide ion. *J. Am. chem. Soc.* 100: *312-313* (1978).

Sedlak, J. & Lindsay, R.H. Estimation of total protein-bound and non-protein sulfhydryl group in tissue with Ellman's reagent. *Analyt. Biochem.* 25: *192-205* (1968).

Spector, A. & Kinoshita, J.H. The incorporation of labeled amino acids into lens proteins. *Invest. Ophthal.* 3: *517-522* (1964).

Weekers, R., Delmarcelk, Y. & Luyckx, J. Biometrics of the crystalline lens, in Cataract and Abnormalities of the Lens (ed. Bellows, J.G.), Grune and Stratton, New York, 1975, p. 139.

Author's Address:
Laboratory for Ophthalmic Research
Department of Ophthalmology
Emory University
Atlanta, Georgia 30322 USA

Docum. Ophthal. Proc. Series, Vol. 18

FACTORS AFFECTING LIGHT TRANSMISSION IN NORMAL AGING LENSES, BROWN NUCLEAR, CORTICAL AND MIXED CATARACTS

SIDNEY LERMAN & RAYMOND F. BORKMAN

(Atlanta, U.S.A.)

ABSTRACT

UV-visible transmission spectroscopy and fluorescence spectroscopy was performed on normal aging lenses, nuclear, cortical and mixed cataracts immersed in saline and glycerol solutions. These experiments demonstrated that glycerol caused a marked increase in light transmission and the transparency of cortical cataracts, and a moderate improvement in the transparency of mixed cataracts. Aging normal lenses and nuclear cataracts were unaffected by glycerol treatment. The fluorescence emission intensities (at 440 and 520 nm) obtained from all these lenses correlated well with values previously reported, and they were not altered by glycerol treatment. These data provide further evidence that the nuclear brown cataract is simply an accelerated aging phenomenon in which there is little if any configurational change or aggregation of lens proteins. Cortical cataracts appear to be caused by marked changes in protein aggregation and/or configuration and these can be reversed in vitro by removing water from such lenses.

INTRODUCTION

Utilizing ultraviolet (UV) and visible light transmission measurements on normal human lenses aged 6 months to 82 years, we have demonstrated that a relatively high percent of UV light (300-400 nm) is transmitted in the 6 month to 8 year old lenses (over 75%) while the corresponding transmission of UV light in lenses above 25 years of age drops markedly to less than 20% (Lerman & Borkman, 1976). These data are consistent with the relative lack of 360 nm excited fluorescence as the lens ages (Lerman et al., 1976). Accompanying the measured increase in lens fluorescence and the decrease in UV light transmission, there is a concomitant increase in the yellow color of the lens as it ages. This lens pigmentation is believed to be generated photochemically and is confined mainly to the lens nucleus because of the relative lack of glutathione (free radical scavenger) in this region of the lens as compared with the lens cortex (Lerman, 1976; Borkman & Lerman, 1977). The increase in concentration of fluorescent material with age is paralleled by an increase in the concentration of water insoluble proteins in the lens (Clark et al., 1969; Lerman et al., 1976; and Lerman, 1972). It has been proposed that the fluorescent compounds may be involved in some protein aggregation mechanism perhaps functioning as a cross-linking agent(s). This hypothesis would explain our observation that lenses from patients with senile brown cataracts show abnormally high levels of fluorescence emission (at 360 nm excitation, 440 nm emission, and at 435 nm excitation, 520 nm emission) as well as marked increases in the relative concentration of insoluble protein. A third specific aging parameter related to the generation of the insoluble protein in the lens is an increase in S-S bonds with age (Lerman, 1972; Lerman & Borkman, 1978). The fact that the secondary configuration of the lens protein is mainly in the anti parallel beta-pleated configuration (Jones & Lerman, 1971; Li & Spector, 1967; Schachar & Solin, 1975; and Yu & East, 1975) would be amenable with the proposed mechanism involving the polymerization and insolubilization of the previously soluble lens polypeptides with age, associated with fluorogen and disulfide bond formation. The secondary structure of the lens proteins does not alter significantly with age or following exposure to monochromatic UV light at 300-320 nm (Lerman & Borkman, 1978; Yu et al., 1976). Thus the aging changes in the lens appear to be mainly due to the accumulation of fluorescent compounds rather than to any marked configurational changes of the lens proteins. These compounds are also responsible for the increasingly yellow and eventually brown to black color of the lens nucleus as it ages and for the decreased transmission of visible light. The extreme example of such an aging process is the brown or black nuclear cataract in which marked discoloration of the lens nucleus leads to an absorption of most of the visible light, thereby significantly reducing visual acuity in a manner analogous to placing a dark colored filter in front of the eye.

In contrast to brown nuclear cataracts, lenticular fluorescence is not significantly altered in anterior cortical cataracts (Lerman & Borkman, 1976 & 1978). Furthermore, the fluorescence spectra of cortical cataracts show a marked degree of light scattering compared to normal lenses and/or brown nuclear cataracts. Thus while the nuclear cataract appears to be an accelerated form of the normal aging process in which visual reduction is mainly due to an increased pigmentation of the lens, it is likely that cortical opacities are derived by different mechanisms, namely, an alteration of protein configuration and protein aggregation. The constituent lens proteins are arranged in a high degree of spatial order within the intact fibers. The proteins are densely packed in the lens and there is little change in the density of proteins throughout the lens, resulting in a transparent organ. As Benedek has pointed out (Benedek, 1971; Miller & Benedek, 1973), when lens proteins are extracted and mixed with water the constituent proteins are now dispersed throughout the water. The proteins are no longer tightly packed and the density of proteins fluctuates markedly about its average value, hence the solution appears milky or turbid. In a similar manner the accumulation of water within the lens can result in a decrease in transparency. Or localized alterations of the density of packing of lens proteins due to significant protein configurational changes and/or aggregations may lead to changes in transparency; that is, cortical opacities will develop which generally appear as white opaque areas. Tanaka & Benedek (1975) and Tanaka et al. (1977) have suggested that the cold cataract phenomenon is due to a phase separation of the protein-water binary mixture within the lens. We have previously proposed that gamma-crystallin acts as the cryoprotein responsible for the cold cataract phenomenon (Lerman et al., 1966). That is, as the temperature is lowered, the gamma-crystallin will tend to go out of solution because of the presence of a considerable number of amino acids with nonpolar side chains. It is well known that the solubility of hydrophobic molecules increases with increasing temperature and decreases as the temperature is lowered. This can account for the reversible cold precipitation of the isolated gamma-crystallin as well as the cold cataract phenomenon within the whole lens. Thus the cold cataract can be regarded as developing because of changes in the physiocochemical state of the lens proteins, leading to localized alterations in the density of packing of these proteins sufficient to induce turbidity (alterations in transparency). If the pathogenesis of white cortical opacities is due to a similar mechanism, it should theoretically be possible to increase the transparency of such lenses by placing them in a solution which would withdraw water until the relative density of packing of the lens proteins returns to relatively normal values. Clark et al. (1977) and Clark et al. (1978) have demonstrated that when cortical cataracts are placed in a 50% glycerol solution (0.137 M NaCl, 0.03 M KCl, 0.016 M Na_2HPO_4, pH 7.4) they recover a significant amount of their transparency.

METHODS

In order to further evaluate the proposed differences in the pathogenesis of the brown nuclear cataract versus the cortical opacities we utilized human lenses obtained from donor eyes (Georgia Lions Eye Bank – Atlanta) and from the Department of Ophthalmology at Emory University. These lenses included normal lenses, nuclear cataracts, white cortical cataracts and mixed (nuclear and cortical) cataracts. All the lenses were immediately photographed, the percent UV and visible transmission and the 440 and 520 nm fluorescence intensity were measured as described in previous communications (Lerman et al., 1976; Lerman & Borkman, 1976). The lenses were then placed in the 50% glycerol solution for two hours and UV-visible transmission spectroscopy was repeated. The lenses were then removed from the glycerol solution, rinsed with normal saline, photographed and repeat fluorescence spectroscopy was performed.

RESULTS

The UV visible transmission data and the 440 and 520 nm fluorescence emission intensities obtained from the normal lenses remained unchanged when the lenses were placed in 50% glycerol solution. Figure 1 shows the appearance of a normal 88 year old human lens prior to being placed in glycerol and 2 hours after it had been kept in glycerol. There was no change in the yellow color of the nucleus nor was there any change in the fluorescence emission intensity or in the percent UV and visible transmission (Fig. 2 & Table I). Similar experiments on a brown nuclear cataract derived from

185

a 77 year old individual showed a marked diminution in the percent transmission of light through this lens (less than 10%) which remained unchanged after two hours incubation in the glycerol medium (Figs. 1 & 2). The fluorescence emission (440 and 520 nm) also remained unchanged (Table I). However, when a white cortical cataract derived from a 20 year old patient (metabolic cataract) was placed in the glycerol solution there was a very rapid increase in the transparency of this lens (Fig. 1). While the fluorescence intensity remained unchanged and was at a level comparable with that for normal human lenses at this age group, the percent transmission of UV and visible light showed a marked increase in the glycerol treated lens (Table I and Fig. 2). Prior to its immersion in glycerol the percent transmission of visible light in this white cortical cataract was less than 20% but it increased dramatically to a level comparable to a normal lens from the second or third decade (Fig. 4). In the case of mixed cataracts, glycerol did improve the percent transmission of these lenses by markedly increasing the transparency of the lens cortex but the fluorescence intensity of such lenses remained unchanged as did the yellow color of the nucleus (Figs. 1 & 3).

DISCUSSION

The results of the foregoing experiments can be correlated with our previous

Table I.

Specimen	$I_F \dfrac{440*}{332}$		$I_F \dfrac{520**}{332}$	
	Before Glycerol	After Glycerol	Before Glycerol	After Glycerol
A-88 year Normal Lens	0.52	0.48	0.40	0.47
B-77 year Brown Nuclear Cataract	0.72	0.68	1.02	1.10
C-20 year Mature Cortical Cataract	0.12	0.13	0.00	0.02
D-81 year Mixed Cataract	0.40	0.36	0.43	0.36
E-62 year Mixed Cataract	0.47	0.49	0.42	0.40

* The ratio $I_F \dfrac{440}{332}$ refers to the fluorescence intensity of the lens chromophore(s) excited at 360 nm divided by the fluorescence intensity of protein bound trytophan in the lens (excited at 290 nm).

** $I_F \dfrac{520}{332}$ refers to the fluorescence intensity of the lens chromophore(s) excited at 435 nm divided by the fluorescence intensity of protein bound tryptophan in the lens.

observations relating to the different mechanisms involved in brown nuclear cataracts compared with cortical and mixed cataracts. We have proposed that the brown nuclear cataract is merely an accelerated form of the aging phenomenon in which there does not appear to be any significant configurational change in, or marked aggregation of, the proteins. Thus glycerol would not be expected to affect these lenses in any way and this was borne out by the results of the present experiments. However, the cortical cataracts are probably caused by changes in the configuration and/or aggregation of the lens proteins resulting in alterations in the density of packing of these

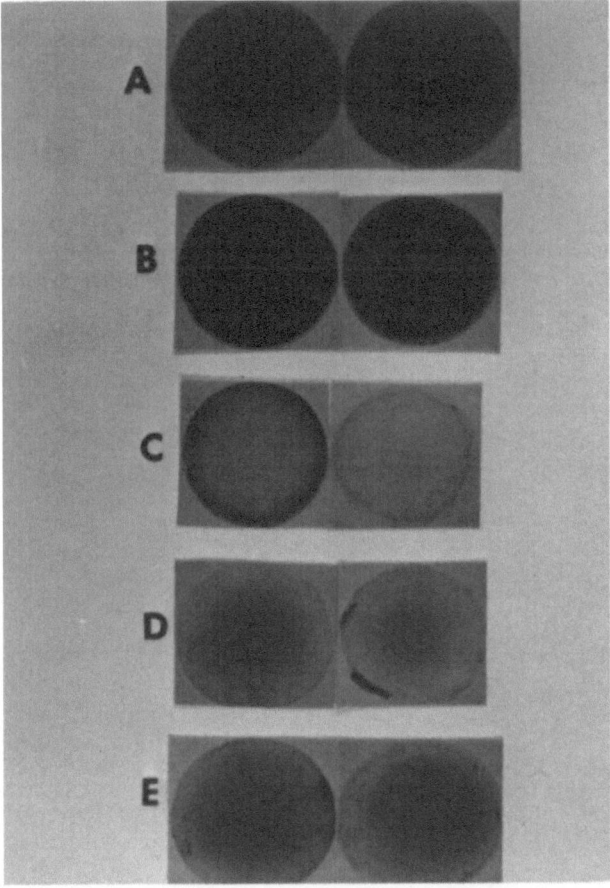

Fig. 1. A = 88 year normal lens before (left) and after glycerol treatment (right).
B = 77 year brown nuclear cataract before (left) and after glycerol (right).
C = 20 year mature cortical cataract before (left) and after glycerol (right).
D = 81 year mixed cataract before (left) and after glycerol (right).
E = 62 year mixed cataract before (left) and after glycerol (right).

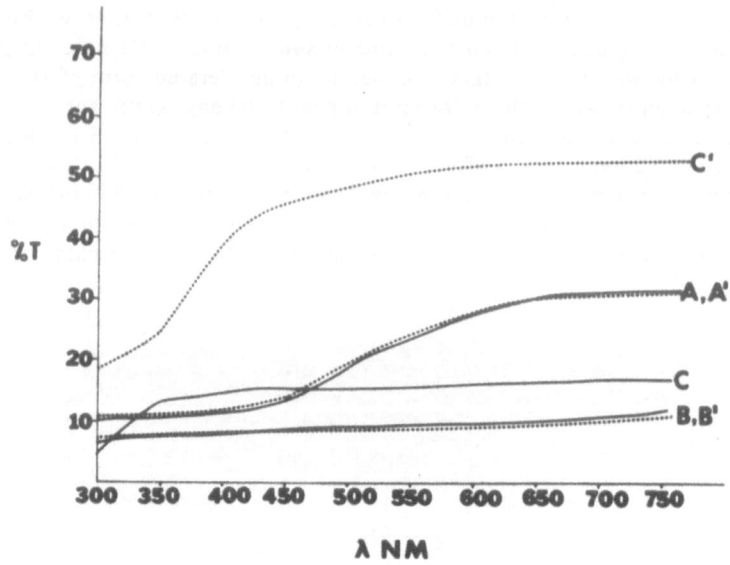

Fig. 2. Percent transmission before (——) and after glycerol treatment (.....). Letters A, A', B, B', C, C' refer to lenses shown in Figure 1 (before and after glycerol).

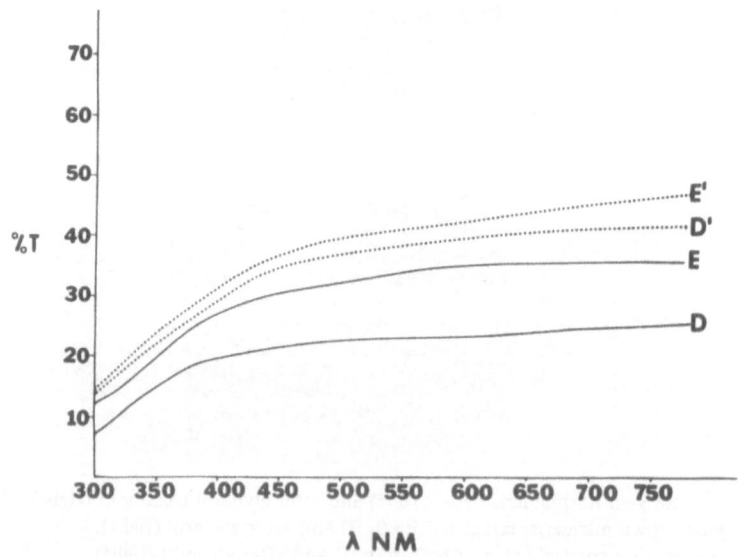

Fig. 3. Percent transmission before (——) and after (.....) glycerol. Letters D, D' and E, E' refer to lenses shown in Figure 1 (before and after glycerol).

macro-molecules and opacification as proposed by Benedek (1971 & 73). By withdrawing a sufficient amount of water from such lenses we were able to increase their transparency and the percent transmission of light to normal levels while the fluorescence emission intensities remained unaffected. The mixed cataracts would be predicted to show an intermediate change; that is, an improvement in the transparency of the cortical portion of the lens while the yellow color of the nucleus should be unchanged and the fluorescence intensity should also not be affected. The experiments with the mixed cataracts confirmed these predictions.

We have previously noted that fluorescence spectra obtained on cortical cataracts showed marked light scattering compared with spectra from normal and brown lenses. A similar situation prevailed in these studies; the normal lenses and the brown cataracts showed minimal light scattering, while cortical and mixed cataracts showed much greater light scattering. However, when these latter cataracts were placed in glycerol solution for 2 hours the scattered light intensity was greatly reduced.

The present experiments tend to support our proposal that the decrease in visual acuity in a brown nuclear cataract is due to the accumulation of fluorescent pigments, which absorb most of the visible light, rather than to any significant aggregation and/or configuration changes in the lens proteins. However, in the cortical and mixed cataracts the changes in the cortical portions of the lens are probably due to significant changes in lens protein configuration and aggregation resulting in a marked light scattering and a decrease in the transmission of light due to scattering. An analogy can be drawn with the case of normal corneas versus edematous corneas as suggest-

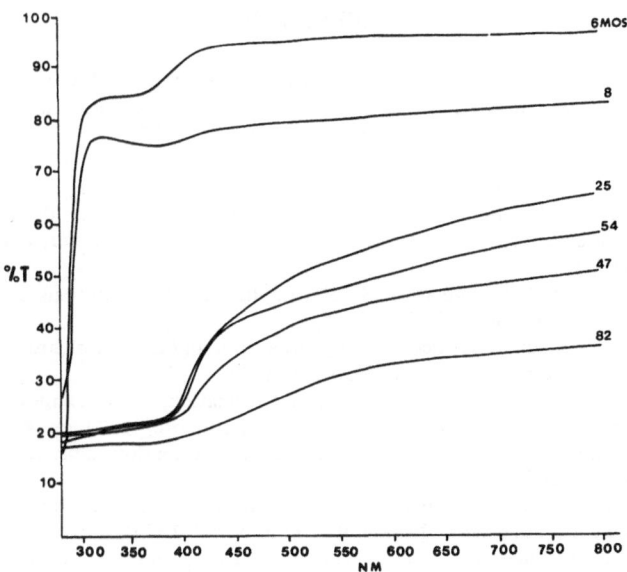

Fig. 4. Percent transmission of normal lenses from 6 months to 82 years of age.

ed by Miller & Benedek (1973). They noted that electron micrographs of edematous corneas contained regions (lakes) where no collagen was present. They suggested that the region of these lakes represented a very large fluctuation in the collagen density and was therefore capable of scattering light very effectively. Furthermore, the dimensions of the lakes were generally comparable to or larger than the light wavelength. In the normal cornea they proposed that the transparency of this tissue is related to the uniform density of the scattering particles (collagen fibrils) throughout the medium. Similarly in the normal lens the constituent lens proteins are densely packed and there is very little change in the density of scattering particles as one moves from point to point in the lens; thus the lens is transparent. However, if protein aggregates tend to form in an irregular pattern adjacent to or surrounded by 'water lakes', the marked changes in refractive index in these regions would result in enhanced light scattering, the density of the proteins would fluctuate markedly about its average value, and the lens would appear opaque or turbid. Such a situation can easily be visualized in the cortical cataract and one could predict that removal of a sufficient amount of water from such a lens should result in denser and more regular packing of the protein molecules and increased transparency.

ACKNOWLEDGEMENTS

This work was supported by NIH Grant EY 01575. The assistance of the Georgia Lions Eye Bank — Atlanta in obtaining human lenses is gratefully acknowledged.

REFERENCES

Benedek, G.B. Theory of transparency of the eye. *Appl. Opt.* 10: *459*-000 (1971).

Borkman, R.F. & Lerman, S. Evidence for a free radical mechanism in aging and UV irradiated ocular lenses. *Expl. Eye Res.* 25: *303-309* (1977).

Clark, J., Serralach, E. & Benedek, G.B. In press, Proc. R. Soc. June (1978).

Clark, J., Serralach, E., Mengel, L., Benedek, K., Sauke, T., Brigham, S. & Benedek, G. Reversible opacification of calf and human lenses. Presented at the fifth conference on biochemistry of the eye, Oakland University, Rochester, Michigan, October (1977).

Clark, R., Lerman, S. & Zigman, S. Studies on the structural proteins of the human lens. *Expl. Eye Res.* 8: *172-182* (1969).

Jones, H.A. & Lerman, S. Optical rotatory dispersion and circular dichroism on ocular lens proteins. *Can J. Biochem.* 49: *426-430*, 1971.

Lerman, S. Lens proteins in aging and cataract formation, in Contemporary Ophthalmology (ed. Bellows, J.), Williams and Wilkins, Baltimore, 1972, pp. *467-493*.

Lerman, S. Lens fluorescence in aging and cataract formation. *Doc. Ophthal. Proc. Series*, 8: *241-260* (1976).

Lerman, S. & Borkman, R.F. Spectroscopic evaluation and classification of the normal, aging and cataractous lens. *Ophthal. Res.* 8: *335-353* (1976).

Lerman, S. & Borkman, R.F. Photochemistry and lens aging, in *Interdiscipl. Topics Geront.*, 12: *000-000* (1978).

190

Lerman, S., Kuck, J.F.R., Borkman, R. Saker, E. Induction, acceleration and prevention (in vitro) of an aging parameter in the ocular lens. *Ophthal. Res.* 8: *213-226* (1976).

Lerman, S., Zigman, S. & Forbes, W.F. Properties of a cryoprotein in the ocular lens. *Biochem. biophys. Res. Comm.* 22: *57* (1966).

Li, L.K. & Spector, A. The optical rotary dispersion and circular dichroism of calf lens alpha-crystallin. *J. biol. Chem.* 224: *3234-3236* (1967).

Miller, D. & Benedek, G.B. Intraocular light scattering, in theory and clinical application. Charles C. Thomas, Springfield, (1973), pp. *21-22*.

Schachar, R.A. & Solin, S.A. The microscopic protein structure of the lens with a theory for cataract formation as determined by Raman spectroscopy of intact bovine lenses. *Invest. Ophthal.* 14: *380-396* (1975).

Tanaka, T. & Benedek, G.B. Observation of protein diffusivity in intact human and bovine lenses with application to cataract. *Invest. Ophthal.* 14: *449-456* (1975).

Tanaka, T., Ishimoto, C. & Chylack, L.T. Phase separation of a protein water mixture in cold cataract in the young rat lens. *Science* 197: *1010-1012* (1977).

Yu, N-T. & East, E. Laser Raman spectroscopic studies of ocular lens and its isolated protein fraction. *J. biol. Chem.* 250: *2196-2202* (1975).

Yu, N-T., East, E.J., Chang, R.C.C. & Kuck, J.F.R. Raman spectroscopic analysis in intact lens of constituents affected by aging, UV, etc. Abstract, ARVO Meeting, Sarasota, Florida, 1976, p. *11*.

Authors' address:
Department of Ophthalmology
Emory University School of Medicine
Atlanta, Georgia 30322, U.S.A.

13. Lenton & Keene, J. & R. Pankratov & Selkov E. Adsorption, desorption and penetration kinetics of Na ions into ... the membrane. O. Med. B. ... 4: 275–226 (1971).

14. ... J. Zaagsma, ... & Kenber, W. A. A series of β-adrenergic ... p-substituted ... membrane. Biochim. Biophys. Acta ... 23: 37 (1966).

15. J. P. R. Sze, ... A. The critical ... Quantum Anharmonic oscillator. J. Comp. Phys. ...

16. ... Pardee, G.B. Intramolecular coupling in ... linking into the ... depenetration. Pharm. Mol. B. ... Pharm. Biol. 13: 3 (1976).

17. Saludes, T. & J. Melius, A. ... ... Structure ... ... with a probe Computer-controlled ... data utilizing ... data ... Structure interior copy of intact membrane. Mol ... Pharmacol. 14: 1183–1186 (1959).

18. ... β-adrenergic ... conformation of protein. Interaction in native ... and ... Acta ... 103: 314–... ... ... J. Comp. ... Chem. (1983).

19. ... L. ... & Clymer, J. & J. ... computation of protein ... interaction in contact areas of the ... crystal ... Acta. 92: 31917... ... (1971).

20. ... & Peter, R. Laser Raman spectroscopic studies of simple ... and interaction ... protein. J. Mol. Biol. ... 85: 257–377 (1982).

21. ... ... Fair, Bloor, M.C. ... & Tyen, J. C. ... ... based ... of cases studied ... ... & ... Schroder. (1976) (trans.)

Docum. Ophthal. Proc. Series, Vol. 18

STUDIES ON LENS PROTEINS II.
Soluble and membrane proteins in normal and cataractous lenses

M.K. MOSTAFAPOUR & V.N. REDDY

(Rochester, Michigan U.S.A.)

ABSTRACT

The composition of lens proteins and the changes in these constituents due to aging and cataractogenesis were investigated. Water soluble and urea- or deoxycholate-insoluble (membrane) fractions were analyzed on gradient polyacrylamide gels. The membrane proteins display nine noncrystallin polypeptides with estimated molecular weights ranging from 37,000-230,000 daltons. Lens fiber membranes also contain crystallins as part of their structure. Gel patterns of lens serial sections from the periphery of the cortex to the center of the nucleus show a gradual decrease in proteins. Such a decrease was more pronounced in older lenses. Loss of proteins was also observed in human senile cataract or in cataracts induced experimentally by X-ray or tryptophan deficiency in rabbits and rats, respectively.

INTRODUCTION

The purpose of this investigation is to provide data about the composition of the water soluble crystallins and membrane proteins of fibers in different regions of the lens and to assess the changes in these parameters as a function of age and in cataract formation. The major proteins of the lens can be broadly classified into two groups: water soluble and urea insoluble. The former consists of α, β and γ-crystallins (Moerner, 1894) while the latter is considered as lens fiber membranes (Dische, Hairstone & Zelmenis, 1967; Lasser & Balazs, 1972). Although the crystallins of the lens have been extensively investigated (see review by Harding & Dilley, 1976), only limited information is available concerning the nature of the proteins of the plasma membranes (Bloemendal et al., 1972; Broekhuyse & Kuhlman, 1974; Alcalá, Lieska & Maisel, 1975) and there is uncertainty as to whether crystallins are an integral part of lens membrane architecture.

It is known that there are changes that occur with age both in the chemistry and the architecture of lens fibers (Harding & Dilley, 1976). Since such changes may have a bearing on cataract development, a knowledge of the nature of plasma membranes is important to our understanding of the basic mechanisms involved in lens opacification.

We have employed gradient slab gel electrophoresis for direct analysis of proteins in different areas of the lens. The methodology provides both a qualitative and quantitative approach for comparison of cortical and nuclear regions of a normal lens or of clear and opaque parts of a cataractous lens.

The present report is concerned with the study of human senile cataract and experimentally-induced cataracts in rabbits and rats with X-ray and tryptophan deficiency, respectively.

MATERIALS AND METHODS

Methods described here are essentially the same as used previously (Mostafapour & Reddy, 1978) with slight modifications.

Preparation of water soluble proteins of lens cortex

Lenses from young rabbits (about 3 months in age) were decapsulated and frozen on dry ice. Nucleus and cortex were separated with a # 2 cork borer as described previously (Reddy, Klethi & Kinsey, 1966). The removed nuclear region was approximately 25-30% of the total lens weight. Routinely, about 1 g of the cortical material was stirred in the cold with 2 ml of a hypotonic buffer consisting of 0.05 M Tris, 0.1 mM EDTA and 10mM dithiothreitol (TED buffer). After stirring for about 2 hr the resulting turbid solution was centrifuged at 30,000 g for 30 min. at 4°C. The supernatant was designated the water soluble proteins of the lens.

Preparation of membrane proteins of the lens

Whole decapsulated lenses were homogenized in TED buffer in an all glass hand homogenizer and centrifuged at 30,000 g for 30 min. This process was repeated once. The resulting pellet was the water insoluble fraction. One half of the pellet was homogenized in 10 ml of 8 M urea in TED buffer for 10 min. and centrifuged. This step was repeated once with the urea solution and finally with TED buffer. The final pellet was used as the urea insoluble lens fiber membrane preparation. The remaining half of the water insoluble pellet used the same procedure substituting 1% deoxycholate (DOC) for urea. Traces of deoxycholate were removed from the final pellet by extraction with one 10 ml acetone wash.

SDS*-polyacrylamide gel electrophoresis

Protein samples from various preparations were dissociated into component polypeptides by dissolving in the dissociation buffer. This buffer was a modification of Laemmli's SDS-buffer (Laemmli, 1970) and consisted of 1% SDS, 20 mM DTT, 1% mercaptoethanol, 10% glycerol (W/V), 10% sucrose (W/V), and 0.05 M Tris, pH 6.8, to a final protein concentration of 5-20 mg/ml and by boiling for 2-3 minutes in a 100°C water bath. Acrylamide solutions and electrophoresis buffers were also made up according to Laemmli (1970). 5-20% gradient acrylamide slab gels, containing 1% SDS were prepared using the Model 200 slab gel apparatus (Bio-Rad Laboratories). The gradient was

* Sodium dodecyl sulfate

poured from a gradient maker consisting of two 15 ml plastic syringes connected by a short length of polyethlylene tubing. A 5% or 3.5% stack was layered on top of the gradient before polymerization had taken place in the resolving gel. The gels were prerun overnight at 10 mA/gel. After applying appropriate amounts of the dissociated protein preparations to the gel by underlayering, electrophoresis was carried out in the cold at a constant current of 10 mA/gel. Gels were stained with a solution of 0.2% Coomassie Blue R250 in H_2O:methanol:acetic acid (46:46:8). Destaining was done in 7.5% acetic acid with 5% methanol both electrophoretically and by several changes of the destaining solutions.

Electrophoretic profiles of proteins across the lens

Decapsulated rabbit and normal human lenses were frozen on dry ice. Each lens was then bisected at the poles with a razor blade. A slice about 1 mm thick was then removed at one of the cut surfaces. A narrow rectangular strip representing a cross section of the lens from pole to pole and going through the nucleus was then obtained. This strip was divided into 6-10 equal size serial sections and each was solubilized in the dissociation buffer for analysis on SDS-acrylamide gels.

Cataractous lenses

Three types of cataractous lenses were studied. X-ray-induced cataract in the rabbit (Giblin, Chakrapani & Reddy, 1978) was decapsulated, homogenized in TED buffer and separated into soluble and urea insoluble fractions for analysis on SDS gels.

Tryptophan deficiency cataracts were produced by placing 60-70 g Sprague-Dawley rats on a diet deficient in this amino acid (Von Sallmann et al., 1959). The control diet contained 0.2% tryptophan. Although very few rats developed frank lens opacities we were able to obtain two lenses with dense nuclear cataracts from animals on the deficient diet after eleven weeks and one with a cloudy nucleus at the end of twenty-five weeks. These, along with clear lenses from animals on control and deficient diets were homogenized directly in the dissociation buffer. Even after boiling with SDS-mercaptoethanol some lens material remained undissolved in both normal and experimental lenses. Insoluble material was removed by centrifugation and the clear supernatants used for gel analysis.

A human senile cataractous lens was obtained immediately after surgery from a 65 year old female patient. The lens was photographed for classification according to the procedure developed by the Cooperative Cataract Research Group (CCRG) (Greiner, Chylack & Grimes, 1976). It was classified as an immature, nuclear sclerotic (yellow) cataract with 25% posterior subcapsular opacity and kept frozen at -80°C. Samples of cloudy and clear cortical areas as well as a sample of the yellow nuclear core were removed after freezing the lens and processed for gel analysis by dissolving directly in the dissociation buffer. An 'eye bank' lens of the same age was used as a control.

RESULTS AND DISCUSSION

Proteins of the rabbit lens

The major proteins of the rabbit lens have been fractionated into water soluble and urea insoluble proteins (UIP) (Fig. 1). We have previously shown that all of the native water soluble crystallins in this lens can be dissociated into ten polypeptides with molecular weights ranging from 11,000-33,000 daltons (lanes C, D and E). A close examination of these lanes reveals several other minor bands with molecular weights below and above those of major crystallins. Actually upon overloading the gels trace amounts of all of the membrane polypeptides can be seen in the water soluble fractions. The membrane proteins (lanes A and B) contain considerable amount of crystallins. The crystallins were present in the membrane preparation despite several washings and homogenizations. Although the occurance of crystallins as

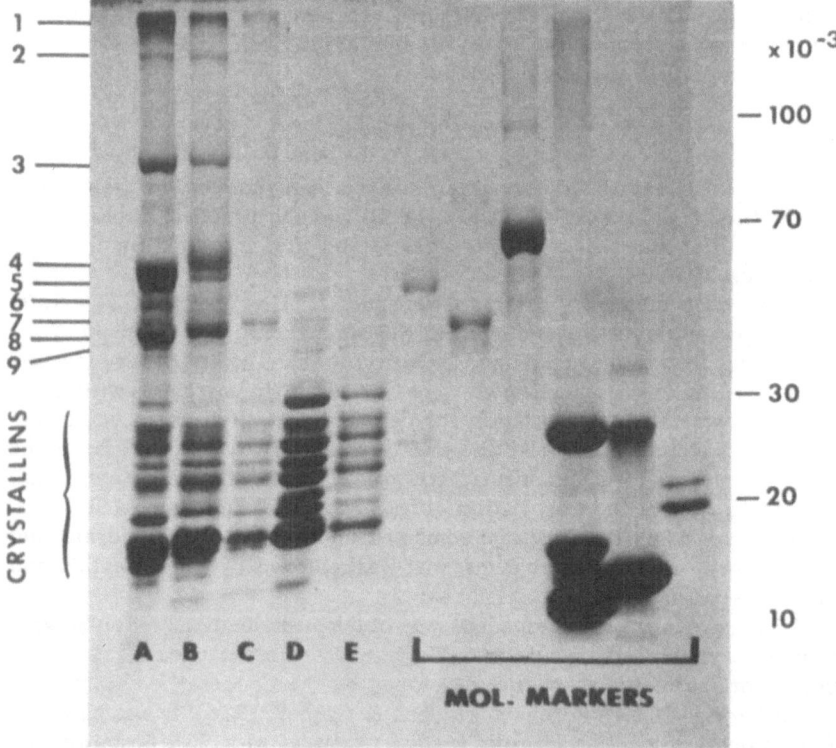

Fig. 1. Resolution of polypeptides from water soluble crystallins and membrane proteins of rabbit lens cortex on polyacrylamide gels.

A – urea insoluble; B – DOC insoluble membrane proteins; C, D and E – different amounts of water soluble fractions.

196

part of membrane proteins has been indicated (Dunia et al., 1974; Alcalá, Lieska & Maisel, 1975), our data clearly demonstrate the presence of almost all of the subunits of crystallins in the membrane structure.

Membrane preparations obtained either by urea or 1% deoxycholate (DOC) treatment yield identical polypeptide patterns as seen from a comparison of lanes A and B of Fig. 1. Therefore, DOC can serve as a suitable substitute for the preparation of lens fiber membranes.

A comparison of water soluble (lanes C, D and E) and urea- or DOC-insoluble (membrane) components of the lens reveals that there are nine prominent non-crystallin membrane polypeptides present in the lens.

Molecular weights of lens membrane polypeptides (Table I) were estimated using a semi-log plot of migration distances of known molecular markers. For the purpose of comparison, the literature values of the polypeptides of ghost erythrocyte membranes are also given (Fairbanks, Steck & Wallach, 1971; Steck, 1974). It is interesting to note that the molecular weights of the slowest moving bands (1 and 2) of the rabbit lens membranes compare well with those of bands 1 and 2 of erythrocyte ghosts. These two bands have been shown to be 'spectrin' (Marchesi & Steers, 1968), a protein which functions as a scaffolding in the membrane structure. Band 3 with an estimated molecular weight of about 90,000 daltons also compares well with its counterpart in the erythrocyte ghost. Band 8 with a molecular weight of around 43,000 daltons is similar to that of band 5 in erythrocytes (Steck, 1974). This is thought to be actin or an actin-like protein (Guidotti, 1972) situated adjacent to the spectrin molecules. Such a proximity would then allow an interaction between spectrin and 'actin' similar to that of muscle actomyosin complex. Against such a background it is conceivable that a similar situation may exist for the lens. Although recent amino acid analyses (Spector, personal communication) of a lens membrane component with a molecular weight of around 40,000 daltons have shown it to have an amino

Table I. Molecular weights of membrane polypeptides of rabbit lens fibers. Published values for ghost erythrocyte membranes are included for comparison.

Lens		Erythrocytes*	
Bands	Mol. Wts.	Bands*	Mol. Wts.
1	230,000	1	240,000
2	190,000	2	215,000
3	90,000	3	88,000
4	68,000	4.1	78,000
5	65,000	4.2	72,000
6	50,000	5	43,000
7	47,000	6	35,000
8	43,000	7	29,000
9	37,000		

* Data and band designation from Steck (1974).

acid composition different from that of actin. Further work is necessary to vigorously establish the presence of spectrin and actin in the lens membrane

Protein profiles across the lens

The innermost fibers of the lens are the oldest and the outermost (epithelial cells) are the youngest lens cells. It was therefore interesting to compare the

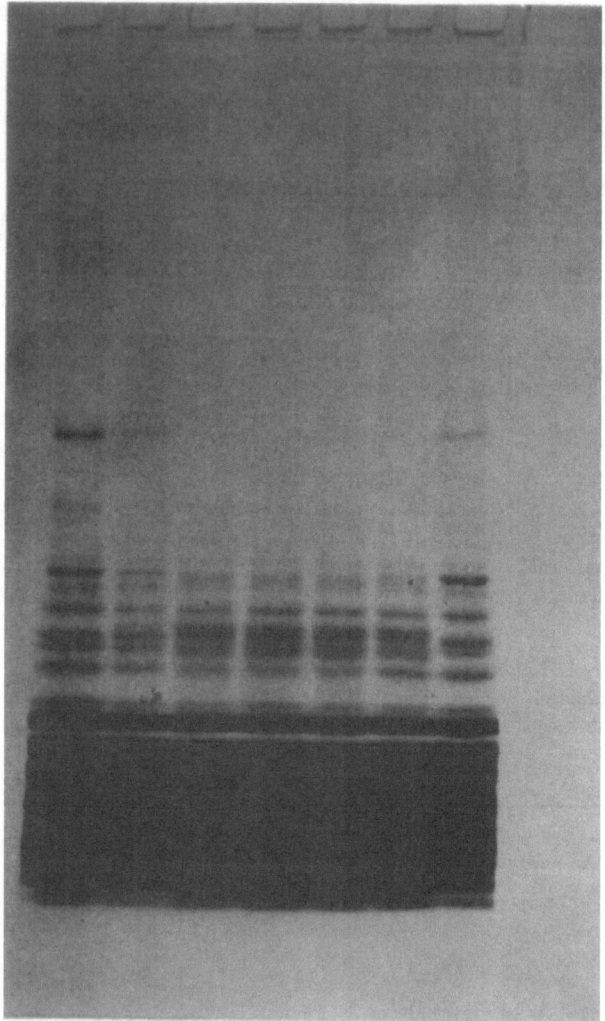

Fig. 2. Polypeptide profiles of a young rabbit lens, serially sectioned from pole to pole going through the center of the nucleus. A decrease in higher molecular weight components is seen towards the center of the lens.

polypeptide patterns of different regions of the lens. For this purpose, serial sections of a narrow rectangular strip, about 1-2 mm wide, representing a cross section of the lens from pole to pole and going through the nucleus were analyzed. Fig. 2 shows the results of such an experiment performed on a young rabbit lens. It can be seen that the bands corresponding to membrane polypeptides tend to decrease towards the center of the lens, but there is no visible change in the amount of crystallins in the young lens. We have evidence (not shown) that in older lenses there is a great loss of membrane polypeptides as well as a decrease in crystallins of the nuclear region. Loss of membrane proteins is better seen from the profile of a 65 year old clear human lens. Another interesting observation is that the preparations from the inner parts of the lens leave a darker background in their electrophoretic tracks. This is not seen with the young rabbit lens (compare Fig. 2 and 4). We have no explanation for this observation except to speculate that it may be due to the yellow colored material present in the nuclear regions of the aging human lens.

It is thus apparent that there is a loss of membrane proteins in the nuclear region due to the aging process. Previous studies have also suggested the loss or redistribution of soluble and membrane proteins with aging and

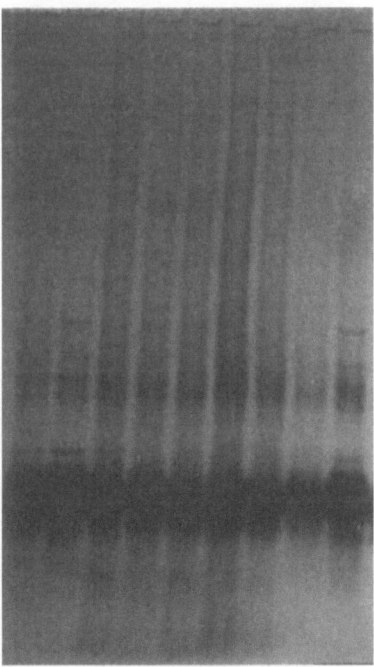

Fig. 3. Polypeptide profiles of a clear 65 year old human lens, serially sectioned from pole to pole going through the center of the nucleus. There is pronounced decrease in high molecular weight components, towards the center of the lens. Notice the darker tracks of the lanes at the center portion.

cataract (Holt & Kinoshita, 1968; Roy & Spector, 1976). Electron microscope studies too have shown that there is disintegration of fiber membranes in the nuclear regions of the lens (Kobayashi & Suzuki, 1975; Kuwabara, T., 1975).

Loss of proteins in cataractous lenses

The polypeptide patterns of clear and opaque cortical regions and the yellow nuclear core of a 65 year old human cataractous lens are shown in Fig. 4. It may be seen that there is a loss of polypeptide in both the cloudy cortex and the nuclear core.

Electrophoretic patterns of soluble and insoluble proteins of X-ray-induced cataract in rabbit together with corresponding pattern from a normal lens are shown in Fig. 5. In this type of cataract loss of crystallins and membrane components is also evident.

Cataractous lenses from rats on a tryptophan deficient diet show a similar loss in membrane proteins and the crystallins (Fig. 6). The two lanes marked

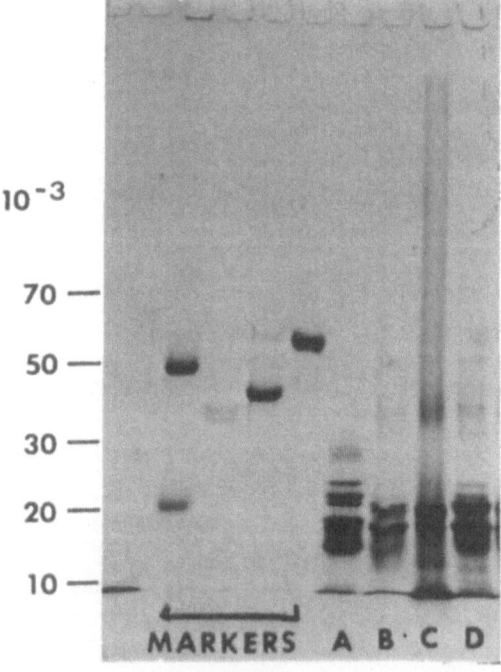

Fig. 4. Polypeptide patterns in clear, opaque and nuclear regions of a human senile cataract removed from a 65 year old patient. A and D — clear cortical regions; B — opaque cortical region; C — yellow nuclear core. The cataract was classified as I-CXE$_{2+}$ — SCP$_{25}$ — NS$_y$.

R are from a rabbit lens cortex directly dissolved and electrophoresed for comparison. Lanes 1-8 are from lenses of control and tryptophan deficient rats. The polypeptide patterns in lanes 5 and 6 are from well developed nuclear cataracts while that in lane 8 is from a lens with a slight nuclear opacity. It may be seen that the slowest moving polypeptide of the crystallins (β_2) is absent in opaque lenses and instead a doublet appears at the fast moving region as indicated by arrows.

In summary, the overall conclusion that can be drawn from the studies reported here is that aging and cataractogenesis are accompanied by the loss of crystallins and fiber membrane components. We do not know, however, if the loss of crystallins that seems to occur simultaneously with the loss of membrane proteins is due to a generalized loss of soluble proteins or due to the disappearance of crystallins associated with membrane structure.

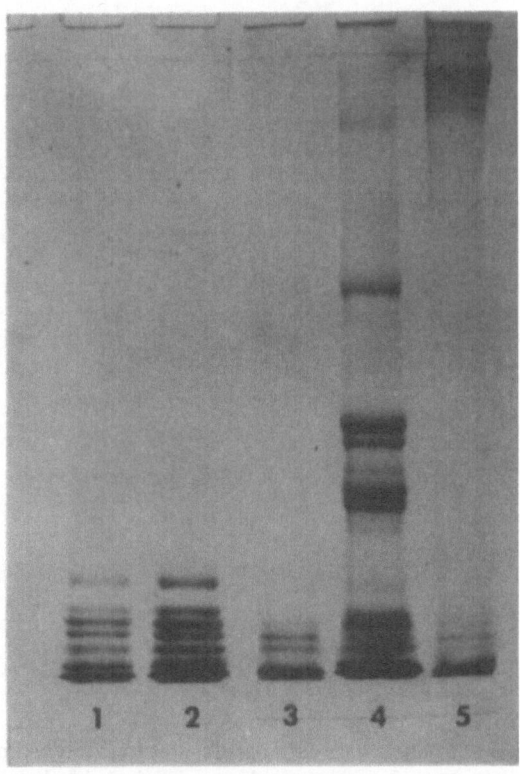

Fig. 5. Comparison of polypeptide patterns of normal and X-ray-induced cataractous lens in rabbits. 1 and 2 — soluble proteins from normal cortex. 3 — soluble proteins from cataractous whole lens. 4 and 5 — from insoluble fractions of normal and cataractous lens respectively.

ACKNOWLEDGMENT

We thank our colleague Dr. Frank J. Giblin for the X-ray-induced cataracts and Ching Peng Lim for her expert technical assistance.

This study was supported by National Institutes of Health Grants EY-00484, EY-02027 and EY-07044, and is also a part of the Cooperative Cataract Research Group's program.

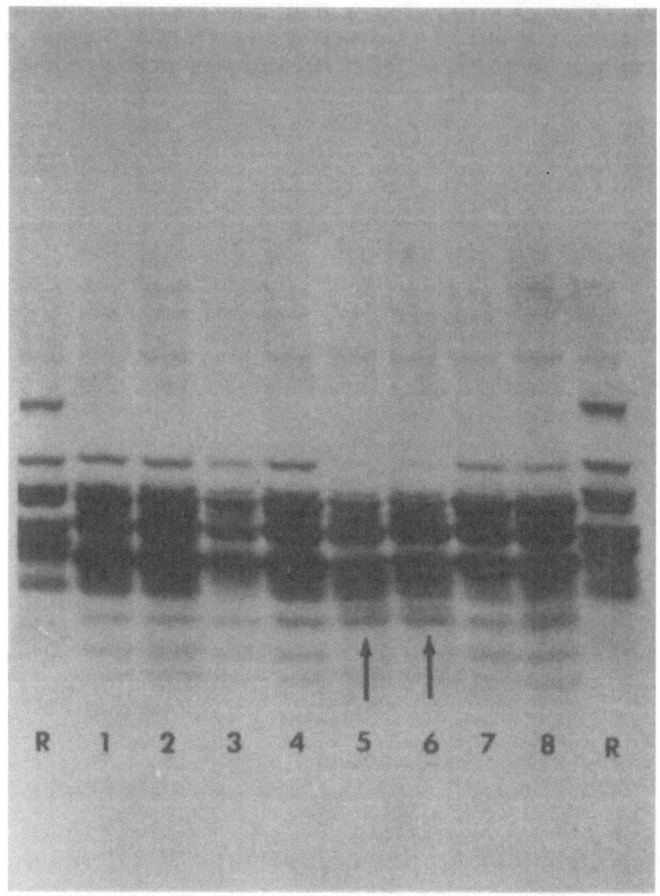

Fig. 6. Comparison of polypeptide patterns of lenses from rats on normal and tryptophan deficient diets. Lane 2 — seven weeks on deficient diet but clear; 4 — eleven weeks on deficient diet but clear; 5 and 6 — eleven weeks on deficient diet with frank nuclear opacities; 8 — twenty-five weeks on diet with a cloudy nucleus. Corresponding controls for the 3 experimental periods are shown in 1, 3 and 7. R — profiles from normal rabbit lens cortex shown for comparison. Arrows show the doublets.

REFERENCES

Alcalá, J., Lieska, N. & Maisel, H. Protein composition of bovine lens cortical fiber cell membranes. *Expl. Eye Res.* 21: *581-595* (1975).

Bloemendal, H., Zweers, A., Vermorken, F., Dunia, I. & Benedetti, E.L. The plasma membranes of eye lens fibers. Biochemical and structural characterization. *Cell differ.* 1: *91-106* (1972).

Broekhuyse, R.M. & Kuhlmann, E.D. Lens membranes. I. Composition of urea-treated plasma membranes from calf lens. *Expl. Eye Res.* 19: *297-302* (1974).

Dische, Z., Hairstone, M. & Zelmenis, G. Glyco- and glycolipoproteins in cell surface from bovine lens fibers, in *Protides of the Biol. Fluids* (ed. Peeters, H.) Vol 15, Elsevier, Amsterdam, 1967, p. 123.

Dunia, I., Sen Ghosh, C., Benedetti, E.L., Zweers, A. & Bloemendal, H. Isolation and protein pattern of eye lens fiber junctions. *FEBS Letters* 45, 139-144, (1974).

Fairbanks, G., Steck, T.L. & Wallach, D.F.H. Electrophoretic analysis of the major polypeptides of the human erythrocyte membranes. *Biochemistry* 10: *2606-2617* (1971).

Giblin, F.J., Chakrapani, B. & Reddy, V.N. High molecular weight protein aggregates in X-ray-induced cataract. *Expl. Eye Res.* 26: *501-509* (1978).

Greiner, J.V., Chylack, L.T. & Pihlaja, D.J. Photomacrography of the crystalline normal and cataractous lens. *Expl. Eye Res.* 22: *281-284* (1976).

Guidotti, G. Membrane Proteins, *Annual Review of Biochem.* 41: *731-752* (1972).

Harding, J.J., & Dilley, K.J. Structural proteins of the mammalian lens: A review with emphasis on changes in development, aging and cataract. *Expl. Eye Res.* 22: *1-73* (1976).

Holt, W.S. & Kinoshita, J.H. Starch-gel electrophoresis of the soluble lens proteins from normal and galactosemic animals. *Invest. Ophthal.* 7: *169-178* (1968).

Kobayaski, Y. & Suzuki, T. The aging lens: ultrastructural changes in cataract, in Cataract and Abnormalities of the Lens. (ed. Bellows, J.G.) Grune & Stratton, New York, 1975, pp. *313-343*.

Kuwabara, T. The maturation of the lens cell: a morphologic study. *Expl. Eye Res* 20: *427-443* (1975).

Laemmli, U.K. Cleavage of structural proteins during the assembly of the head bacteriophage T_4 *Nature* (London) 227: *680-685* (1970).

Lasser, A. & Balazs, E.A. Biochemical and fine structure studies on the water-insoluble components of the calf lens. *Expl. Eye Res.* 13: *292-308* (1972).

Marchesi, V.T. & Steers, E. Selective solubilization of a protein component of the red cell membrane. *Science* 159: *203-204* (1968).

Moerner, C.T. Untersuchung der proteinsubstanzen in den leichtbrechenden medien des auges. Hoppe-Seyler's *Z. physiol. Chem.* 18: *61-106* (1894).

Mostafapour, M.K. & Reddy, V.N. Studies on lens proteins. I. Subunit structure of beta crystallins of rabbit lens cortex. *Invest. Ophthal. & Vis. Science* 17: *660-666*, 1978.

Reddy, D.V.N., Klethi, J. & Kinsey, V.E. Studies on the crystalline lens. XII. Turnover of glycine and glutamic acid in glutathione and ophthalmic acid in the rabbit. *Invest. Ophthal.* 5: *594-600* (1966).

Roy, D. & Spector, A. Absence of low molecular weight alpha crystallin in the nuclear region of old human lenses. *Proc. Natn. Acad. Sci.*, (U.S.A.) 73: *3484-3487* (1976).

Steck, T.L. The organization of proteins in the human red blood cell membrane, *J. Cell Biol.* 62: 1-19, 203 (1974).

Von Sallmann, L., Reed, M.E., Grimes, P.A. & Collins, E.M. Tryptophan deficiency cataract in guinea pigs. *A.M.A. Arch. Ophthalmol.* 62: *662-672* (1959).

Authors' address:
Institute of Biological Sciences
Oakland University
Rochester, Michigan, U.S.A.

Docum. Ophthal. Proc. Series, Vol. 18

POST-SYNTHETIC ALTERATIONS OF BOVINE LENS ENZYMES DEMONSTRATED BY HEAT LABILITY MEASUREMENTS*

CHRISTIAN OHRLOFF, ULRICH TEIMANN & OTTO HOCKWIN

(Bonn-Venusberg, Fed. Rep. Germany)

ABSTRACT

The heat lability of certain enzymes of carbohydrate metabolism was determined in the nucleus and equator of bovine lenses of different age (1, 4-6 and 15 years old).

The crude extract was incubated at $57°C$ and subsequently the activities of phosphofructokinase (EC 2.7.1.11), fructose-1.6-diphosphate-aldolase (EC 4.1.2.13), enolase (EC 4.2.1.11), lactate dehydrogenase (EC 1.1.1.27), and malate dehydrogenase (EC 1.1.1.37) were determined.

Compared with the heat lability in the equator, that of the nucleus is increased in all age groups. With ageing, heat lability increases in the nucleus, while remaining unchanged in the equator.

Increase in heat lability in all tissues is an indication for age dependent modifications of the enzyme molecules and is probably due to postsynthetic protein changes.

INTRODUCTION

The regular intercellular arrangement of the structural proteins, which is requisite for lens transparency, is dependent on the intact metabolism responsible for the cellular environment such as pH or ion concentration. Its smooth running depends on the enzymes catalysing and co-ordinating the single steps. This means that the impact of the ageing phenomenon, i.e. the decrease in functional capacity, first and foremost affects the enzymes. At any rate, whatever the causes of the ageing mechanism, altered enzymes will always be involved. There are already numerous data on single findings and criteria of biochemical alterations of the energy and protein metabolism in the lens during the ageing process.

The most important among these changes are:

1) A general decrease of the energy metabolism with diminished activity of most of the enzymes.

2) Increase in high-molecular and water-insoluble crystallins which are formed by aggregation from low molecular water-soluble protein.

---

* In part presented at the Colloquium 'Molecular and Cellular Models of Ageing' Paris, Centre National de la Recherche Scientifique, 5-7 avril 1978, and 3rd International Congress of Eye Research, Osaka/Japan, May 21-25, 1978.
The investigations were supported by Deutsche Forschungsgemeinschaft (Oh. 32/1).

Due to the methodological difficulties involved, knowledge on conformation and protein structure of the lens enzymes and their possible age changes is still scarce. However, it is certain that even slight modifications of the enzyme protein may affect the conformation of a molecule. These changes in conformation mostly lead to a decrease in activity of the enzyme concerned. Another effect is a changed denaturation process of the enzyme molecule, which can be determined by investigating the influence of heat. Thus, heat lability tests are an indirect method to detect protein changes with respect to the conformation of an enzyme. A parameter for the denaturation by heat is the loss in activity of the enzyme in question.

Due to the appositional lens growth the nucleus represents old tissue while the periphery, i.e. the equator, represents young tissue. Therefore our investigations on the heat lability of lactate dehydrogenase (LDH) (EC 1.1.1.27), malate dehydrogenase (MDH) (EC 1.1.1.37), aldolase (ALD) (EC

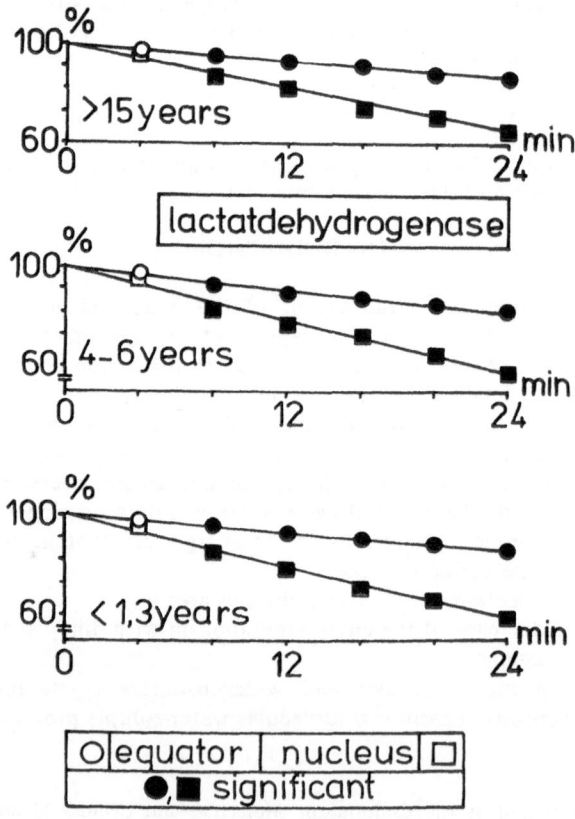

Fig. 1. The course of inactivation of lactate dehydrogenase at 57°C, obtained from equator and nucleus of bovine lenses of different ages. o = equator; □ = nucleus. n = 6; •, ■ = significant, p. ⩽ 0.05.

4.1.2.13), phosphofructokinase (PFK) (EC 2.7.1.11) and enolase (EC 4.2.1.11) used the nucleus and equator separately. Measurements were performed with the crude extract of bovine lenses aged < 1.3, 4-6, and > 15 years.

MATERIAL AND METHODS

Bovine lenses were procured from the local slaughter house. Estimation of age was performed according to Schmutter (1961) from lens wet weight. The lenses were frozen and separated into nucleus and equator after the method of Hockwin & Kleifeld (1965).

The lens tissue was homogenized, 1 g per 20 ml aqua bidest, in an Ultra Turrax, (Jahnke + Kunkel), then centrifuged for 1 hr at 8°C and 20.000 g with a MSE High Speed 18. The supernatant was used for incubation under heat conditions.

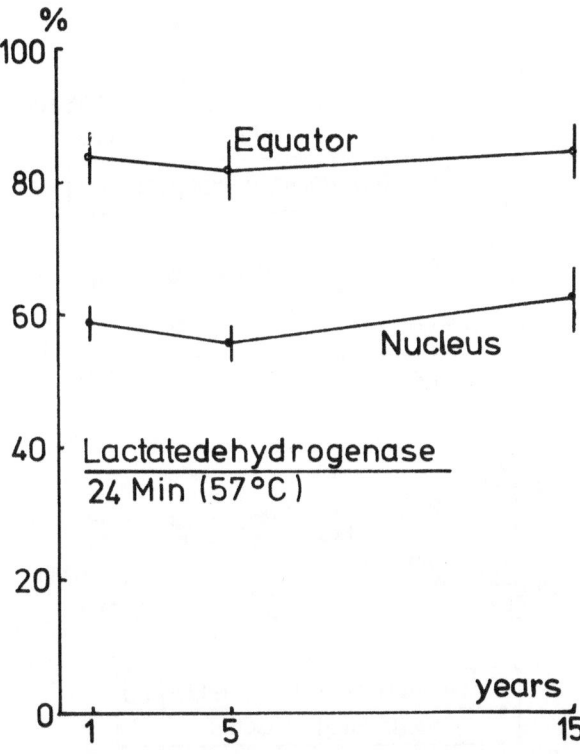

Fig. 2. Heat treatment of extracts from equator and nucleus of bovine lenses (age < 1 year, 4-6 years, > 15 years) for 24 min. at 57°C with subsequent determination of LDH-activity. Values are calculated as percentage of the non-heated controls.

2 x 11 test tubes were filled with 1 ml of the supernatant each. They were closed with parafilm and were incubated at 57°C for 0, 1, 2, 4, 8, 12, 16, 20, 24, 36, 48, or 60 min. in a waterbath (Köttermann). Due to the differences in sensitivity the total time of incubation varied. Subsequent to the respective incubation periods the test tubes were left to cool in a waterbath at 10°C. This extract was used for the measurements of enzyme activity which were performed according to Bergmeyer (1974) for LDH, MDH, ALD, and enolase, and according to Bous (1977) for PFK at 340 nm with a PM Q 2 spectrophotometer (Zeiss). In the case of enolase, however, the extract had to be diluted 1:10 prior to the activity measurements because of the high specific activity.

In a further test the supernatant obtained by centrifugation was diluted in such a way that total enzyme activity was identical for nucleus and equator. Heat incubation was then performed as described above.

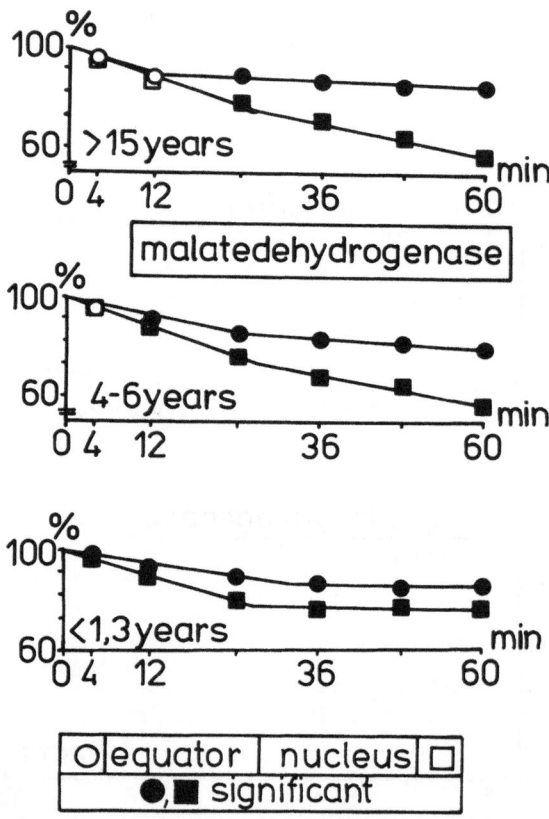

Fig. 3. The course of inactivation of malate dehydrogenase at 57°C, obtained from equator and nucleus of bovine lenses of different ages. o = equator; □ = nucleus. n = 6; •, ■ = significant, p ⩽ 0.05.

Activity values (n = 5) obtained from the single measurements were referred to, b, the non-incubated controls (100 per cent), and plotted semi-logarithmically.

Lactate dehydrogenase

In all three age groups, inactivation through heat was linearly dependent on time in the nucleus as well as in the equator (Fig. 1). In the nucleus, the enzyme was less stable (40 per cent inactivation after 24 min.) than in the equator (about 18 per cent inactivation after 24 min.) With older age, however, there was no increase in heat lability (Fig. 2).

The linear course of the inactivation is rather surprising since this phenomenon is usually typical for an enzyme consisting of homogenous molecules. With respect to LDH, however, the presence of isoenzymes is well known.

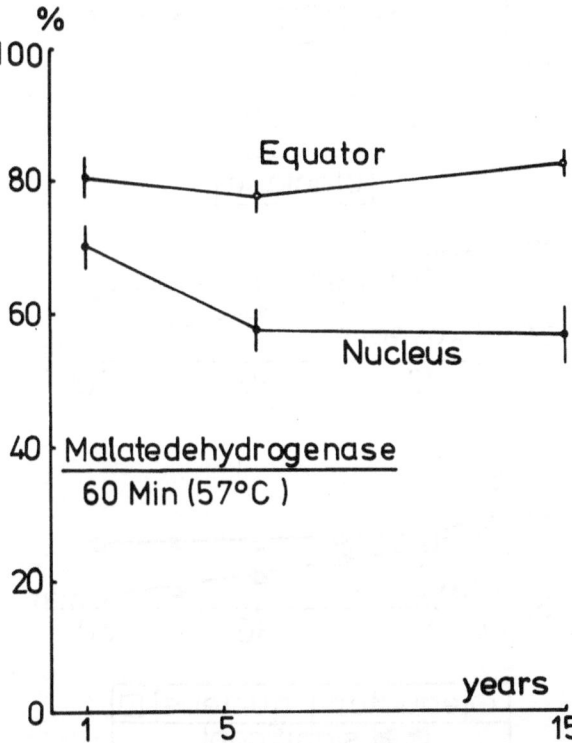

Fig. 4. Heat treatment of extracts from equator and nucleus of bovine lenses (age < 1 year, 4-6 years, > 15 years) for 60 min. at 57°C with subsequent determination of MDH-activity. Values are calculated as percentage of the non-heated controls. The increase of heat-lability in the nucleus between 1 and 4-6 years is significant.

To exclude a possible inactivation of certain enzyme structures by cold we repeated the tests with unfrozen lenses, and obtained the same results. Probably the high portion of LDH$_5$ (Bours et al., 1977) is responsible for the greater part of the total activity, thus determining the curve.

Malate dehydrogenase

Here the inactivation curve in dependence on time was not linear but showed a biphasic course (Fig. 3). In the nucleus and equator of all three age groups the loss in activity occured mostly within the first 24 min., after that time the decrease in activity was less evident. In general such a curve in- dicates that the enzyme consists of two forms, one of them less heat stable than the other. If the flatter segment of the curve (Fig. 3) is extrapolated to

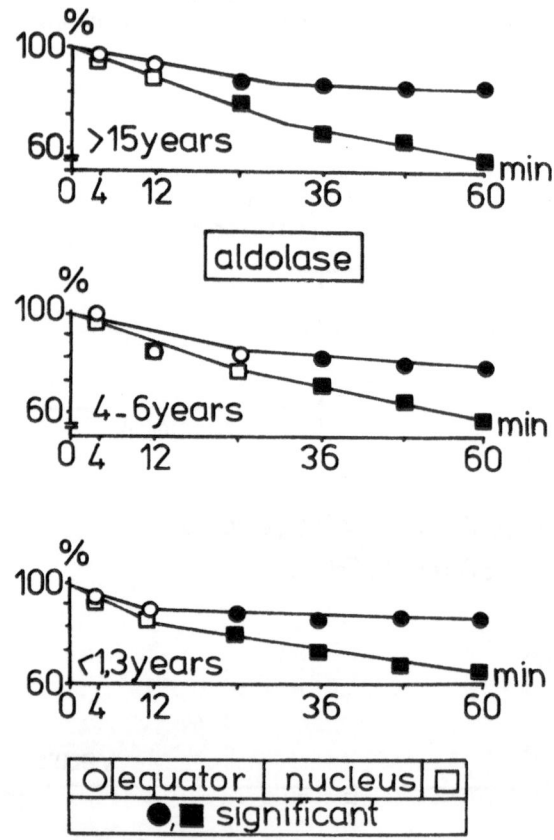

Fig. 5. The course of inactivation of aldolase at 57°C, obtained from equator and nucleus of bovine lenses of different ages. ○ = equator; □ = nucleus. n = 6; ●, ■ = significant, p ≤ 0.05.

210

t = 0, the portion of the less stable enzyme form is, independent on age, 15 per cent in the equator and about 25 per cent in the nucleus. The decrease of the half-life value of heat inactivation of the stable part in the nucleus is rather striking between the groups aged 1.3 and 4-6 years, it falls from 360 min. to 130 min. Fig. 4 shows the significant increase in heat lability between these two groups. As concerns *aldolase*, the heat lability is also higher in the nucleus than in the equator (Fig. 5). The heat inactivation curve shows that in both lens regions there are two enzyme forms, one of them less stabile than the other. The latter amounts to about 10-15 per cent in the nucleus and equator of all three age groups. As Fig. 6 shows, the heat lability present in the nucleus and equator does not increase with age.

Phosphofructokinase

Phosphofructokinase is rather heat labile and the better part of its activity is already gone after 25 min. Here too, inactivation runs biphasic and is most evident in the lens nucleus (Fig. 7).

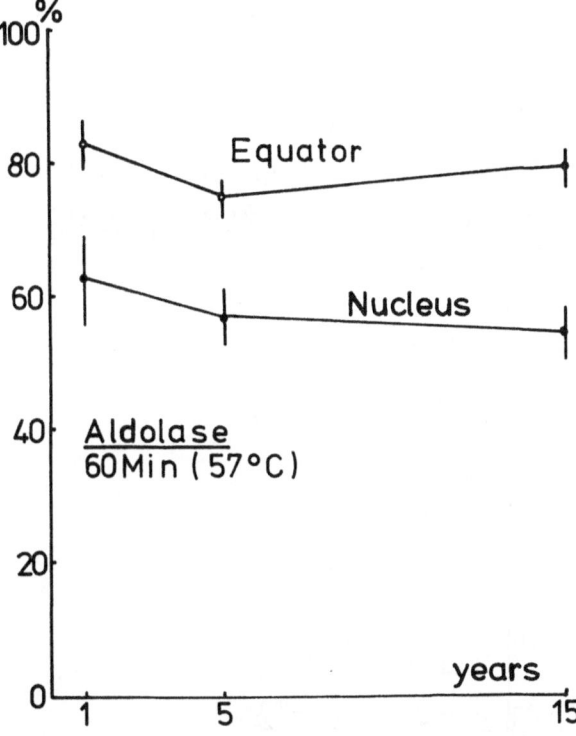

Fig. 6. Heat treatment of extracts from equator and nucleus of bovine lenses (age < 1 year, 4-6 years, > 15 years) for 60 min. at 57°C, with subsequent determination of ALD-activity. Values are calculated as percentage of the non-heated controls.

While the half-life time of the labile enzyme parts for the youngest group is 10 min., it is only 5 min. for the eldest group, the labile part now forming 70 per cent instead of 50 per cent, (the more stable part extrapolated to t = 0 min.) Fig. 8 shows that in the nucleus there is a significant increase in heat lability with ageing, which does not hold true for the equator.

Enolase

Enolase is the most heat labile of the enzymes investigated; its activity was decreased to 7-30 per cent after 6 min. (Fig. 9). The heat inactivation curve differs from that of the other enzymes, its first half running flatter, its second half showing a sharp descent. This course may be interpreted after

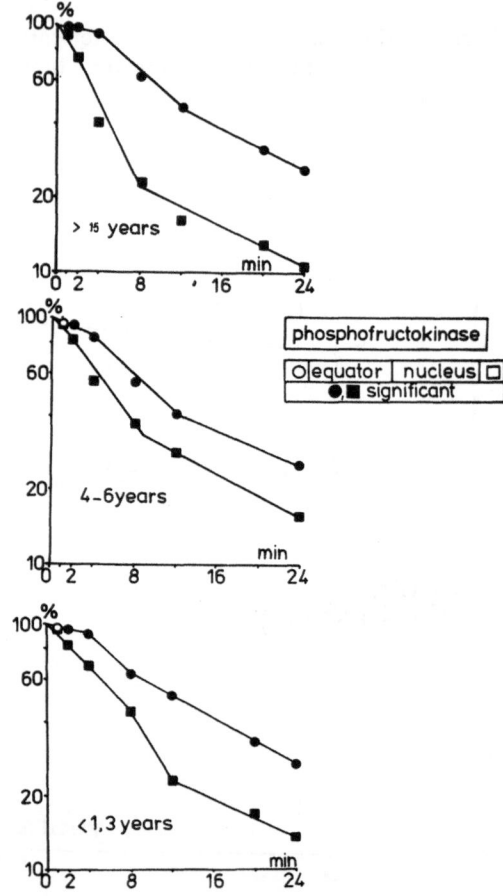

Fig. 7. The course of inactivation of phosphofructokinase at 57°C, obtained from equator and nucleus of bovine lenses of different ages. ○ = equator; □ = nucleus. n = 6; ●, ■ = significant, p ≤ 0.05.

212

the 'multi-hit-theory' known from radiobiology (Dertinger and Jung, 1969). At first the enzyme was only slightly damaged after a brief heat treatment, while after prolonged treatment the damages accumulated which led to a more rapid decrease in enzyme activity. Again heat lability was more evident in the nucleus than in the equator, and there was also a significant increase of heat lability in the nucleus during ageing (Fig. 10).

In general the specific activity was 2-3 times higher in the equator than in the nucleus. To avoid errors in interpretation through the differences in initial activities, tests were performed bringing the activity of the equator up to that of the nucleus. As concerns the enzymes in question, no differences from the aforementioned results could be found.

DISCUSSION

Increased heat lability of numerous enzymes is known for various ageing tissues, such as liver, muscle, fibroblasts, nematodes, and erythrocytes. The

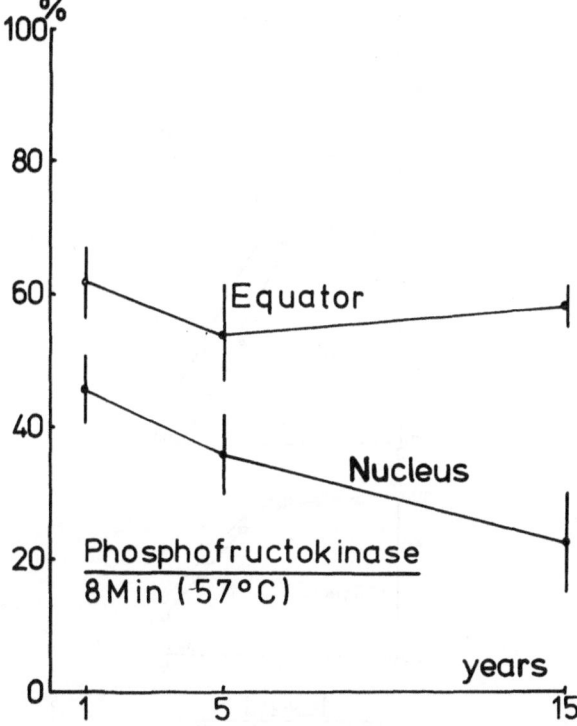

Fig. 8. Heat treatment of extracts from equator and nucleus of bovine lenses (age < 1 year, 4-6 years, > 15 years) for 8 min. at 57°C, with subsequent determination of PFK-activity. Values are calculated as percentage of the non-heated controls. There is a significant increase of heat-lability between 1 and 15 years in the nucleus.

relevant investigations have been performed mainly with the crude extract (Holliday & Tarrant, 1972; Gershon & Gershon, 1976; Hilz, 1975) as well as with the purified enzyme (Reiss & Rothstein, 1975). Up to now, in the ageing human lens only glutathione-reductase is known to show an increased heat lability (Harding, 1973). Chylack (1974) reported heat lability changes in hexokinase.

Increased heat lability is generally a sign for age-related modifications of the enzyme proteins affecting the stability of the conformation and thereby influencing the denaturation process. This is either due to errors in protein-synthesis in accordance with the error-catastrophe theory of Orgel (1963) or to changes in the respective molecules, such as postsynthetic alterations.

In our investigations we found with all enzymes concerned that heat lability was significantly higher in the older tissue, i.e. the nucleus, than in

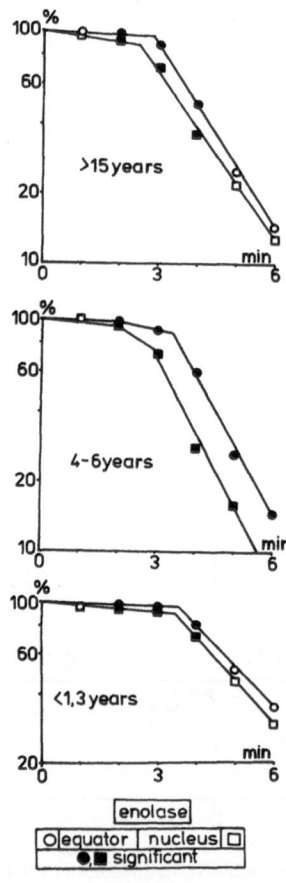

Fig. 9. The course of inactivation of enolase at $57°C$, obtained from equator and nucleus of bovine lenses of different ages. $\circ$ = equator; $\square$ = nucleus. n = 6; $\bullet$, $\blacksquare$ = significant, $p \leqslant 0.05$.

the younger tissue, i.e. the equator where protein synthesis is located. Further, in the case of MDH, PFK, and enolase the heat lability in the nucleus increased during ageing. It remained unchanged for all enzymes in the equator of the age groups investigated, which indicates that even to a great age protein synthesis in the lens takes place normally and without formation of altered molecules. It seems that postsynthetic changes, as found for the structural proteins and particularly for the α-crystallin (van Kleef et al., 1976) also occur in enzyme proteins in the nucleus. In some of the enzymes these postsynthetic changes continually increase with ageing.

It is well-known that in the lens nucleus all enzymes suffer a remarkable loss of activity, some of them, such as PFK (Bous et al., 1977), and HK (Chylack, 1974, Hockwin et al., 1977) even changing their substrate affinity.

It is obvious that the enzyme proteins of the lens change during the ageing process to a different degree. Slight protein changes may be determined through an increase in heat lability; more profound modifications of the conformation affect either the substrate affinity or even cause loss of the

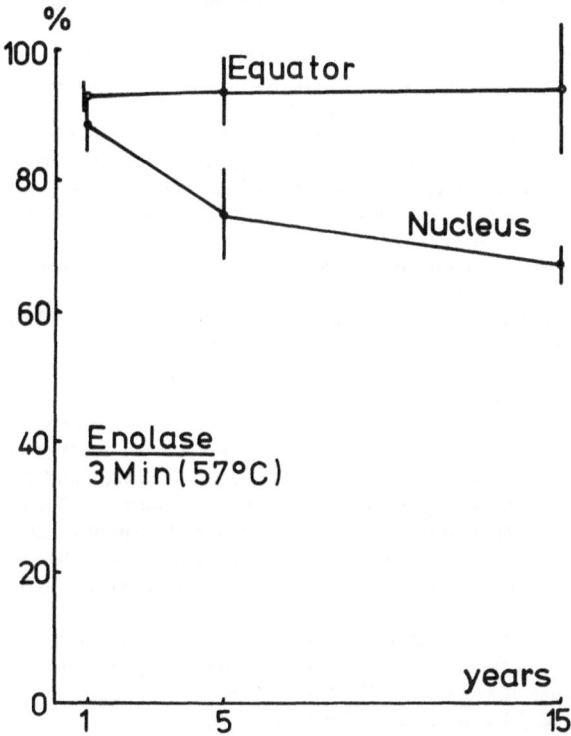

Fig. 10 Heat treatment of extracts from equator and nucleus of bovine lenses (age < 1 year, 4-6 years, > 15 years) for 3 min. at 57°C with subsequent determination of enolase activity. Values are calculated as percentage of the non-heated controls. There is a significant increase of heat-lability between 1 and 4-6 years in the nucleus.

catalytic ability. Such postsynthetic changes through non-enzymatic deamidation and amino acid cleavage represent a mechanism which plays an important role in the ageing of the lens. Their influence is the more profound if enzymes, as forming the engine of metabolism, are affected.

The smooth functioning of the lens fibre, i.e. maintaining the arrangement of the structural proteins ensuring lens transparency, is dependent on an intact energy metabolism keeping the cell balance. If protein changes occur which disturb the kinetic properties such as specific activity and substrate affinity of single enzymes, the metabolism of maintenance is drastically reduced. Subsequent changes in the cell environment lead to altered conformation of the structural proteins, which then form larger aggregates. This phenomenon is well-known for the ageing and the cataractous lens.

Summarizing we may state, in accordance with Strehler (1976) that ageing implies an increase in entropy and therefore a loss of energy.

REFERENCES

Bergmeyer, H.U. Methoden der enzymatischen Analyse, 3. Aufl. Bd.l, Verlag Chemie, Weinheim/Bergstr. 1974.

Bours, J., Neuhaus, H., Hockwin, O. The thin-layer isoelectric focusing of lactate dehydrogenase isoenzymes in rabbit lens parts and intraocular tissues. *Albrecht v. Graefes Arch. klin. exp. Ophthal.* 203: *9-19* (1977).

Bous, F., Hockwin, O., Ohrloff, C., Bours, J. Investigations on phosphofructokinase in bovine lenses in dependence on age, topographic distribution and water soluble protein fractions. *Expl. Eye Res.* 24: *383-389* (1977).

Chylack, L.T. Jr.: Soluble, insoluble and latent hexokinase in the mammalian lens. *Ophthal. Res.* 6: *93-106* (1974).

Dertinger, H., Jung, H.: Molekulare Strahlenbiologie, Springer-Verlag HTB: Bd. 57/58, Berlin-Heidelberg 1969.

Gershon, D., Gershon, H.: An evaluation of the 'error catastrophe' theory of ageing in the light of recent experimental results. *Gerontology* 22: *212-219* (1976).

Harding, J.J.: Altered heat-lability of a fraction of glutathione reductase in ageing human lens. *Biochem. J.* 134: *995-1000* (1973).

Hilz, H.: Fehlerhafte Enzyme – Ursache oder Folge des Alterungsprozesses. In: Verhandlungen der Deutschen Gesellschaft für Pathologie 59: *21-26* (1975).

Hockwin, O.: Age changes of lens metabolism. In: H. Bredt and J.W. Rohen eds. Ageing and Development, Vol. 1, pp. *95-129*, F.K. Schattauer, Stuttgart 1971.

Hockwin, O., Fink, H., Ohrloff, C.: Carbohydrate metabolism of the lens depending on age. Evaluation of factor analysis. 5th Eurp. Symp. Basic Res. in Gerontology, Weimar, GDR, 1976 p. *632-645*, ed. by U.J. Schmidt et al., Verlag Dr. Straube, Erlangen (1977).

Hockwin, O., Kleifeld, O. Das Verhalten von Fermentaktivitäten in einzelnen Linsenteilen unterschiedlich alter Rinder und ihre Beziehung zur Zusammensetzung des wasserlöslichen Eiweißes. In: J.W. Rohen (Hrsg.), Die Struktur des Auges, II Symp. 395-401, F.K. Schattauer Verlag, Stuttgart (1965).

Holliday, R., Tarrant, G.M.: Altered enzymes in ageing human fibroblasts. *Nature* (Lond.) 238: *25-30* (1972).

Kleef, van, F.S.M., Willems-Thijssen, W. & Hoenders, H.J.: Intracellular degradation and deamidation of α-crystallin subunits. *Eur. J. Biochem.* 66: *477-483* (1976).

Orgel, L.E.: The maintenance of the accuracy of protein synthesis and its relevance to ageing. *Proc. Natn. Acad. Sci. US* 49: *517-521* (1963).

Reiss, U., Rothstein, M.: Age-related changes in isocitrate lyase from free living nematode, Turbatrix aceti. *J. Biol. Chem.* 250: *826-830* (1975).

Schmutter, J.: Untersuchungen über die Altersabhängigkeit des Gewichtes und Volumens der Rinderlinse. Dissertation, Bonn, 1961.

Strehler, B.L.: Elements of unified theory of ageing: Integration of alternative models. In: Alternstheorien, Hrsg. D. Platt, F.K. Schattauer Verlag, Stuttgart 1976.

Authors' address:
Division Biochemistry of the Eye
Institute of experimental Ophthalmology
D 5300 Bonn-Venusberg
Fed. Rep. Germany

EFFECT OF VARYING MEDIUM POTASSIUM ON LENS VOLUME

JOHN W. PATTERSON

(Farmington, Connecticut, U.S.A.)

ABSTRACT

Potassium in varying amounts was substituted for sodium in a 305 mOsm saline plus glucose medium. Rat lenses were incubated for 24 hours in the media and the effects on sodium and potassium concentration and on water, sodium and potassium content were determined. Cation potentials and the potential differences across the lens membranes were calculated from the Nernst and Goldman equations. Changes in lens volume are accounted for by changes in the content of potassium with accompanying anion and water. The change in potassium content with increasing potassium in the medium involves two processes – one saturable and identified with the Na, K-pump and one nonsaturable and evident when the pump is saturated. Increases in net potassium content are viewed as being the result of temporary preponderance of potassium influx over efflux that occurs between steady states. A model of volume regulation is described that is consistent with the premises of the double-Donnan model and the data on volume regulation reported for duck red cells.

The process by which cells and the lens maintain a relatively constant volume is of current interest and receiving an increasing amount of attention. A recent review (Macknight & Leaf, 1977) cites over 400 references and supports the double-Donnan hypothesis for the maintenance of cell volume. This model, however, is recognized as having limitations especially when the medium contains a high concentration of potassium.

The double-Donnan model starts with the view that the concentration of permeable intracellular cations and anions is determined by the Gibbs-Donnan equilibrium. Thus, there is an osmotic excess of intracellular ions and protein which is viewed as being balanced by an external Donnan effect that is produced by extracellular sodium being maintained outside the cell by the Na, K-pump.

Before our knowledge of the pump developed, the membranes were considered to be impermeable to sodium. The classical study by Dr. Harris and his colleagues (Harris, Gehrsitz & Nordquist, 1953) on cation changes in lenses during refrigeration and during recovery at normal temperatures dispelled this view and helped to establish the concept of a relative physiological impermeability based on metabolism. Thus, it is a pleasure to recall this work and make this contribution to a volume published in honor of Dr. John Harris.

The concept of membrane impermeability introduced two ideas which do not follow from the double-Donnan model. The first is that the lens acts as a 'perfect osmometer' (Kinoshita, Merola & Hayman, 1965 and Cotlier, Kwan & Beaty, 1968) when incubated in anisotonic media. According to the model the concentration of intracellular cations and anions should vary with the extracellular concentration and the countering extracellular Donnan effect produced·by the pump should balance the excess osmolarity associated with a Donnan equilibrium. There should be little change in volume with a change in osmolarity. This has been demonstrated for rat lens (Patterson & Fournier, 1976). The second is that a special volume related change in potassium permeability is required to change from one osmotic steady state to another (Kregenow, 1977). This concept is not necessary if the change is from one Donnan equilibrium to another.

This study is concerned with volume changes in the presence of high potassium concentrations in the medium.

METHODS

Lenses were obtained from male Sprague-Dawley rats weighing 100 ± 20 gms. Lenses were removed by a posterior approach as previously described (Schenck, Fournier & Patterson, 1976). Lenses were harvested after 24 hours of incubation in a saline medium containing (mM): 0.5 NaH_2PO_4; 0.8 Na_2HPO_4; 1.0 $MgSO_4$; 1.5 $CaCl_2$; 11.0 $NaHCO_3$; 6.7 glucose and variable mixtures of NaCl and KCl to provide the desired concentration of potassium. The osmolarity was 305 mOsm and the pH 7.4. Dry weights were determined by drying to constant weight in a 95°C oven. Sodium and potassium levels were determined with a Perkin-Elmer atomic absorption spectrophotometer on 5% trichloroacetic acid extracts of dried lenses. A correction of 6 percent of lens water was made for extracellular space and values were normalized to reflect levels in lenses having a 10 mg dry weight.

RESULTS

The content of water, potassium and sodium in lenses incubated in 305 mOsm medium for 24 hours with varying concentrations of potassium are shown in Figure 1. Each point represents the mean ± S.E. for a minimum of six lenses except that there were only five at 0.5 mM-K.

The line describing changes in potassium content is typical of that obtained when two processes are involved, one saturable and the other unsaturable. Similarly the line describing the volume of lens water is a straight line in the higher range of potassium concentration. However, in the lower range the points tend to fall above this line.

Since the osmolarities inside and outside the lens are equal, a simple calculation indicates that the gain in potassium content per mM increase in medium potassium, at the higher levels, is 1.94. When this is doubled to allow for accompanying anion it represents a change in volume of lens water equal to 0.13 mg per mM of potassium increase in the medium. This agrees with the slope found for the change in lens water at higher levels of medium potassium. Thus the increase in volume associated with the unsaturable process can be related to an increase in the content of potassium and an accompanying anion.

The change in sodium content with increasing medium potassium is what would be expected for a saturable process. The portion of the curve above 20 mM-K is flat indicating little change in sodium content when large amounts of potassium are substituted for sodium in the medium. At concentrations of medium potassium below 20 mM the fall in sodium content is matched by a somewhat greater increase in potassium content.

The changes in concentration of sodium and potassium are shown in Table I. Also shown are the calculated values for the potassium (E_K) and the sodium (E_{Na}) potentials and the potential difference across the lens membrane (P.D.). The cation potentials are calculated by use of the Nernst equation.

$$E = -58 \log_{10} \frac{[\text{Ion}] \text{ inside}}{[\text{Ion}] \text{ outside}}$$

This potential is the equilibrium potential at which the tendency of an ion to diffuse down a chemical gradient will be counteracted by the membrane potential. The chloride ion has been shown to have a high permeability in the rabbit lens (Kinsey & Hightower, 1976) so that it is distributed passively. Therefore, the potential difference (P.D.) across the membrane can be calculted with a simplified Goldman equation assuming that potassium is 100 times as permeable as sodium (Hodgkin, 1957).

$$P.D. = -58 \log_{10} \left(\frac{[K]_i + 0.01 [Na]_i}{[K]_o + [Na]_o} \right)$$

The relative permeability of sodium to potassium as reported for toad lens is 0.067 (Duncan & Croghan, 1969) and for rabbit lens four times this value

Table I. Values of potential difference (P.D.), potassium potential (E_K) and sodium potential (E_{Na}) calculated from concentrations of sodium and potassium inside and outside the lens (305 mOsm).

$[K]_o$	$[K]_i$	$[Na]_o$	$[Na]_i$	P.D.	E_K	E_{Na}
	meq/liter			mV	mV	mV
0.5	48	146.5	113	−81	−115	+ 6
1.5	93	144.5	69	−87	−104	+19
7.0	121	139	32	−67	− 72	+37
14.0	135	132	25	−55	− 57	+42
21.0	136	125	19	−46	− 47	+47
34.0	150	112	20	−37	− 35	+43
61.0	152	85	17	−23	− 23	+41
75.0	149	71	19	−17	− 17	+33

(Kinsey, 1973). Relative permeabilities in muscle and nerve are about 0.01 (Hodgkin & Horowicz, 1949, Hodgkin, 1957). Trauma associated with the removal of lenses from the eye can introduce changes from which the lens seems to recover only after several hours of incubation (Kinsey, 1973 and Kinsey & Hightower, 1976). The calculated P.D. of -67 mV at 7 mM-K for rat lens compares reasonably with -68 mV found for rabbit lens (Kinsey & Hightower, 1976), -68 to -74 mV found for rabbit lens (Paterson et al., 1975), -65 mV found in toad lens (Duncan, 1969) and -77 mV found for frog lens (Rae, 1973). The latter two workers also demonstrated that the lens becomes progressively depolarized with increasing levels of potassium in the medium.

Graphs of the lens content of sodium and potassium (Figure 2) and of the lens concentration of sodium and potassium (Figure 3) against P.D. change the scale along the abscissa and thus emphasize certain variations that are not obvious when plotted against the concentration of potassium in the medium.

DISCUSSION

The changes in potassium content with increasing levels of potassium in the medium indicate that two processes are at work. The curve depicting the changes (Figure 1) is the same shape as that found for changes in potassium influx in horse (Shaw, 1955) and human (Glynn, 1956) erythrocytes as the level of potassium in the medium is increased. This is not surprising inasmuch as these workers showed that the change in influx was the initial change in going from one steady state to another and inasmuch as changes in content reflect net changes in potassium flux. The two processes are evident at different levels of medium potassium. At concentrations above 20 mM-K_o the process is nonsaturable and potassium content increases with increasing levels of medium potassium, while at concentrations below 20 mM-K_o the process appears to be saturable and is more readily characterized if the effects of the nonsaturable process are subtracted from the total. Glynn (1956) showed that the saturable process fitted a Michaelis equation with a Km of 2.2. This is consistent with what is found for the Na,K-pump. With a similar treatment the content of potassium in the rat lens can be described by the equation:

$$K_c = \frac{161\,[K]_o}{0.48 + [K]_o} + 1.93\,[K]_o$$

The first term describes the saturable process and the second the nonsaturable process. The equation indicates for the saturable process a maximum potassium content of 161 meq/kg of dry weight and a Km of 0.48 mM-K. This is about half that found for the active transport of potassium by the pump (Kinsey & McLean, 1970).

The changes in sodium content with increasing potassium in the medium are the reciprocal of the changes in the potassium content that are associated

222

with the saturable process. The mean ± S.E. of the sum of the two cation contents for eight different points equals 191 ± 3. If it is accepted that the sodium efflux which is against the electrochemical gradient is almost entirely active then the reciprocal response of sodium and potassium with changes in medium potassium suggests that in the rat lens the sodium and potassium effects of the pump are linked and that the potassium gained is equal to the sodium lost on a 1:1 basis. These two conclusions differ from those reached by Kinsey (1973) for rabbit lens, but the latter agrees with the finding of Duncan & Croghan (1969) for toad lens.

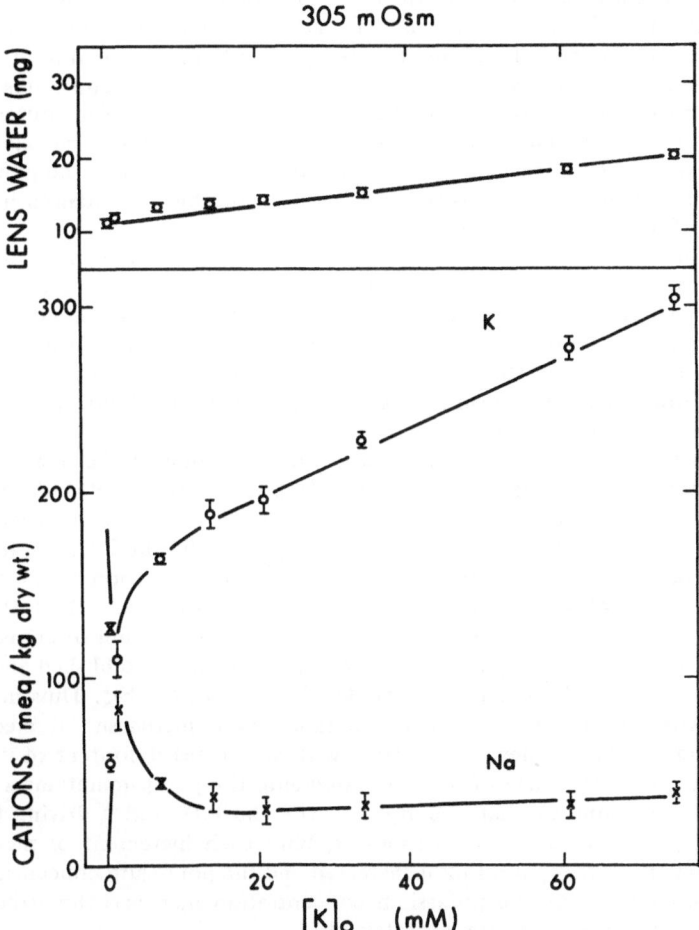

Fig. 1. The effect of medium potassium on water potassium and sodium content of rat lenses after incubation in a saline plus glucose medium for 24 hrs at 37° and pH4. Each point is the mean ± S.E. of values on six or more lenses except that there were only 5 lenses at 0.5 mM-K_0.

The Na, K-pump is stimulated by potassium in the medium as indicated by the replacement of sodium with potassium as the level in the medium is raised. This is consistent with the observation in red blood cells that the pump is only stimulated by extracellular potassium and by intracellular sodium (Whittam & Ager, 1965). A correlation of pump activity in the lens with the concentration of intracellular sodium has been noted in this laboratory (Patterson, 1978) and also by others (Kinsey & Hightower, 1978). It has been reported that the pump discharges 3 ions of sodium for every two ions of potassium that are pumped into the lens (Kinsey, 1973). This has been the basis for proposing that the pump is electrogenic (Paterson et al., 1975 and Hightower & Kinsey, 1977). If the pump has a sodium-potassium pumping ratio of 3:2 then it would be expected that lens volume would decrease with increments of pump activity. The data do not support this view for rat lens, but rather show a net increase in volume and potassium content as medium potassium is increased above 0.5 mM. The content of potassium when the pump is unsaturated is greater than would be expected if the result were determined by the forces that are active when the pump is saturated (Figure 2) and passive forces are responsible for changes in the content of potassium.

The increase in lens volume as medium potassium is increased is clearly related to an increase in the content of potassium with an accompanying anion. Changes in sodium content at external potassium levels below 20 mM-K result in a replacement of intracellular sodium by potassium and at levels above 20 mM-K, the content of sodium is relatively constant (Figure 2). Therefore, the mechanism for explaining changes in volume must center around a net change in potassium content.

Following an incremental increase in medium potassium a new steady state is achieved and changes are noted in $[K]_o$, $[K]_i$, E_K and P.D. (Table I). Consider first changes in the high range of medium potassium when the pump is saturated. At 21 mM-K the E_K is -47 mV and the P.D. is -46 mV or very nearly a steady state with a saturated pump. As soon as the K_o is changed to 34 mM-K the E_K falls to -35 mV which is below the P.D. and establishes an inward driving force for potassium. The content of potassium is increased. After the $[K]_i$ increases a new steady state is established and the P.D. equals -37 mV which is essentially the same as the E_K. Thus in this range, with the activity of the pump fixed, each increment of medium potassium results in a new steady state with an increased content of potassium. In the lower range of medium potassium the pump maintains a high level of potassium so that the E_K exceeds the P.D. and a driving force favoring potassium efflux is maintained. With each increment of medium potassium the potassium influx is increased and the potassium concentration and content rises. As the potassium concentration increases the efflux increases until a new steady state is attained.

The major changes in lens volume come after the potassium concentration is approaching the limit imposed by osmolarity and the pump is saturated. Under these conditions a relative preponderance of influx over efflux results in a net increase of potassium, anion and lens water. This causes the

224

lens to swell and as this happens the concentration of fixed solute within the lens is diluted and the concentration of potassium can increase until a new steady state is attained. While the concentration of potassium can increase at the expense of sodium this process is not necessary. Therefore, small increments of medium potassium in the physiological range may not produce much volume change. This could account for the fact that the lens volumes in the range of 7 and 14 mM-K are the same.

As a working model the lens volume is viewed as being determined by a Donnan-equilibrium with the Na,K pump providing the energy to maintain a steady state. The pump produces large sodium and potassium gradients which along with the excess ions and colloidal osmotic pressure arising with

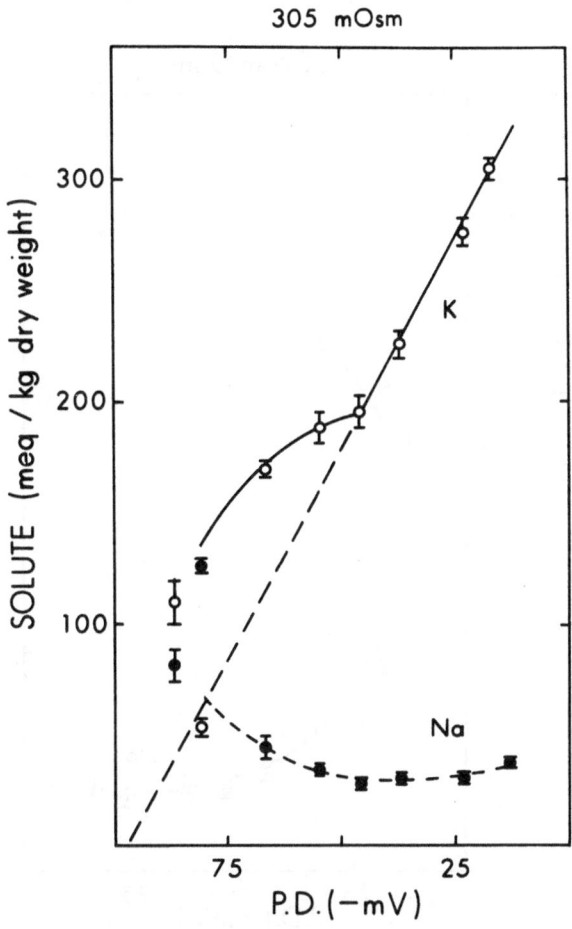

Fig. 2. Values for potassium and sodium content plotted against calculated values for the potential difference across the lens membranes (means ± S.E.).

the Donnan equilibration create a very unsteady state which must be balanced by other forces. The electrochemical gradient controls the sodium influx which is balanced by the pump. The level of intracellular sodium affects pump activity (Kinsey & Hightower, 1978) and is in turn affected by the pump so that this provides a feed-back mechanism that maintains a relatively constant concentration of intracellular sodium. Under physiological conditions the influx of potassium is determined largely by the pump along with some passive diffusion against the electrochemical gradient. The potassium efflux, which balances the influx, is in the direction of the electrochemical gradient and the efflux varies with the concentration of potassium so that this serves as a feed-back mechanism and maintains a steady state. The concentration of potassium, in turn, affects the P.D. and this completes the cycle by influencing the influx of sodium.

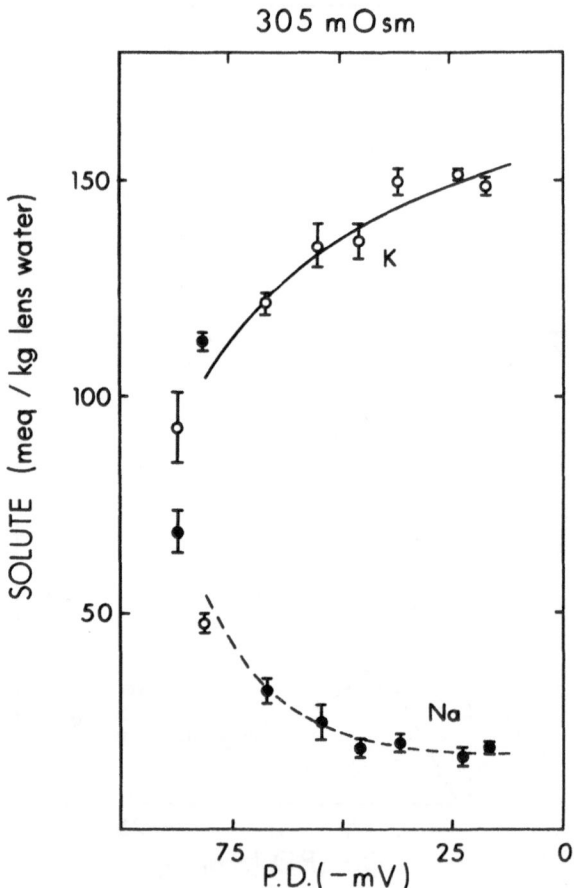

Fig. 3. Potassium and sodium concentrations plotted against the calculated potential difference across the lens membranes (means ± S.E.).

226

This study was not designed to test the role of the Donnan equilibrium. The fact that the concentration of Na plus K is 18 meq per liter greater in the lens water than it is in the medium indicates that it plays a part. Other studies now in progress support the concept that the major changes in lens cation content associated with changes in osmolarity follow a change in the concentration of permeable ions in the medium.

This study offers an explanation for the increase in potassium content and lens water that occur as the concentration of potassium is increased in the medium. The proposed model explains why the concentration of sodium remains relatively unchanged at different steady states with the volume of lens water determining sodium content and why the concentration and content of potassium may vary at different steady states. It is suggested that the excess of internal solute arising from Donnan equilibration becomes part of the total ionic content and is affected by the mechanisms proposed in the model for maintaining ionic balance. The concentration of potassium in the medium is seen as having the key role in maintaining the balance that is superimposed on the results of Donnan equilibration, because it affects the influx of potassium and of sodium. At a steady state the levels of the effluxes are viewed as being equal to and determined by the levels of influx.

The proposed model offers an alternative mechanism for explaining the changes in potassium efflux in anisosmotic media as reviewed by Kregenow (1977) and is consistent with the general provisions of the double-Donnan model (Macknight & Leaf, 1977).

ACKNOWLEDGEMENT

The author is grateful to Drs. Salvador Fernandez and Ramadan Sha'afi for serving as helpful 'sounding boards' and to Miss Janis Langston for essential technical assistance. Gratitude is also expressed to the National Eye Institute, National Institutes of Health, Bethesda, Maryland for research grant EY-00904.

REFERENCES

Cotlier, E.B. Kwan & C. Beaty. The lens as an osmometer and the effects of medium osmolarity on water transport, ^{86}Rb efflux and ^{86}Rb transport by the lens. *Biochim. Biophys. Acta* 150: *705-722* (1968).

Duncan, G. The site of the ion restricting membranes in the toad lens. *Expl. Eye Res.* 8: *406-412* (1969).

Duncan, G. & P.C. Croghan. Mechanisms for the regulation of cell volume with particular reference to the lens. *Expl. Eye Res.* 8: *421-428* (1969).

Glynn, I.M. Sodium and potassium movements in human red cells. *J. Physiol., Lond.* 134: *278-310* (1956).

Harris, J.E., L.B. Gehrsitz & L. Nordquist. The in vitro reversal of the lenticular cation shift induced by cold or calcium deficiency. *Am. J. Ophthal.* 36: *39-50* (1953).

Hightower, K.R. & V.E. Kinsey. Studies on the crystalline lens. XXIII electrogenic potential and cation transport. *Expl. Eye Res.* 24: *587-593* (1977).

Hodgkin, A.L. Ionic movements and electrical activity in giant nerve fibres. *Proc. R. Soc.* B 148: *1-37* (1957).

Hodgkin, A.L. & P. Horowicz. The influence of potassium and chloride ions on the membrane potential of single muscle fibres. *J. Physiol. Lond.* 148: *127-160* (1959).

Kinoshita, J.H., L.O. Merola & S: Hayman. Osmotic effects on amino acid concentrating mechanisms in the rabbit lens. *J. biol. Chem.* 240: *310-315* (1965).

Kinsey, V.E. Studies on the Crystalline Lens. XIX Quantitative aspects of active and passive transport of sodium *Expl. Eye Res.* 15: *699-710* (1973).

Kinsey, V.E. & K.R. Hightower. Studies on the Crystalline lens. XXII characterization of chloride movement based on the pump-leak model. *Expl. Eye Res.* 23: *425-433* (1976).

Kinsey, V.E. & K.R. Hightower. Studies on the crystalline lens. XXVI kinetic study showing saturation of the sodium pump. *Invest. Ophthal.* 17: *186-190* (1978).

Kinsey, V.E. & I.W. McLean. Studies on the crystalline lens. XVI Characterization of active transport and diffusion of potassium, rubidium and cesium. *Invest. Ophthal.* 9: *769-784* (1970).

Kregenow, F.M. Transport in avain red cells, in membrane transport in red cells. (ed. J.C. Ellory and V.L. Lew) Academic Press, N.Y. 1977.

Macknight, A.D.C. & A. Leaf. Regulation of cellular volume. *Physiol. Rev.* 57: *510-573* (1977).

Paterson, C.A., M.C. Neville, R.M. Jenkins II & J.P. Cullen. An electrogenic component of potential difference in the rabbit lens. *Biochim. Biophys. Acta* 375: *309-316* (1975).

Patterson, J.W. Effects of amino acid loading on 'Volume Regulation' in rat lenses. submitted to *Expl. Eye Res.* (1978).

Patterson, J.W. & D.J. Fournier. The effect of tonicity on lens volume. *Invest. Ophthal.* 15: *866-869* (1976).

Rae, J.L. The Potential Difference in frog lens. *Expl. Eye Res.* 15: *485-494* (1973).

Schenk, D., D.J. Fournier & J.W. Patterson. Tissue culture of rat lenses. *Proc. Soc. Exper. Biol. Med.* 153: *444-448* (1976).

Shaw, T.I. Potassium movements in washed erythrocytes. *J. Physiol., Lond.* 129: *464-475* (1955).

Whittam, R. & M.E. Ager. The connection between active cation transport and metabolism in erythrocytes. *Biochem. J.* 97: *214-227* (1965).

Authors' address:
Department of Physiology
University of Connecticut Health Center
Farmington, Connecticut 06032
U.S.A.

Docum. Ophthal. Proc. Series, Vol. 18

CATARACT – A SEMANTIC TRAP

ALBERT M. POTTS

(Louisville, U.S.A.)

ABSTRACT

The medieval word 'cataract' signifying a single disease entity preceded our modern dilemma with lens disease. In this dilemma we have multiple morphological types of lens turbidity and multiple postulated causes without a clear connection between causes and morphological types.

The sorting-out process has finally begun with a single contribution from electron microscopy. Additional multiple contributions from biochemistry and biophysics promise, for the first time, to allow us to connect cataract morphology with cataract etiology.

By using the single word 'cataract' for what we well know to be fifteen or twenty disease entities, we trap ourselves into thought processes which are selfdefeating.

The very word 'cataract' is a curiosity out of the past. It comes not from antiquity but from the middle ages. It was coined by Constantine the African who studied medicine at the famous school of Salerno and who spent his later years at the monastery of Monte Cassino translating Arabic medical writers into medieval Latin. *Cataracta* introduced by him dates from the end of the eleventh century. Its Greek roots mean something that comes down precipitously like a cliff, or figuratively like a portcullis. It signifies the curtain that comes down over vision as lens turbidity progresses (*Constantine* in Pansier, 1933).

Cataract was so poorly understood that until the introduction of the ophthalmoscope by Helmholtz (1851) entities like retinal detachment and optic nerve disease were called black cataract – 'schwarzer star' (German).

With the ophthalmoscope and particularly with the slit lamp introduced by Gullstrand (1902), the situation was entirely reversed. Attention could now be paid to what we understand today as true 'cataract', i.e., loss of transparency of a portion or all of the lens. (Not 'lens opacity' as ophthalmological jargon has it.) Instead of a paucity of findings we were confronted with a plethora of configurations that the loss of transparency assumed. What could be more logical than to believe that for each configuration a corresponding etiology could be found. That was certainly true in 1905 when Hess (1905) wrote his chapter for the Graefe-Saemisch Handbuch. It was still true when Bellows' (1944) book appeared. Yet, here we sit 34 years later than that with a basket of 'characteristic configurations' on the one hand and a second basket of etiological factors on the other with no real capacity for matching one with the other.

Consider the congenital cataracts which can be anterior polar, posterior polar, reduplicated, zonular or uniform. Consider the cortical spokes characteristic of senile cataract and the snowflake opacity said to be characteristic of diabetic cataract but, in actuality, extremely rare. Consider the posterior subcapsular location of steroid cataract, ecothiophate cataract, traumatic cataract and some senile diseases. Infrared cataract can show radial striae and exfoliation of the anterior capsule. Cataract in retinitis pigmentosa tends to be in the posterior subcapsular area.

These are examples which could be multiplied but they are sufficient to show how similar morphology does not mean similar etiology. Neither does morphology as such give a clue to mechanism.

The known mechanisms of cataractogenesis are few enough but should be described. Perhaps the best established mechanism is that for sugar cataracts. Here the parallel researches of Kinoshita and co-workers (Kinoshita et al., 1962; Kinoshita, 1974) and of Pirie and van Heyningen (van Heyningen, 1962; Pirie & van Heyningen, 1964) are definitive. These workers showed that in galactose fed rats (or in galactosemic infants) the high level of sugar activates aldose reductase. This causes accumulation of dulcitol in the lens and, because the sugar alcohol does not diffuse readily through the lens capsule, it causes an increase in hydration associated with loss of transparency. In diabetes mellitus the elevated glucose is reduced in part to sorbitol by a similar mechanism and diabetic cataract results.

There are similarities in the appearance of cortical spokes in experimental naphthalene cataract in rabbits and in senile cataract in man. Van Heyningen & Pirie (1967) showed that the more proximal toxic agent in naphthalene cataract was 1,2 naphthoquinone. For this reason van Heyningen (1976) sought oxidizable phenols that might occur in the human diet whose oxidation to quinones might be responsible for senile cataract. A series of possible candidates tested on explanted lenses did not cause cataract. Once again no correlation was found between morphology and cause.

In dinitrophenol cataract an early morphological finding is posterior subcapsular opacity (Horner, 1941). We can be reasonably sure that the well-known uncoupling of oxidation from phosphorylation caused by dinitrophenol is responsible for its toxicity in the lens. No such mechanism seems likely for the other subcapsular cataracts.

If the truth be known, we have only the haziest notions about the physics of lens turbidity, i.e., cataract. Classical histological techniques have contributed little of substantive value. The changes of liquefaction of lens cortex, fragmentation of lens fibers, irregularity of subcapsular epithelium, and 'nuclear sclerosis' as expounded by a standard textbook of ophthalmic pathology (Hogan & Zimmerman, 1962) merely confirm what is seen by the slit lamp. One may question equally whether the electron microscopic changes observed, e.g., in the formation and reversal of galactose cataract (Unakar, et al., 1978) are causally connected with the loss and recovery of transparency or are merely parallel phenomena. One must question whether

230

any technique which requires initial dehydration will give significant information on the cataracts where small hydration changes may play a role.

The one outstanding exception to the failure of electron microscopy is in the rare disease myotonic dystrophy. The cataract that accompanies this disease is typically stellate, relatively symmetrical axially and is located in the posterior cortex. In addition, there is an 'iridescent dust' in a thin layer of anterior and posterior cortex just interior to the capsule. Two recent reports (Dark & Streeten, 1977; Eshaghian, et al., 1978) agree that a consistent finding in the lens with electron microscopy is a series of vacuoles containing whorls of multilaminated membranes. It is the diffraction by the laminae that appears to be responsible for the iridescence.

This finding suggests that the non-progressive coronary cataract may derive its color from a similar configuration.

Our knowledge of optics tells us that the structural changes that would cause a change in transparency of the lens or any other structure must be of an order of magnitude somewhere near the wavelength of the incident light. No structure observable in the light or electron microscope fulfills this requirement. Certainly the lens fibrils are much too large and their contents appear to be amorphous by transmission electron microscopy.

The logical modulators of light in the lens are the protein molecules themselves. Only in recent years has there been an attempt to deal with lens transparency on this basis. Benedek (1971) suggested that as with the cornea, the normal lens was transparent to visible light because the Fourier components of the density fluctuations in both tissues have wavelengths less than half the wavelength of transmitted light. Benedek postulated the creation of high molecular weight protein aggregates in cataract which cause light-scattering and hence turbidity. Jedziniak et al. (1973) found high molecular weight aggregates in protein solutions from lenses. Tanaka & Benedek (1975) using the width of the scattered light spectrum from whole lens measured Brownian movement of the protein molecules and hence the diffusivity of the molecules. On cooling calf lenses the cold cataract in the lens appeared at nearly the same temperature as that at which the diffusivity reached zero, indicating phase separation of protein-water mixtures. In the human cataract the diffusivity was approximately 5.5 times less than in normal human lens, again suggesting high molecular weight aggregates.

Schachar & Solin (1975) viewed the matter of transparency from another aspect. They emphasized the findings on examination of the lens in polarized light made by earlier researchers. That work was in agreement that the lens behaves like a uniaxial crystal. This finding suggested orderly orientation of protein molecules and they investigated the polarized Raman spectra of beef lens to explore this possiblity. On the basis of their findings they concluded that the proteins of the lens have an anti-parallel β-pleated sheet structure. Schachar and Solin went on to suggest that there might be a microhexagonal arrangement of protein sheets corresponding to the hexagonal outline of the lens fibers and with predominant arrangement of the CONH peptide bonds orthogonal to the lens axis. This hypothesis would explain the uniaxial behavior of the lens between crossed polarizers. It would also explain the similar behavior of lens and cornea to point pressure. They each develop opacity instantly at the point of pressure and become transparent instantly when pressure is released. The most logical explanation for such a phenomenon is distortion of an elastic and ordered microstructure which is returned to its original order by its elasticity. Finally, this type of hypothesis would best fit loss of transparency after increased hydration as in sugar cataract.

The point of all the foregoing is to suggest that we may finally have both the vision and the tools to break out of the semantic trap of the word 'cataract'. The application of the advanced biochemistry described above and the application of physical techniques that operate at the level of the modulators of visible light to each category of 'cataract' may truly sort out multiple disease entities. This, rather than slit lamp morphology, may eventually allow us to give a rational name to each of the confusing configurations we now lump under the name of 'cataract'.

REFERENCES

Bellows, J.G. Cataract and anomalies of the lens. Mosby St. Louis, 1944.

Benedek, G.B. Theory of transparency of the eye. *Appl. Opt.*, 10: *459-473* (1971).

Constantini Monachi Montecassini. Liber De Oculis in: Collectio Ophthalmologicum Veterum Auctorum. (ed. Pansier, P.) Balliere Paris, 1933.

Dark, A.J. & Streeten, B.W. Ultrastructural study of cataract in myotonia dystrophica. *Amer. J. Ophthal.*, 84: *666-674* (1977).

Eshaghian, J., March, W.F., Goossens, W., & Rafferty, N.S. Ultrastructure of cataract in myotonic dystrophy. *Invest. Ophthal. Vis. Sci.*, 17: *289-293* (1978).

Gullstrand, A. Demonstration eines Instrumentes zur Erzeugung von Strahlengebilden um leuchtende Punkte. Ber. Versamm. ophthal. Ges., Heidelberg (1902) *290-292* (1903).

Helmholtz, H. Beschreibung eines Augen-Spiegels. Berlin: Förstner (1851).

Hess, C. Pathologie und Therapie des Linsensystems, in Handbuch der Gesamten Augenheilkunde, 2nd ed., 6: Abt. 1, Chapt. IX. W. Engelmann Leipzig: 1905.

Heyningen, van R. The sorbitol pathway in the lens. *Expl. Eye Res.* 1: *396-404* (1962).

Heyningen, van R. Experimental studies on cataract. *Invest. Ophthal.*, 15: *685-697* (1976).

Heyningen, van R. & Pirie, A. The metabolism of naphthalene and its toxic effect on the eye. *Biochem. J.*, 102: *842-852* (1967).

Hogan, M.J. & Zimmerman, L.E. Ophthalmic Pathology, 2nd. ed. Saunders Philadelphia/London: 1962.

Horner, W.D. A study of dinitrophenol and its relation to cataract formation. *Trans. Amer. Ophthal. Soc.*, 77: *405-437* (1941).

Jedziniak, J.A., Kinoshita, J.H., Yates, E.M., Hocker, L.O. & Benedek, G.B. On the presence and mechanism of formation of heavy molecular weight aggregates in normal and cataractous lenses. *Expl. Eye Res.*, 15: *185-192* (1973).

Kinoshita, J.H. Mechanisms initiating cataract formation. *Invest. Ophthal.* 13: *713-724* (1974).

Kinoschita, H., Merola, L.O. & Dikmak, E. Osmotic changes in experimental galactose cataracts. *Expl. Eye Res.* 1: *405-410* (1962).

Pirie, A. & Heyningen, van R. The effect of diabetes on the content of sorbitol, glucose, fructose and inositol in the human lens. *Expl. Eye Res.* 3: *124-131* (1964).

Schachar, R.A. & Solin, S.A. The microscopic protein structure of the lens with a theory for cataract formation as determined by Raman spectroscopy of intact bovine lenses. *Invest. Ophthal.*, 15: *380-396* (1975).

Tanaka, T. & Benedek, G.B. Observation of protein diffusivity in intact human and bovine lenses with application to cataract. *Invest. Ophthal.*, 14: *449-456* (1975).

Unaker, N.J., Genyea, C., Reddan, J.R. & Reddy, V.N. Ultrastructural changes during the development and reversal of galactose cataracts. *Expl. Eye Res.* 26: *123-133* (1978).

Author's address:
Department of Ophthalmology
University of Louisville
301 East Walnut Street
Louisville, Kentucky 40202
U.S.A.

Steichen, R.A. & Hart, R.A. ... ... phase quantities ... ... in a ... ... of ... information ... determined by X-ray diffraction ... ... Garden Cress. ... 1:1-3, 197-200 (197..)

Tidwell, ... & Baker, C.J.E. Observation of ... ... with ... pump and ... ...

... ... C. ... J.R.R. ... ... for ... ... and ... ...

Author's Address

...
... ... Street
Cambridge, ...

THE REVERSAL OF TRIPARANOL-INDUCED CATARACT IN THE RAT. VI. ULTRASTRUCTURAL CHANGES***

GERHARD SCHLÜTER, OTTO HOCKWIN,
JOHN E. HARRIS & LOUISE GRUBER

(Bonn, F.R.G., Minneapolis, U.S.A.)

ABSTRACT

The morphology of triparanol-induced cataracts in the rat has been investigated using electron microscopy. The findings are as follows. Although in controls the cytoplasm of the hexagonal configurated lens fibers appears finely granular and fibrillar showing a homogeneous electron density, fibers of cataractous lenses are swollen and irregularly outlined. Moreover, inside the cytoplasm the granular material aggregated to flocculent globules which were localized in a very light matrix. These altered fibers correspond to light microscopically visible vacuoles, situated in the transitional zone between lens cortex and nucleus. During the cataract clearing process, these ultrastructural changes almost disappear. Occasionally, however, more pronounced alterations of fibers are also found. In these fibers, the limiting cell membrane frequently becomes disrupted and the altered cytoplasmic content leaks into the intercellular spaces. These alterations which were predominantly observed in severe cataracts were sometimes still found during the clearing phase.

INTRODUCTION

Triparanol, a cholesterol-reducing drug, causes cataracts in rats following an ingestion period of about 10 weeks (Harris & Gruber, 1969, 1972). These cataracts are characterized by a true reversal if the rat is continued on a diet devoid of triparanol. In addition to different biochemical alterations during the cataractous stage (Bours et al., 1978; Harris & Gruber, 1972; Rathbun et al., 1973, 1978) severe morphological changes have also been observed. These consist of large vacuoles forming in the transitional zone between lens cortex and nucleus.

The origin and nature of these vacuoles are still unknown, and until the present study, the question of whether these vacuoles are localized intracellularly or extracellularly had not been investigated. To get a better understanding of these morphological alterations, the present study was concerned with ultrastructural observations of lens fibers during the cataractous and clearing stages of the triparanol-induced cataracts in the rat.

*** This investigation was supported in part by U.S. Public Health Service grant EY-01200 and by grant of Deutsche Forschungsgemeinschaft (Schl 166/1). This paper was included in this special issue without the prior knowledge of John E. Harris.

MATERIALS AND METHODS

Weanling Wistar rats were fed a diet of 0.075% triparanol (W.S. Merrel Co.) for a period of 60-80 days (Harris & Gruber, 1969, 1972). For the purpose of the present study, lenses were divided into 3 groups: 1. controls, 2. cataractous, and 3. cataractous with subsequent clearing.

For electron microscopy, pieces of lenses were first fixed in a modified Karnovsky mixture (2% paraformaldehyde, 2.5% glutaraldehyde in 0.2 M cacodylate buffer) for 3 hrs. After a short rinse in buffer solution, the tissue was postfixed in 1.3% OsO_4 (in 0.2 M cacodylate buffer) for a further period of 2 hrs. After dehydration in a graded series of ethanol, the tissue was embedded in a soft Durcupan mixture (Fluka, 4 parts epoxy resin, 3 parts hardener) via propylene oxide.

RESULTS

Since it is known from light microscopic studies (Harris & Gruber, 1969) that vacuolar transformation occurs in the lens cortex bordering the nucleus, only portions of the lens periphery were investigated.

Fig. 1 illustrates by light microscopy, the normal lens cortex as compared to those altered by administration of triparanol. Whereas in normal lenses the typical hexagonal configuration of fibers is seen, cataractous lenses are characterized by the development of large vacuoles localized in the transitional zone between lens cortex and nucleus. Moreover, it is evident that the typical hexagonal arrangement of lens fibers is lost. Instead, they appear swollen and are irregularly outlined.

In electron microscopic sections of normal lenses, the hexagonal form of the fiber was also observed. The fine structure corresponded to that previously described by other authors (Cohen, 1965; Tanaka & Iino, 1967; Kuwabara, 1968; Dickson & Crock, 1972; Maisel & Perry, 1972; Farnsworth et al., 1974). The superficial fiber layers were joined by complex interdigitations; the extracellular space was limited. Fibers contained a nucleus, few mitochondria, and microtubules. The distribution of these structures varied inside each fiber and seemed to be related to the position of the fiber within the lens.

In more longitudinal sections of the deeper part of the cortex (Fig. 2), the fibers were very closely attached; an intercellular space was not observed. The cytoplasm was filled with a finely granular and fibrillar material, possibly representing the different kinds of crystallins. Although this material showed a different osmiophilic density, it appeared to be distributed in a very homogeneous manner. At higher magnifications, the closely attached fibers were coupled by typical 5 layered gap junctions, which could be followed over long distances (Fig. 3). Tight junctions, as previously described to occur by Maisel & Perry (1972), were not observed.

Fig. 4 demonstrates the fine structural aspect of lens fibers in a triparanol-induced cataractous lens in the region of the vacuolar transformation. As compared to controls, the cytoplasm of these fibers stained lightly and the

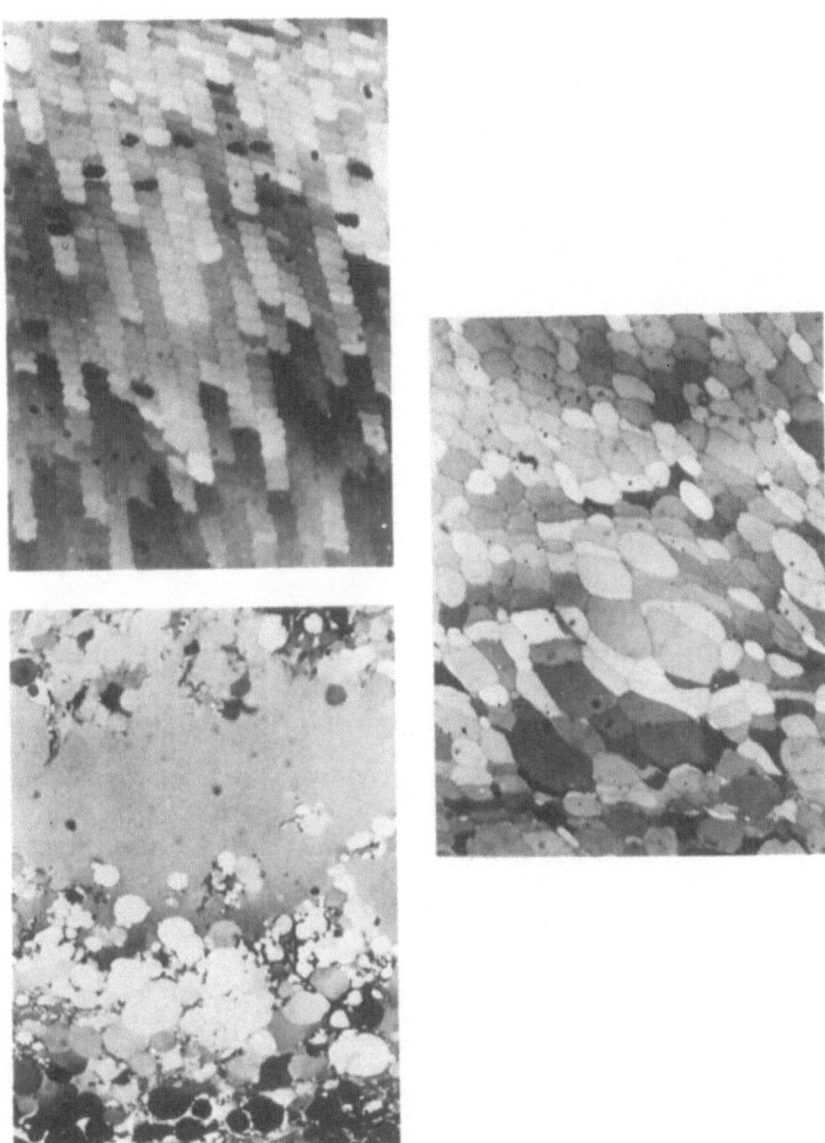

Fig. 1 a-c. Light microscopic views of normal and triparanol altered lens tissue.
a. In controls the lens fibers are hexagonal shaped, showing a different staining pattern.
b. Transitional zone between lens cortex and nucleus in a cataractous lens. Large vacuoles are the predominant feature in this area. c. The typical hexagonal configuration of lens fibers is lost in the most peripheral region.
1 μ semi-thick sections of plastic embedded material, stained with toluidine-blue-pyronine.
Magn.: 360 x

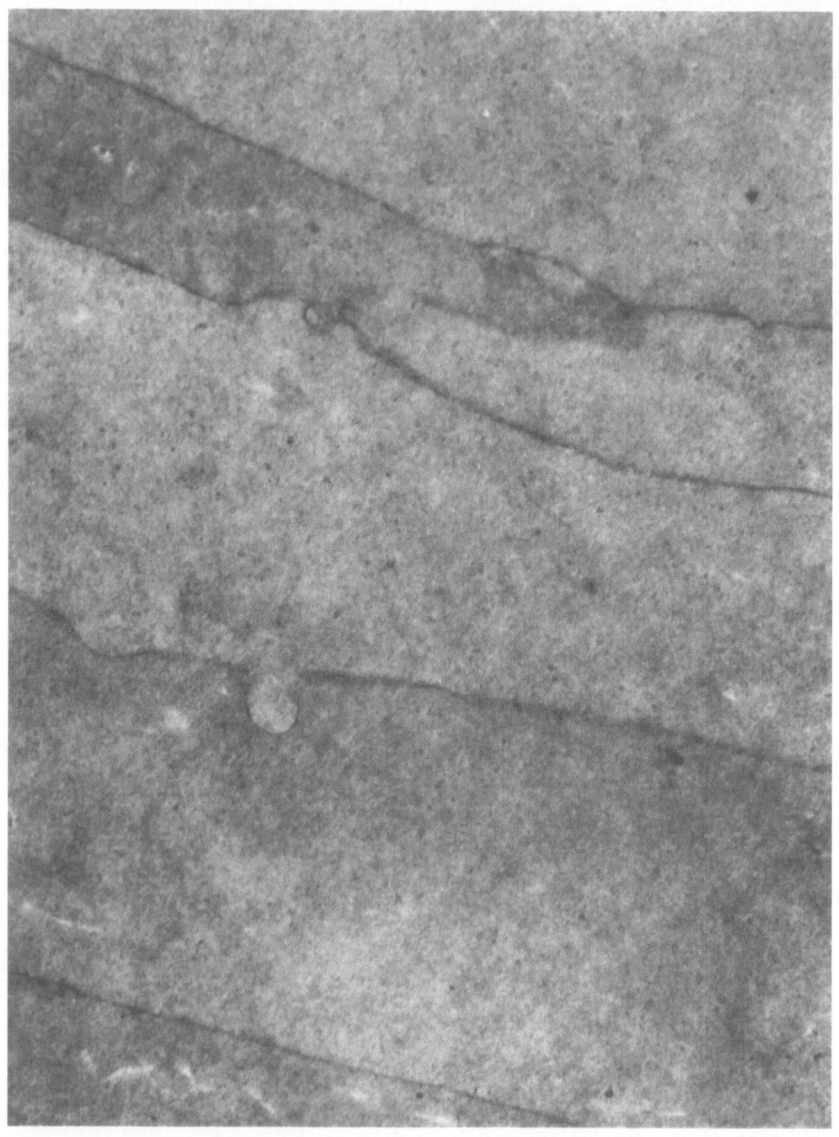

Fig. 2. Low magnification of normal lens fibers. The fibers are closely attached, and the cytoplasm is filled with a fine granular and fibrillar material, showing a homogeneous density.
Magn.: 8.000 x

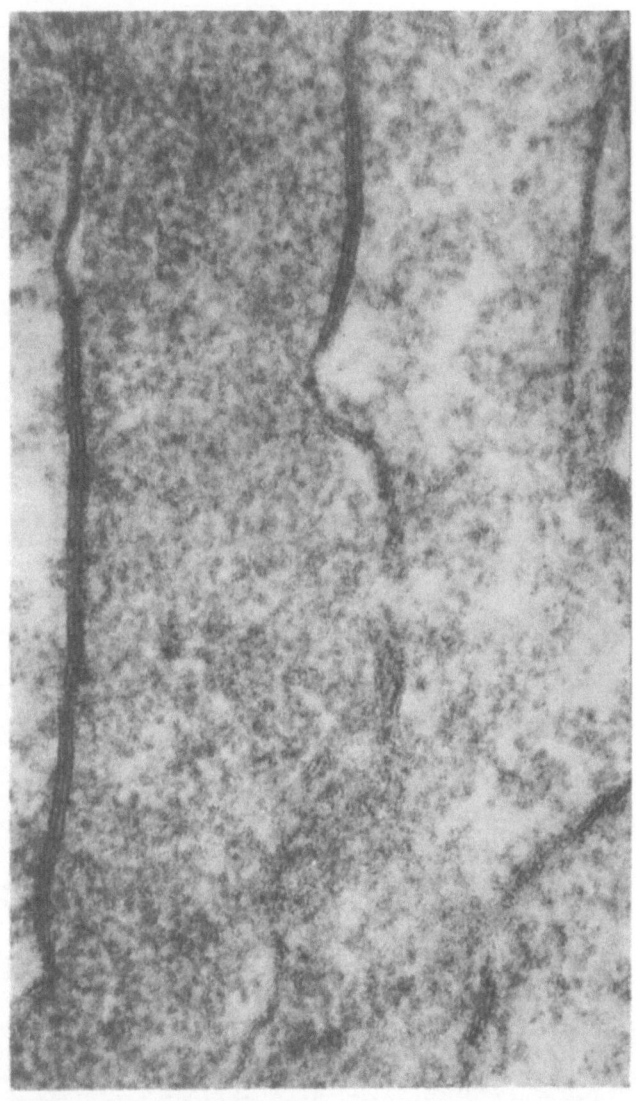

Fig. 3. Junctional complex of neighbouring normal lens fibers at higher magnification. The fibers are always coupled by long stretches of 5-layered gap junctions.
Magn.: 160.000 x

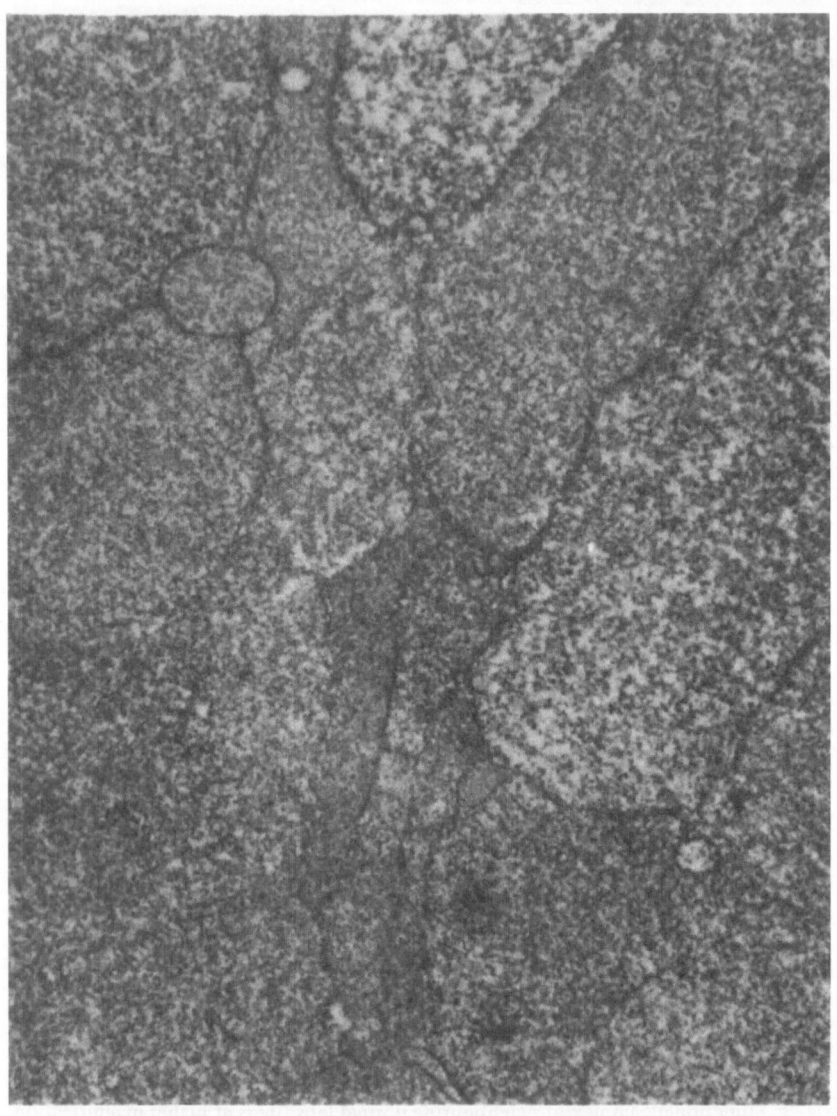

Fig. 4. Low magnification of cataractous lens fibers. The cytoplasm has aggregated to flocculent globules, embedded in a very light matrix. No alterations are seen concerning the closely attached cell membranes and the intercellular spaces.
Magn.: 8.000 x

homogeneity of the granular and fibrillar materials disappeared. Instead, aggregates of flocculent globules were seen. As seen from the integrity of the limiting cell membranes, which were still in close apposition and formed typical junctional complexes, no changes were observed in the intercellular spaces. These ultrastructural alterations of lens fibers were similar in all cataractous lenses and were independent of the cataract severity.

Some fibers were found which showed more pronounced alterations (Fig. 5). Those fibers were characterized by numerous fractures of the limiting cell membrane, leading to leakage of the cytoplasmic contents into the intercellular spaces. The material inside the fibers also exhibited marked alterations. It became aggregated to form coarse globules which were embedded in an electron-microscopically empty matrix. These degenerations, predominantly seen in the more severe stages of cataracts, were occasionally also found in lenses during the process of clearing. The ultrastructural aspect of the majority of fibers, however, normalized during the clearing process and did not differ from that of normal lenses.

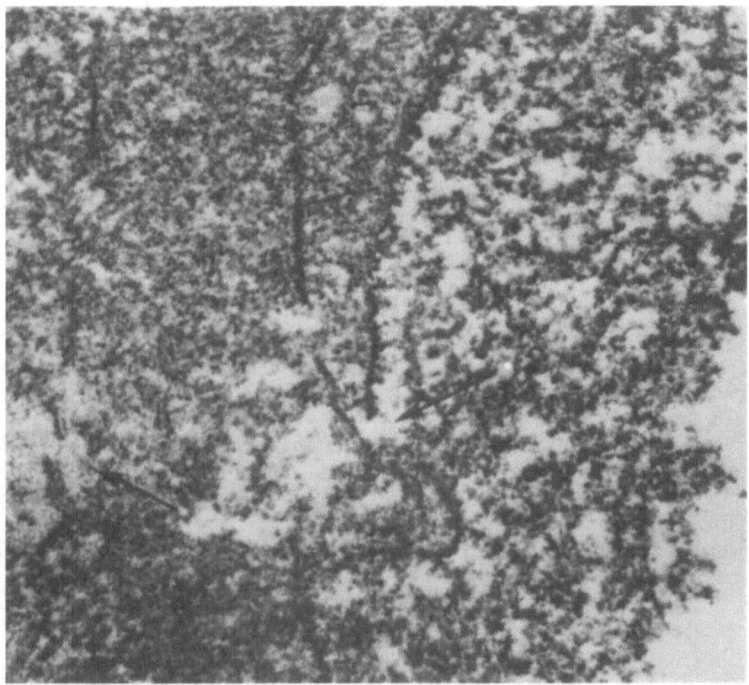

Fig. 5. Degeneration of fibers in a cataractous lens. The limiting membrane has become broken and the altered cytoplasmic content leaks out into the now widened intercellular space (↑).
Magn.: 40.000 x

DISCUSSION

The present study has shown that, in triparanol-induced cataracts in the rat, fine structural alterations occur. These alterations consist of a marked swelling of lens fibers, leading to an irregular outline of the fibers. Moreover, the normally homogeneous dispersed granular and fibrillar material of the cytoplasm becomes concentrated, forming flocculent globules localized in a very light matrix. From the findings that the limiting membranes of neighbouring fibers are morphologically intact and closely attached it can be concluded that these alterations are intracellular in nature and probably are caused by an inflow of water.

The swollen and therefore lightly staining fibers correspond to the light-microscopically visible vacuoles localized in the transitional zone between lens cortex and nucleus. These vacuoles are known to occur regularly in triparanol-induced cataracts (Harris & Gruber, 1969). The observed changes usually disappear during the clearing phase and lead to a normal ultrastructural aspect of lens fibers. Thus, it appears that these observed cytoplasmic alterations are reversible in nature.

However, sometimes degenerative and irreversible changes of lens fibers are found. These changes, characterized by numerous disruptions of the limiting fiber membrane, are possibly caused by an excessive intracellular swelling. Thus, the altered cytoplasmic content leaks out into the now widened intercellular spaces. Although these changes are found in stages of severe cataracts, they are also occasionally seen during the clearing phase.

It may be stated that triparanol probably causes changes of the cell membrane of lens fibers which lead to a reversible inflow of fluids. However, consistent alterations of the fiber membrane were not found by electron microscopy.

REFERENCES

Bours, J., Grube, L., Hockwin, O. & Harris, J.E. The crystallins of the rat lens with triparanol-induced cataracts, also related to ageing. *Interdiscpl. Topics Geront.* 12 (1978, in press).

Cohen, A.J. The electron microscopy of the normal human lens. *Invest. Ophthal.* 4: *433-466* (1965).

Dickson, D.H. & Crock, G.W. Interlocking patterns on primate lens fibers. *Invest. Ophthal.* 11: *809-815* (1972).

Farnsworth, P.N., Fu, S.C.J., Burke, P.A. & Bania, J. Ultrastructure of rat eye lens fibers. *Invest. Ophthal.* 13: *274-279* (1974).

Harris, J.E. & Gruber, L. The reversal of triparanol-induced cataracts in the rat. *Doc. Ophthal.* 26: *324-333* (1969).

Harris, J.E. & Gruber, L. Reversal of triparanol-induced cataracts in the rat. II. Exchange of ^{22}Na, ^{42}K, and ^{86}Rb in cataractous and clearing lenses. *Invest. Ophthal.* 11: *608-616* (1972).

Kuwabara, T. Microtubules in the lens. *Arch. Ophthal.* 79: *189-195* (1968).

Maisel, H. & Perry, M.M. Electron microscope observations on some structural proteins of the chick lens. *Expl. Eye Res.* 14: *7-12* (1972).

Rathbun, W.B., Harris, J.E., Vagstad, G. & Gruber, L. The reversal of triparanol-induced cataracts in the rat. IV. Reduced sulfhydryl groups in soluble protein and glutathione. *Invest. Ophthal.* 12: *388-390* (1973).

Rathbun, W.B., Hough, M., Gruber, L. & Harris, J.E. The reversal of triparanol-induced cataract in the rat. V. Activity levels of ATPase, and three enzymes of glutathione metabolism. *Interdiscpl. Topics Geront. 12* (1978, in press).

Tanaka, K. & Iino, A. Zur Frage der Verbindung der Linsenfasern im Rinderauge. *Z. Zellforsch.* 82: *604-612* (1967).

Author's address:
Anatomical Institute
University of Bonn
Nussallee 10, 5300 Bonn
F.R.D.

Docum. Ophthal. Proc. Series, Vol. 18

STAPHYLOCOCCAL CENTRAL CORNEAL ULCER

ROBERT P. BURNS & ZINA STEPHAN

(Portland, Oregon U.S.A.)

ABSTRACT

A review of staphylococcal central corneal ulcers has shown that the staphylococcus is the commonest bacterium isolated at the University of Oregon Health Sciences Center. One-third of central corneal ulcers cultured Staphylococci; one-third of these were Staphylococcus aureus. These ulcers occurred in immunodepressed or otherwise previously diseased patients, but not as a primary disease entity. Penicillin resistance was a common characteristic of the isolated Staphylococci. Prognosis for retention of the eye was good.

INTRODUCTION

It is often advisable for different institutions to review their local statistics on frequency of disease, since these vary from area to area. Because corneal ulcer is a common and potentially very serious disease, threatening blindness or loss of the eye, we have recently analyzed the occurrence of Staphylococci cultured from corneal ulcers at the Department of Ophthalmology of the University of Oregon Health Sciences Center (UOHSC).

There is a marked discrepancy in different literature reports of the incidence of Staphylococci in corneal ulcers. Thus, Thygeson (1948) reported no corneal ulcers due to Staphylococci in San Francisco in 1947. Suie et al. (1959) listed coagulase positive Staphylococci in four of fifty consecutive corneal ulcers. Duke-Elder (1965) dismissed Staphylococcus as only an 'occasional' cause of corneal ulcer. However, Pettit (1963) from Los Angeles, California found 25% of corneal ulcers were caused by Staphylococci. Smith & Rose (1967) in Vancouver, Canada, said Staphylococcus aureus was present in nine of fifty central corneal ulcers. Wilson (1976), of Atlanta, Georgia cultured Staphylococci in six of fifty-seven ulcers, and from Europe, Witmer (1974) described 12% of corneal ulcers as due to Staphylococcus aureus. Finally, Locatcher-Khorazo (1972), over a thirty year period in New York, cultured Staphylococci from 49% of a series of several thousand corneal ulcers.

MATERIALS & METHODS

The Department of Ophthalmology at the UOHSC maintains a Microbiology Laboratory in the center of the department. An especially trained full-time technician operates the laboratory. When a central corneal ulcer is diagnosed clinically by biomicroscopy, immediate scraping for Gram and Giemsa stains is performed and cultures are inoculated directly on blood, chocolate agar plates and mannitol salt agar, as well as in thioglycolate broth tubes for aerobic and anaerobic organisms. Special cultures are carried out as indicated. Bacterial cultures are isolated and identified according to standard methods (Buchanan & Gibbons, 1974).

If a Gram-positive coccus, identified on a scraping of a corneal ulcer, is grown in culture, it is considered a Streptococcus if catalase negative, and Staphylococcus if catalase positive. Only rarely is an anaerobic Staphylococcus (Peptococcus) isolated. An aerobic Staphylococcus requires glucose, whereas a Micrococcus does not. Finally, a coagulase test is performed, either by slide typing or tube coagulation. Only coagulase positive, Gram positive cocci are considered Staphylococcus aureus.

We studied only central corneal ulcers. Excluded was the much more common occurrence of Staphylococcal blepharo-conjunctivo-keratitis in which Staphylococci grow in the lid margins, inhabiting the sebaceous glands of the eyelid and Meibomian glands. These Staphylococci secrete exotoxins into the tear film, and are responsible for the resultant conjunctivitis and marginal corneal infiltrates (Fig. 1). These have been excluded from consideration, as not being true ulcers.

RESULTS

A review of the central corneal ulcers cultured in 1977 listed 67 patients as having cultures performed. Cultures were negative for bacteria in thirty-one of sixty-seven; of the thirty-six positive, Staphylococci were isolated in twenty-five, a frequency of almost 2/3rds. Eight of these were coagulase positive Staphylococcus aureus and seventeen were coagulase negative Staphylococcus albus. The role of Staphylococcus albus in disease production is not clear.

The records of the patients with central corneal ulcers from which Staphylococcus aureus was isolated were reviewed. Clinical diagnosis was nonspecific. None of these patients had primary infections of the cornea without antecedent disease, or followed minimal trauma such as an abrasion or corneal foreign body. Staphylococcus aureus central corneal ulcers occur in compromised hosts. Most commonly these are adrenocorticosteroid treated patients, particularly those on chronic steroid and anti-viral treatment of herpes simplex keratitis (Fig. 2). Other factors noted in the eight patients included corneal anesthesia and neurotrophic keratitis in two patients who developed Staphylococcus aureus superinfection. Immunocompromised patients with atopic dermatitis, who also had steroid therapy, were candidates for Staphylococci cultured from their typical shield-shaped corneal ulcer (Fig. 3). Corneal exposure from inadequate lid closure was found in some patients. The presence of a foreign body, including a loose nylon suture in a corneal transplant, was another predisposing factor (Fig. 4). Hypopyon occasionally occurred, but was not prominent (Figure 5).

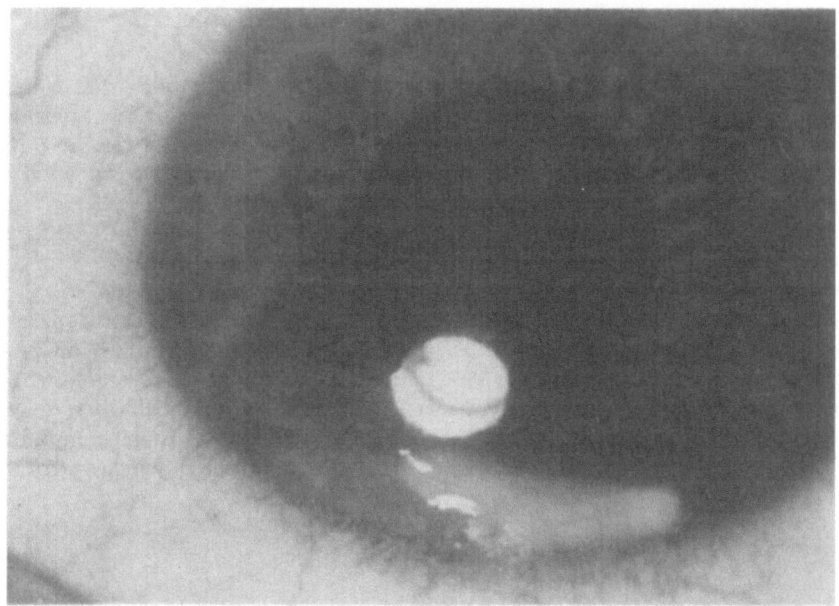

Fig. 1. Marginal corneal infiltrate, due to hypersensitivity reaction to Staphylococcus toxin.

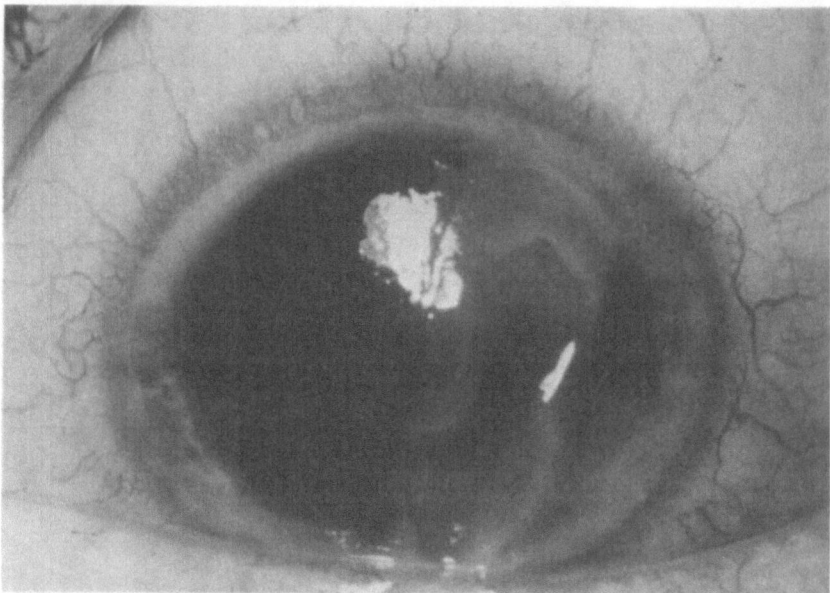

Fig. 2. Sudden sloughing of cornea due to Staphylococcic superinfection, in idoxuridine and steroid treated herpes simples stromal keratitis.

A review of predisposing factors in these eight cases implies that other methods of therapy, apart from ordinary antibiotics, are necessary. Steroids should be decreased or stopped, if possible, and adequate lid closure provided. None of these patients were contact lens wearers (Brown et al., 1974).

A general classification of corneal ulcers devised by Jones (1973) was used in planning therapy. A Grade I corneal ulcer is less than two mm. in diameter, not in the visual axis, and in the superficial one-third of the cornea. These patients are treated as an outpatient with topical drops or ointment. A Grade II ulcer is between two and six mm. in size, in the superficial third of the stroma. This patient is hospitalized and treated with antibiotic drops very frequently, as well as subconjunctival antibiotics, daily to the point of tolerance. A Grade III corneal ulcer is greater than six mm. in diameter and involves the inner third of the stroma, or one in which perfora-

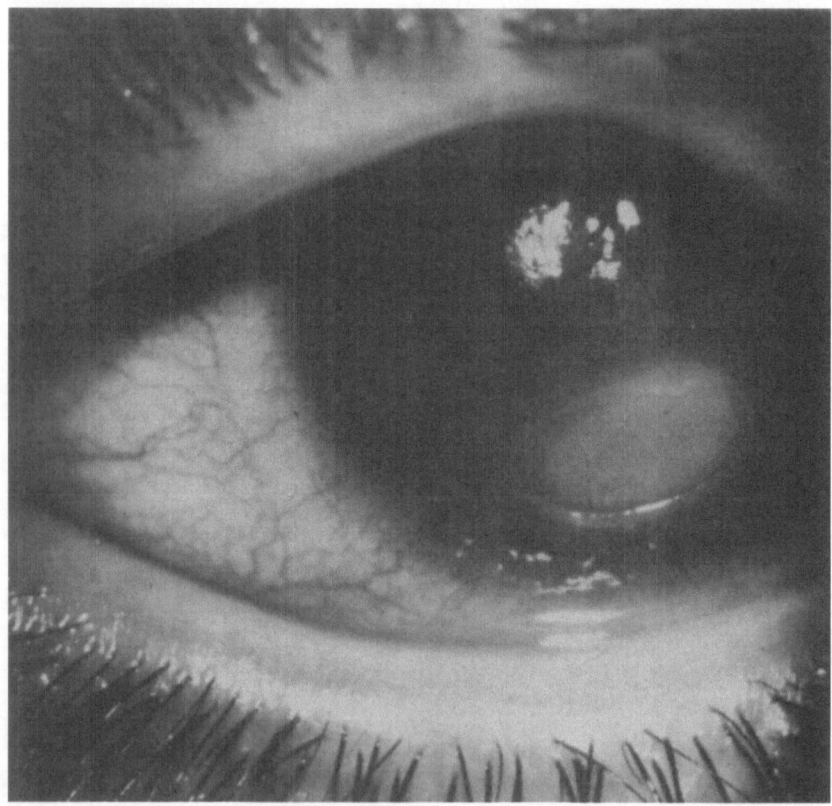

Fig. 3. Atopic dermatitis patient on chronic steroid therapy, with corneal ulcer from which Staphylococcus aureus was grown.

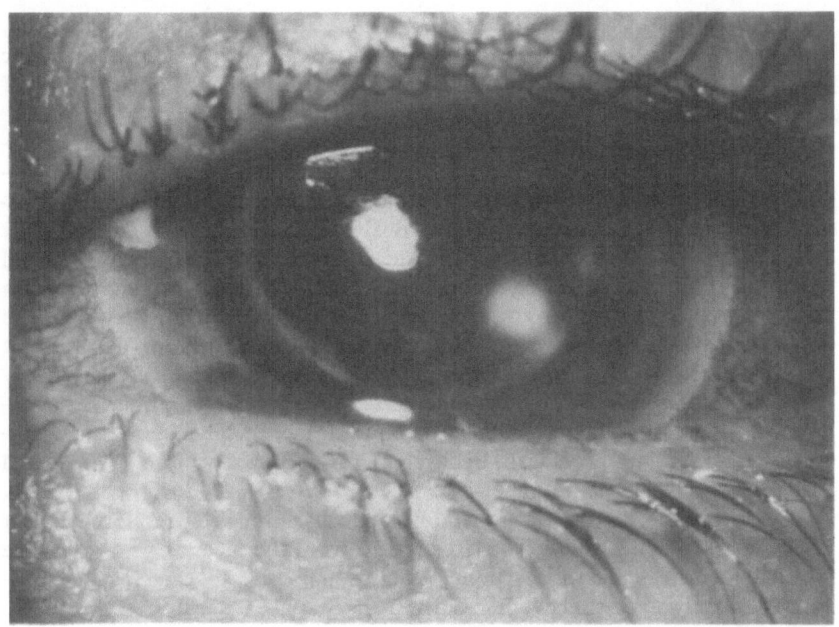

Fig. 4. Abscess which became ulcer at site of eroded nylon suture in patient on steroid therapy after keratoplasty.

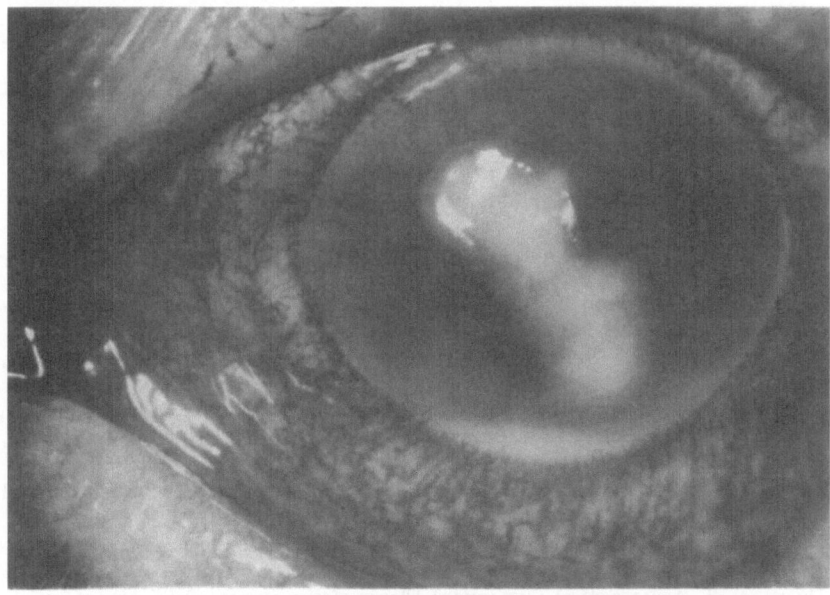

Fig. 5. Minimal hypopyon in Staphylococcal central corneal ulcer.

tion is threatened. A Grade III corneal ulcer patient should be hospitalized, examined with the slit lamp twice daily, and treated with frequent antibiotic drops and subconjunctival injections to tolerance. Probably pulsed doses of intravenous antibiotics should be added.

Topical systemic antibiotic therapy depends upon isolation of the Staphylococcus on culture and determination of antibiotic sensitivities. Kupferman & Leibowitz (1977) found five antibiotics equally effective in supressing the growth of a single strain of Staphylococcus aureus. In our eight cases, only one of the cultures showed a Staphylococcus sensitive to all twelve antibiotics that are commonly used in Kirby-Bauer testing for Gram positive pathogens. Six of the eight cultures were penicillin resistant, and one was penicillin sensitive but chloromycetin resistant. None of the eight Staphylococci tested were gentamicin resistant. Thus, penicillin G probably would not be indicated for subconjunctival or parenteral treatment. Subconjunctival injections of methicillin or cephaloridine, in 50 to 100 mgm. dosages, would be more logical. Bacitracin was frequently used as a topical antibiotic, as well as gentamicin.

The prognosis for the eye in Staphylococcus aureus central corneal ulcer was invariably good. The patient recovered from the ulcer and no eyes were lost from corneal ulceration alone. Debilitating corneal scars ensued, however. The only eyes that we have lost from Staphylococcal infections were those that have had bacteria enter into the eye, such as through a filtering bleb or surgical wound.

REFERENCES

Allen, H.F., Current status of prevention, diagnosis and management of bacterial corneal ulcers. *Ann. Ophthal.* 3: *235-245*, (1971).

Brown, S.I., Bloomfields, S., Pearce, D.B. & Tragakis, M. Infections with the therapeutic soft lens. *Archs. Ophthal.* 91: *275-277*, (1974).

Buchanan, R.E. & Gibbons, N.E. Bergey's manual of determinative bacteriology, Eighth Ed. Williams & Wilkins, Baltimore, 1974, pp. *483-489.*

Duke-Elder, W.S. System of ophthalmology, Vol. 8, Disease of the Outer Eye. Henry Kimpton, London, 1965, p. *773.*

Jones, D.B. Early Diagnosis and therapy of bacterial corneal ulcers. *Int. Ophthalmol. Clin.* 13: *1-29,* (1973).

Kupferman, A. & Leibowitz, H.M. Topical antibiotic therapy of staphylococcal keratitis. *Archs. Ophthal.* 95: *1634-1637,* (1977).

Locatcher-Kohrazo, D. & Seegal, B. Microbiology of the eye, C.V. Mosby, St. Louis, 1972, p. *69.*

Petit, T.H. Management of bacterial corneal ulcers, in Symposium on ocular therapy, Vol. 8, (ed. Leopold, I.H. & Burns, R.P.) John Wiley & Sons, New York, 1976, pp.*57-65.*

Smith, E.L. & Rose, H.A. Medical and surgical management of deep central corneal Ulcers and Descemetoceles. *Can. J. Ophthalmol.* 2: *115-121*, (1967).

Suie, T., Blatt, M.M., Havener, W.H. *et al.* Bacterial Corneal Ulcers. *Am. J. Ophthal.* 48: *775-777,* 1959.

Thygeson, P. Acute central (hypopyon) Ulcers of the cornea. *Calif. Med.* 69: *3-10* (1948).

Wilson, L.A. Bacterial corneal ulcers, in: Clinical Ophthalmology, Vol. 4, Chapter 18, (ed. Duane, T.D.) Harper & Row, Hagerstown, Md., 1976, pp. *1-19*.

Witmer, R. Corneal ulcers, in Round Table Discussion, Ocular inflammatory disease, (ed. Golden, B.) Charles C. Thomas, Springfield, 1974, pp. *274-281*.

Authors' address:
John E. Weeks Institute of Ophthalmology
University of Oregon Health Sciences Center
3181 SW Sam Jackson Park Rd.
Portland, Oregon 97201 U.S.A.

Docum. Ophthal. Proc. Series, Vol. 18

METABOLIC HETEROGENEITY OF KERATAN SULFATE IN BOVINE CORNEA AND ITS ROLE IN THE MAINTENANCE OF CORNEAL COLLAGEN STRUCTURE

ZACHARIAS DISCHE, GERTRUD CREMER-BARTELS,
GORDON I. KAYE, NANCY W. KAYE & ERHARDT BUDDEKE

(New York, U.S.A., Munster, F.R.G.)

ABSTRACT

On sequential extraction of bovine corneas with 0.155 M NaCl and 1 M CaCl$_2$ two macromolecular fractions were obtained in a ratio of 0.7-1.5, both containing glycosaminoglycans and a hexosamine containing non-glycosaminoglycan subfraction.

Electron microscopy revealed that the NaCl extraction has no effect on the form, the diameter, the course of the collagen fibrils or their distance from each other. Unlike previous studies, CaCl$_2$ extraction leads to only minimal disruption of lamellar organization or collagen fibrils. This incomplete extraction is probably attributable to the presence of an intact epithelium which is necessary for the incorporation experiments below.

Incubation of bovine cornea in the presence of l-^{14}C glucosamine results in a specific labeling of all hexosamine-containing compounds. The chondroitin sulfate preparations isolated from the saline and CaCl$_2$ extracts had equal specific radioactivity. However, the specific radioactivities of the keratan sulfates isolated from the NaCl extract was 3-5 times higher than that of the keratan sulfate prepared from the CaCl$_2$ extract.

In a pulse-chase experiment no shift in the ratio of the specific radioactivities of the two keratan sulfate preparations was observed. From these results it is concluded that two metabolically independent keratan sulfate fractions in two topographically different sites may be present in the stroma. The less labeled keratan sulfate and its proteoglycan, respectively, are thought to be involved in the maintenance of corneal collagen structure.

INTRODUCTION

Keratan sulfate (KS) and chondroitin sulfate (CS) containing proteoglycans and collagen are known to be essential components of the corneal stroma and to contribute substantially to the macromolecular organization of the extracellular matrix. However, on sequential extraction of bovine cornea by NaCl and CaCl$_2$, only a part of the structural components becomes soluble, each extract containing proteoglycans and a small portion of collagen (Dische et al., 1973). These results suggest the existence of two different groups of proteoglycans which significantly differ in their extractibility. A

Supported in part by Grants EY-00210, CA-2075, BSRG 05394 from the NIH, USPHS and by a grant from the Deutsche Forschungs Gemeinschaft.

study of the specific labeling of proteoglycans by ^{14}C-glucosamine would be expected to give valuable information as to whether the proteoglycans are related to metabolically independent pools or whether a precursor-product relationship exists between the proteoglycan fractions obtained by extraction with NaCl and CaCl$_2$. The results presented and an electronmicroscopic control of the extraction procedure suggest the existence of two different and metabolically independent proteoglycan pools, one of them being involved in the maintenance of the structure of collagen fibrils.

MATERIALS AND METHODS

Materials: Bovine corneas were obtained from the local slaughter house, immediately placed in ice cold 0.155 M sodium chloride solution, and kept in this solution for up to 90 min, until the incubation experiments started.

All chemicals used for biochemical studies were of analytical grade and were purchased from Boehringer, Mannheim G.m.b.H. (Mannheim, Germany), Merck (Darmstadt) and Serva Heidelberg. l- ^{14}C-glucosamine hydrochloride (specific activity 55 mCi/mMol) was obtained from the Radiochemical Centre (Amersham, England).

Analytical methods: Total hexosamines were determined after hydrolysis in 6 N HCl for 4 h at 100°C (Boas, 1953), uronic acids by the carbazol borate reaction (Bitter & Muir, 1962) and hexoses by the anthron method.

Separation and identification of the individual glycosaminoglycans on an analytical scale was by thin layer chromatography according to Humbel & Chamoles (1973).

Radioactivity measurements: 10 ml Instagel^R (Packard Instruments, Frankfurt/M) or Unisolve^R were added to 0.1-0.5 ml aqueous solutions for measurement of radioactivity in a Packard scintillation spectrophotometer (Model 3025).

Incubation experiments in vitro: 30 bovine corneas (15 pairs of adult corneas) were distributed equally into 3 experimental sets, each set weighing about 5.6 g. Incubation was under a gas phase of 95% O$_2$/5% CO$_2$ at 37°C in 10 ml Binotal^R for the following periods.

1. Pulse experiments: 30 min. in the presence of 50 uCi l- ^{14}C glucosamine.
2. Pulse-chase experiment: 30 min. in the presence of 50 uCi l- ^{14}C glucosamine after which time the corneas were transferred for an additional 5 1/2 h incubation into a new flask without glucosamine.
3. Continuous labeling experiment: 6 h in the presence of 25 uCi l- ^{14}C glucosamine. The incubation was stopped by rinsing the cornea three times with ice cold Ringer's solution.

In all of the incubations the corneas were intact, i.e. they had been dissected at the limbus and the epithelium and, presumably, the endothelia were still present.

Extraction procedures: After incubation, each set of corneas was extracted four times, 24 hrs each, with 20 ml 0.155 M NaCl at 4°C under gentle shaking. The incubation medium, the wash water, and the NaCl extracts were pooled and dialyzed against tap water for 48 h and 2 changes of

254

distilled water for 24 h each. The sodium chloride extraction was followed by four extractions of the corneas with 20 ml. 1.O M $CaCl_2$, pH 8.0, under otherwise identical conditions. The precipitates formed during dialysis were separated by centrifugation at 20,000 g for 30 min. (fractions 1b and 2b). The supernatants (fractions 1a and 2a) were lyophilized and redissolved in 6 ml distilled water for analysis and further experiments.

Pronase degradation: 3 mg pronase (Merck, 70,000 PUK/g) and 0.33 ml Tris buffer (pH 7.6) containing 0.1 M $CaCl_2$ were added to 3 ml of fraction 1a and 2a and incubated at 37°C for 24 h. The digest was centrifuged at 20,000 g for 30 min., dialyzed against distilled water twice for 24 h and an aliquot submitted to Sephadex G-50 chromatography. The glycosamino-glycans were precipitated by addition of 2 1/2 volumes of ethanol and potassium acetate (1%).

RESULTS

1. Sequential extraction of macromolecular bound hexosamine

About 20% of the total hexosamine of bovine corneas becomes soluble as a result of incubation in buffered Ringer's solution for the initial period of time and subsequent repeated extraction with 0.155 M NaCl (Table 1). In the course of the NaCl extraction most of the hexosamines come out in the first extraction, the solubilized amounts decreasing sharply to a low level in the following extraction steps.

The extracted hexosamine-containing compounds may be separated by dialysis against distilled water into a precipitate (fraction 1b) accounting for about 40% of the extracted hexosamine and a fraction (1a) soluble in distilled water. Electron microscopy after the NaCl extraction revealed that the

Table 1. Recovery and chemical composition of hexosamine containing macromolecules (fraction 1a - 2b) obtained from bovine corneae by sequential extraction with 0.155 M sodium chloride and 1.0 M calcium chloride followed by dialysis of the extractions. The values given for extracted hexosamine are means with standard deviations of 6 experiments. The collagen content was calculated from the hydroxyproline content. The analytical data for tissue residue are calculated on the basis of dry weight of the tissue. The latter was determined after exhaustive dialysis of the extracted cornea against distilled water and lyophilization.

Subfraction	μMol hexosamine extracted/g wet weight	g/100 g total hexosamine	μMol/mg substance			μg collagen/ mg substance
			HexN	Uronic acid	Hexoses	
0.155 M NaCl 1a	1.3 ± 0.24	11.5	0.24	0.04	0.06	9
1b	0.9 ± 0.11	7.5	0.21	0.21	0.03	25
1.0 M $CaCl_2$ 2a	2.6 ± 0.26	22.0	0.36	0.09	0.85	6
2b	0.7 ± 0.09	6.8	0.19	0.19	0.02	21
Tissue residue 3	11.5 ± 1.88	51.0	0.16	0.09	0.03	863

stroma still retains its lamellar organization and the collagen fibers retain their normal length, diameter, apparent density and spacing.

There is, however, considerable loss of density in the ground substance and the 64 nm periodicity of collagen becomes more readily seen even at low magnification (Fig. 1). In some preparations there appears to be an interlamellar swelling and/or separation. Subsequent repeated extraction of the cornea with 1.0 M $CaCl_2$ yields about 30% of the hexosamine in solubilized form; a quarter of it is obtained as a precipitate on dialysis against distilled water (fraction 2b) while the main bulk remains in solution (fraction 2a). After extraction, the cornea still contains about 50% of its total hexosamine (fraction 3).

Corneas fixed after the $CaCl_2$ extraction still showed recognizable lamellar organization at the light microscopic level (Fig. 2) as well as normal mature collagen fibers at the electron microscopic level (Figs. 3 and 4). There appeared to be no significant difference in degree of extraction between anterior and posterior lamellae.

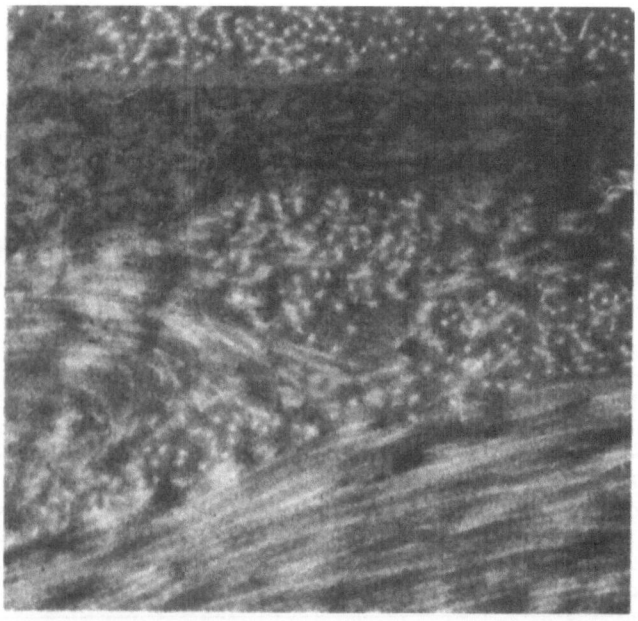

Fig. 1. Sodium chloride extracted steer cornea. Extraction under the conditions of this study, i.e. with cornea intact and epithelium and endothelium present, removes about 20% of the total extractable hexosamine and leaves the gross and fine structure of the cornea intact. Note the regular thick lamellar array of collagen fibers and the remnant of a keratocyte cell process (C) between two lamellae. The periodicity of the collagen is evident in the longitudinally sectioned fibers. An essential negative imaging of the collagen fibers is seen in the cross sectioned lamellae in the epoxy resin embedding procedure. X34,400

Chemical analysis revealed that all fractions contain glycosaminoglycan bound hexosamine as well as nonglycosaminoglycan hexosamine (Table 2), the latter being released as low molecular weight (dialysable) split products on pronase digestion and being separable from the glycosaminoglycans by gel filtration (Fig. 5). On the basis of the data of Tables 1 and 2 it may be calculated that the glycosaminoglycan content of the fractions 1a-2b is between 10 and 15% of the extracted material and accounts for 30-60% of the total hexosamine. In all extracts the ratio of KS/CS was determined by thin layer chromatography and found to be 1.8-2.2.

The NaCl and CaCl$_2$ extracts contain a small portion of soluble collagen (6.5% of total collagen) which precipitates together with a glycosaminoglycan and nonglycosaminoglycan fraction after dialysis. The main bulk of the collagen of the bovine corneas remains unextracted (Table 1; Figs. 3 & 4).

2. ^{14}C-glucosamine incorporation

Incubation of the cornea in vitro in the presence of l-^{14}C glucosamine results in a specific labeling of all fractions.

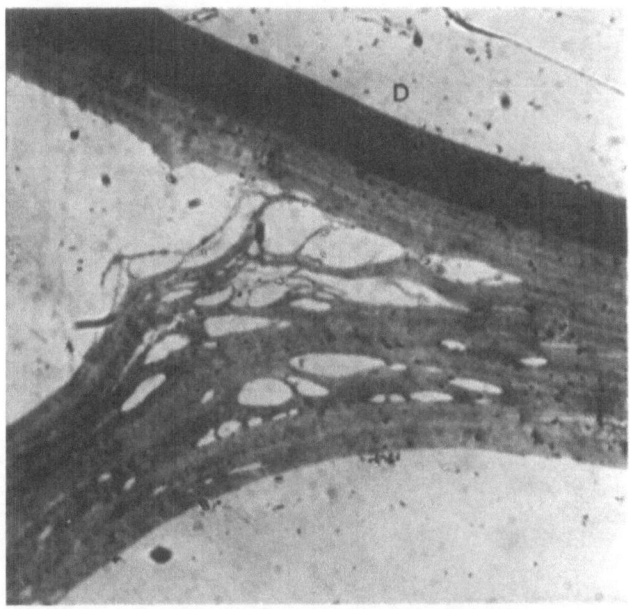

Fig. 2. One micron epon section of NaCl-CaCl$_2$ extracted bovine cornea stained with methylene blue – Azure II. It is evident that in this series of experiments the double extraction left both the fibrillary and lamellar organization of the cornea essentially intact. Although there is some separation of lamellae and interlamellar swelling to the point of some gross distortion of structure, the lamellae closest to Descemet's membrane (D) appear normal as do portions of those at some distance. X320

Table 2. Percent distribution of hexosamine containing macromolecules in individual fractions obtained by stepwise elution of bovine cornea. Keratan sulfate and chondroitin sulfate were isolated 100% from the extracts after pronase digestion and separated by thin layer chromatography. The non-glycosaminoglycan hexosamine refers to the hexosamine which is released in dialysable form after proteolytic digestion and may be separated from the glycosaminoglycans by gel filtration.

Subfraction	CS-hexosamine	KS-hexosamine	non-GAG[1] hexosamine
1a	16	24	60
1b	11	20	69
2a	21	39	40
2b	10	18	72
3	15	31	54

[1] GAG: glucosaminoglycon.

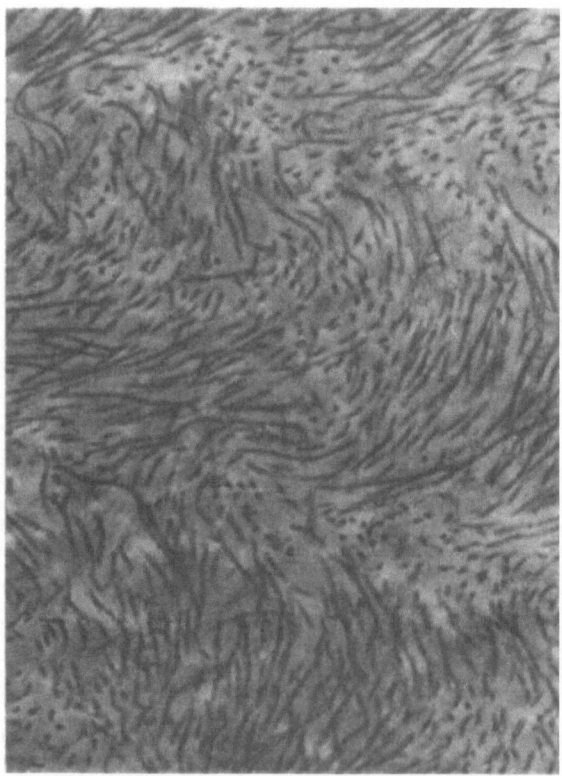

Fig. 3. Electron microscopic examination of NaCl-CaCl$_2$ extracted bovine cornea in this experimental series shows intact, long collagen fibers as well as some indication of the lamellar organization. X34,400

The specific activity of the KS of fraction 1a clearly exceeds that of the KS of fraction 2, the ratio of their specific activities being 3.5-5.0 under either experimental condition. From the data of Table 3 it can be concluded that (a) at least 2 metabolically independent KS fractions exist in the cornea and that (b) there is no precursor-product relationship between the KS of fractions 1a and 2a. This is indicated by the fact that the ratio of the specific activities of KS1a/KS2a found in the pulse experiment undergoes no change during the chase. Taking into consideration that the quantity of KS 2a is about twice as high as that of KS 1a and that the newly synthesized labeled material is diluted by the KS already present, it turns out that after continuous labeling the total radioactivity incorporated into the KS 1a fraction is higher by about 50% as compared with that incorporated into KS 2a.

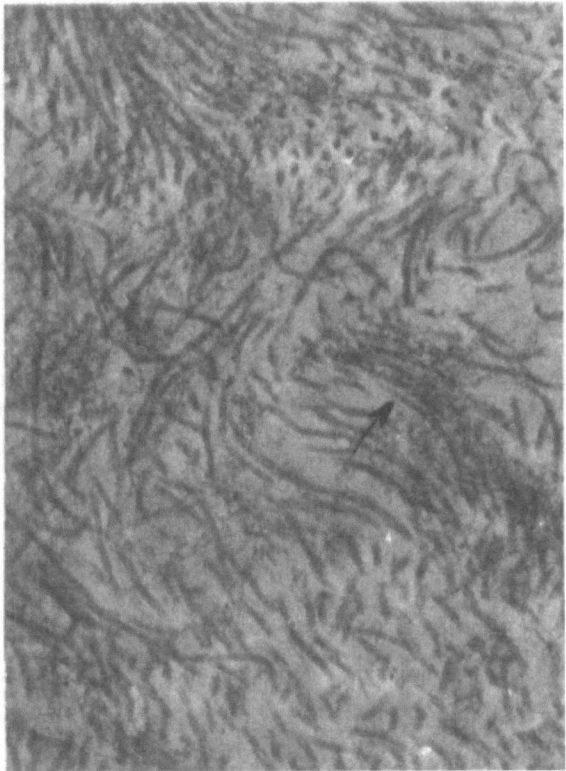

Fig. 4. Higher magnification electron micrograph of NaCl-CaCl$_2$ extracted bovine cornea showing evident periodicity of longitudinally sectioned collagen fibers as well as uniformity of fiber diameter in both longitudinal and cross section fibers. Fine fibrillar material associated with some bundles of collagen fibers may represent unextracted glycoprotein or the basal lamina-like material reported in previous studies (Kaye, et al., 1974; 1976) X51,600

259

On the basis of this calculation a higher rate of synthesis of KS 1a can be assumed.

The possibility of the existence of different pools for the synthesis of the non-glycosaminoglycan fractions of 1a and 2a is suggested by the nearly 10 times greater labeling of the hexosamine in fraction 1a in all experiments.

In contrast to KS and the non-glycosaminoglycan hexosamine the specific radioactivies of CS fractions 1a and 1b in the cornea are approximately the same in all experiments, thus suggesting a single or common site for the biosynthesis of all CS fractions.

DISCUSSION

Previous studies from this group (Cremer-Bartels & Dische, 1975; Kaye, et al., 1974; Kaye, et al., 1976; Dische, et al., 1977) have shown that extraction of pre-swollen, minced or homogenized bovine corneas with 0.155 M NaCl can remove up to 80% of the total extractable hexosaminoglycans without affecting significantly the capacity of the remaining interfibrillary matrix to support the collagen fibrils in their spatial arrangement and their longitudinal course. Subsequent extraction with 1.0 M $CaCl_2$ removed nearly 95% of the remaining extractable hexosaminoglycans and produced profound morphologic effects visible at the electron microscopic level. The organization of the collagen into thick banded fibers of indeterminate length was totally disrupted and there remained only short (0.05-0.1 μm) fibers of about half the diameter of the collagen fibers remaining after NaCl extraction. It was suggested that this phenomenon may be explained by the existence of two proteoglycan types with different functional properties: the NaCl soluble fraction (Fraction 1a) not being involved in the maintenance of collagen structure while the $CaCl_2$ soluble macromolecules are closely associated with the collagen fibers. This assumption is supported by the observation of Smith & Frame (1969) who found that there is an electron-dense material which surrounds each collagen fibril and sends out microfibrils which attach themselves to certain discrete points on adjacent

Table 3. Specific ^{14}C-radioactivities of keratan sulfate, chondroitin sulfate and non-glycosaminoglycan fractions after incorporation in vitro of 1 - [14]C glucosamine into bovine cornea. The specific labeling was performed in a pulse experiment (0.5 h), a pulse-chase experiment (0.5 h pulse, 5.5 h chase) and by continuous labeling for 6 h under conditions specified in 'Methods'.

| Subfraction | Specific radioactivity (cpm x10⁻³/μMol hexosamine) | | | | | | | | |
| | Pulse-experiment | | | Pulse-chase experiment | | | continuous labeling experiment | | |
	KS	CS	nonGAG	KS	CS	nonGAG	KS	CS	nonGAG
1a	2.0	1.5	12.5	10.6	15.2	69.9	50.1	63.4	100.0
2a	0.6	1.2	1.0	2.8	15.0	2.0	10.0	84.1	26.0
3	1.5	2.5	0.5	7.4	8.0	1.5	28.2	49.5	8.3

collagen fibrils. After extraction of NaCl soluble proteoglycans the residual proteoglycans apparently prevent the collapse of the fibrillary structure of the stroma by forming bridges between adjacent fibrils at certain strategic points and offering adequate resistance to shearing forces by a firm attachment to the collagen fibrils and a high, probably structural, viscosity.

The low yield on extraction in the present series of experiments is presumably due to the essentially intact state of the corneas during extraction. In each instance the epithelium and, presumably, the endothelium were present. This condition thereby restricted the surface available for diffusion of the extraction media into the corneal stroma. That the low level of yield is probably associated with an incomplete extraction is supported by the fact that lamellar organization and collagen fibril structure are only minimally affected by the double extraction (Figs. 2-4).

The corneal collagen is generally believed not to show any significant turnover in the adult animal. In our experiments, however, a small portion of collagen is soluble in saline solution and co-precipitates with proteoglycans on removal of the NaCl and $CaCl_2$, respectively. This result suggests that the corneal collagen may exhibit chemical heterogeneity, a minor saline soluble fraction being involved in the formation of proteoglycan aggregates.

The different specific radioactivities of the keratan sulfate fractions 1a and 2a (Table 3) and the constant ratio of these specific radioactivities in the pulse experiments, as well as in the pulse-chase and in the continuous labeling experiments, suggest the existence of two topographically different sites of keratan sulfate biosynthesis, one delivering the NaCl-soluble highly labeled keratan sulfate and the other the $CaCl_2$-soluble keratan sulfate having a lower specific radioactivity. Considering the portions of keratan sulfate present in the NaCl (1a) and $CaCl_2$ (2a) fraction, the differences of the specific radioactivity cannot be related to different rates of biosynthesis from the same precursor pool. No conclusions about the locus of the keratan sulfate synthesis can be drawn from the described experiments. However, since Hay et al. (1972) reported on the biosynthesis of ^{14}C-labeled material in the epithelium from which the product of synthesis was transferred to the stroma and considering the fact that the ^{14}C- and ^{35}S-incorporation into the corneal keratan sulfate drops to very low values after removing the epithelium (Cremer, et al., 1973) a localization of one of the keratan sulfate synthesizing sites in the epithelium cannot be excluded.

REFERENCES

Bitter, F. & Muir, H.M.: Modified uronic acid carbozole reaction. *Analyt. Biochem.* 4: *330-334*, (1962).

Boas, F.: Methods for determination of hexosamine in tissues. *J. biol. Chem.* 204: *553-563*, 1953.

Cremer-Bartels, G. & Buddecke, E.: Factors regulating the keratan sulfate. Biosynthesis in bovine cornea. *Expl. Eye Res.* 14: *171-172*, (1972).

Cremer-Bartels, G. & Dische, Z.: Comparison of glycosaminoglycans of elasmo branch and mammalian corneas. *Archs. Ophthal. (Paris)* 35: *27-32*, (1975).

Dische, Z.: Biochemistry of connective tissue of the vertebrate eye. *Int. Rev. Connective Tissue Res.* 5: *209-274,* (1970).

Dische, Z., Cremer-Bartels, G. & Kaye, G.: v I, *Expl. Eye Res.* (In Press)

Hay, E.D. & Dodson, J.N.: Secretion of collagen by corneal epithelium. *J. Cell Biol.* 57: *190-213,* (1973).

Humbel, G. & Chamoles, B.: Sequential thin layer chromatography of urinary acid glucosaminoglycans. *Clinica Chim. Acta* 40: *209-293,* 1973.

Kaye, G.I., Cremer-Bartels, G., Buddecke, E. & Dische, Z.: Structure of the Eye III Yamada, E., Mishima, S., *Jap. J. Ophthal. Suppl.* 63: *63-76,* 1976.

Smith, J.W. & Frame, J.: Observations on collagen and protein polysaccharide complex of rabbit cornea. *J. Cell Sci.* 4: *421-4336,* (1969).

Authors' address:

Ophthalmology Research

College of Physicians and Surgeons Columbia University

630 West 168th Street

New York, N.Y. 10032 U.S.A.

THE ANTIGENICITY OF NON-VIABLE EXPERIMENTAL CORNEAL XENOGRAFTS

DONALD J. DOUGHMAN, LLOYD MINAAI &
ELIZABETH A. MINDRUP

(Minneapolis, U.S.A.)

ABSTRACT

Chicken corneas were rendered non-viable by repeated freeze-thaw injury for transplantation intralamellarly into rabbits. These non-viable chicken xenografts had a modest, but statistically significant, delayed rejection time when compared to fresh controls. Viable chicken corneas with the epithelium removed prior to transplantation showed a similar delay in rejection time. These data suggest that prolonged survival of non-viable xenografts after freeze-thaw injury or of viable corneas after removal of epithelium is probably secondary to donor hypocellularity.

INTRODUCTION

This laboratory has previously reported prolonged survival of experimental chicken and guinea pig corneal xenografts in rabbits after three weeks of organ culture (Doughman, et al., 1976). Since there is a reduction of the epithelial and stromal cell population during organ culture (Hall, et al., 1975; Summerlin, et al., 1973: Van Horn, et al., 1975) it is possible that reduced viability accounted for this antigenic modification. However, whether or not non-viable corneal tissue can stimulate an immune response was not clear after reviewing the literature. Freeze-dried skin and bone allografts have reduced antigenicity presumably due to loss of histocompatability antigens (Abbott, 1969; Burwell, 1963). Spleen and kidney cells frozen and thawed three times lost their ability to immunize their host (Brent, 1958). Basu & Ormsby (1956), Kornbleuth, et al., (1962), Maumenee (1960) and Silverstein & Khodadoust (1973) found that non-viable corneal tissue is non-antigenic. Others, using freeze-thawed interlamellar porcine corneal xenografts in rabbits, observed no delay in rejection when they were compared to fresh controls (Lorenzetti & Kaufman, 1966). It is the purpose of this paper to investigate the antigenicity of non-viable experimental chicken xenografts in the rabbit.

Supported in part by USPHS Grant 1R01 EY01211, 5T01 EY00027 and Minnesota Lions Eye Bank.

MATERIALS AND METHODS

Recipient Animals

Sixty-five healthy, adult Dutch and New Zealand rabbits of both sexes weighing 2-4 kg were used as recipients after stabilization in our animal facility.

Donor Corneas

Donor corneas came from paired eyes of mixed breed adult chickens of both sexes. All donor corneas were carefully removed from the globe with a 2-3 mm rim of sclera as previously described (Doughman, et al., 1976). Five mm whole-thickness buttons were immediately transplanted from one of the paired corneas as a fresh control, and the other paired cornea was immediately frozen at $-70°C$ for 8-24 hrs and allowed to completely thaw. This cycle of freeze-thaw was repeated two more times, then a 5 mm whole thickness button was transplanted as a non-viable cornea to a recipient animal. Twenty-four animals were in each group. To reduce the cellularity of donor corneas without affecting the viability, the epithelium was completely removed, by scraping with a knife blade, from one of a fresh pair, and the cornea was transplanted immediately. The paired cornea with epithelium intact was then transplanted and served as a control as described above. Eight animals were in each group.

Determination of Viability

Based upon the work of McPherson, et al. (1956) organ culture was selected to assess corneal viability. All donor rims from the fresh, freeze-thaw and epithelium-removed groups were divided and one half explanted in organ culture media as previously described (Doughman, et al., 1976). The other half was placed in formalin for histologic examination. The medium for organ culture consisted of the following ingredients: (1) Minimum Essential Medium (Eagle's) with Earle's salt without L-glutamine; (2) decomplemented calf serum in a 10% final concentration; (3) L-glutamine in a 1% final concentration; and (4) an antibiotic-antimycotic mixture consisting of penicillin (10,000 units/ml), amphotericin (25 ug/ml), and streptomycin (10 mg/ml) added at a concentration of 1% in the final mixture. The donor rims were washed three times in the medium, placed in plastic Petri dishes endothelial side up, covered with medium, and placed in a water-jacketed tissue culture incubator at $37°C$ with an atmosphere of 95% air and 5% CO_2, and with 100% humidity. The medium was changed twice a week. Contaminated donor rims were discarded. The incidence of culture contamination was less than 1%. The explanted rims were examined three times a week for cell growth using an inverted phase microscope. Any sign of cell outgrowth regardless of its origin was considered a sign of viability. All corneas from the freeze-thaw group whose donor rims showed evidence of cellular outgrowth were considered viable and therefore eliminated from the study. If no sign of cell outgrowth from the freeze-thaw donor rims had occurred by the sixth week of culture, the explant was considered non-viable and the donor cornea from which it had come was kept in the non-viable group. Selected non-viable explants were examined histologically at the conclusion of the experiment.

Grafting Technique

One of us (E.M.) performed all the surgery. Only one eye, usually the right eye, of each rabbit was used. Sodium pentobarbital anesthesia was induced via the marginal ear vein, the eye proptosed, and a 6 mm midstromal intralamellar pocket was dissected 1-2 mm from the limbus as previously described (Doughman, et al., 1976; Lorenzetti & Kaufman, 1966). A 5 mm whole-thickness donor cornea was then inserted into the intralamellar pocket and the pocket closed with two 8-0 silk sutures. Except for antibiotic drops at the time of surgery, no medication was used during the experiment. To encourage graft rejection, suture removal was delayed until blood vessels from the limbus had reached the edge of the graft (Silverstein & Khodadoust, 1973, Polack, 1962).

Animal Evaluation

Animals were excluded from the study if there were any operative or post operative complications causing immediate graft opacification.

To avoid confusion with non-immunological causes of graft opacification, xenograft rejection was diagnosed only if the graft was clear postoperatively and at least five days had elapsed from surgery to the onset of rejection, the earliest time noted by others when the corneal xenograft rejection may begin (Silverstein, et al., 1970).

The animals were observed daily with a slit lamp. The grafts were graded in a single blind fashion as described before (Doughman, et al., 1976; Lorenzetti & Kaufman, 1966), on the basis of graft clarity and vascularization. (Fig. 1) Rejection was diagnosed when a score of two or more for either vascularization or clarity occurred. Based upon the clinical characteristics of rejection in our controls as well as data from previous studies (Doughman, et al., 1976; Lorenzetti & Kaufman, 1966), this scoring system readily differentiated rejection from non-rejection. Only xenografts that were adequately exposed to the afferent immune limb, i.e., those that attained vascularization scores of at least 1, were included in this study.

Histological examinations were performed on selected non-viable, epithelium-removed and control xenografts.

RESULTS

All of the control corneas were rejected by day 14. (Table 1) Histologic examination of the controls showed infiltration from the limbus with lymphocytes, polymorphonuclear leukocytes, and blood vessels similar to that previously described by Doughman, et al., (1976) and others (Lee & Basu, 1973; Leibowitz & Luzzio, 1970; Silverstein, et al., 1970). Initially, twenty-four chicken corneas were in the experimental freeze-thaw group. Ten of the donor rims showed evidence of cellular outgrowth in organ culture (Fig. 2) and therefore were excluded from this group. The remaining

Grading

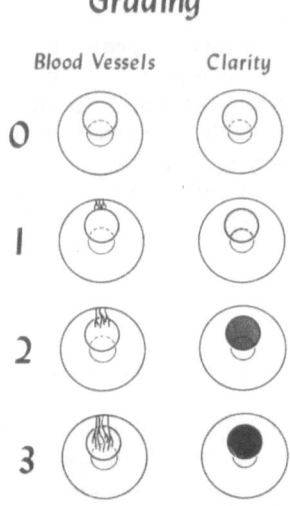

Fig. 1. Schematic grading representation of xenograft reaction based on graft vascularization and clarity. Blood vessel grading: 0, no vessels; 1, vessels to graft edge; 2, vessels into less than 1/2 of graft; 3, vessels into more than 1/2 of graft. Clarity grading: 0, iris and pupil detail clear; 1, slight haze to graft; 2, moderate haze to graft, iris and pupil still visible; 3, iris and pupil not visible.

Table 1. Rejection of Chicken to Rabbit Corneal Xenografts.

Donor Group	Number of Grafts	Percent Rejected	Mean Rejection Time (Day + 1SD)	P Value*
Control**	32	100	8.33 ± 1.97	
Non-viable	14	100	12.78 ± 2.96	< 0.001
Epithelium-removed	8	100	13.75 ± 2.40	< 0.001

* Two tailed vs. Control
** The control group is comprised of pooled controls of the non-viable and epithelium-removed groups. This number is greater than the sum of the experimental grafts as ten from the non-viable group were eliminated because, in organ culture, donor rims were viable.

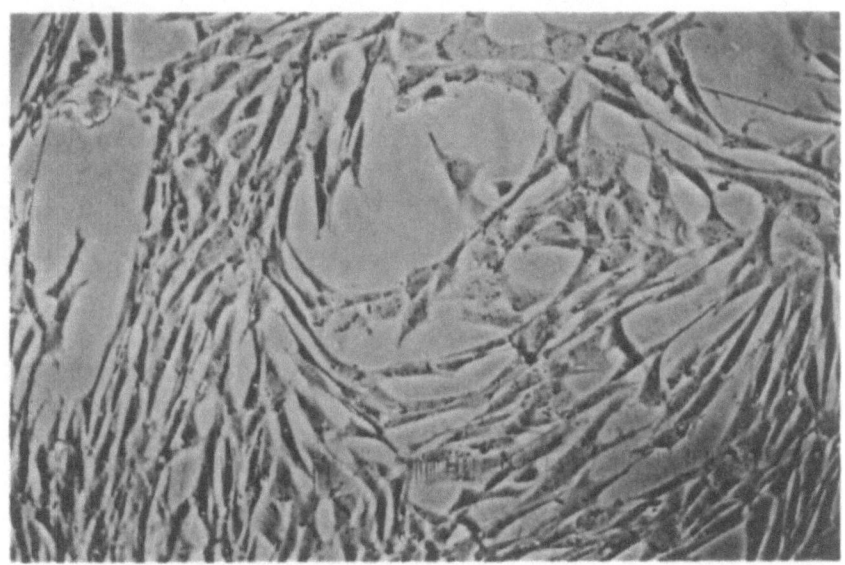

Fig. 2. Three week organ culture rim of donor cornea from freeze-thaw group show-ing outgrowth of fibroblastic cells, presumably stromal in origin, indicating that the cornea was viable. (Phase contrast, original magnification x 100)

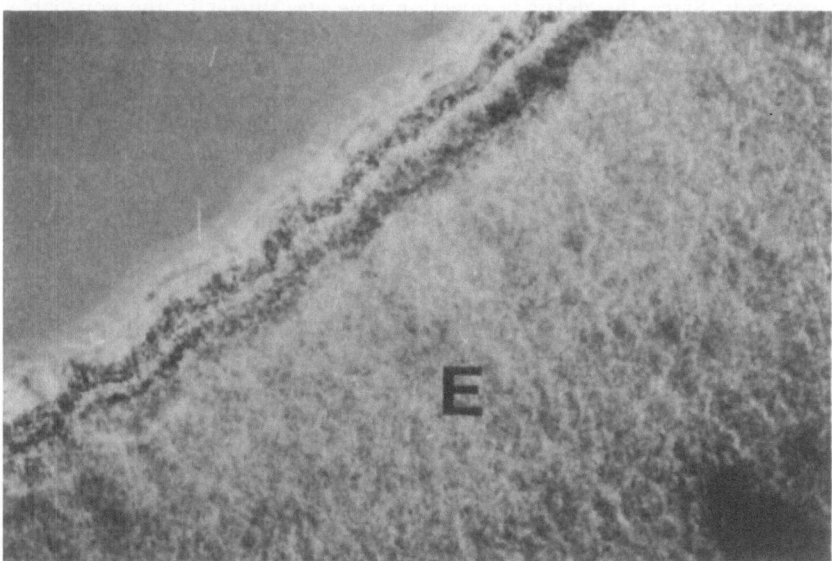

Fig. 3. Six week organ culture rims of donor cornea from the freeze-thaw group showing no outgrowth of cells from the edge of the explant (E) indicating a non-viable cornea. (Phase contrast, original magnification x 100)

14 showed no evidence of cellular outgrowth from the donor rim explant during the six weeks of organ culture (Fig. 3) and comprised the non-viable group. As seen in Table 1, these non-viable xenografts had a statistically significant delay in rejection time. A similar delay was seen when fresh, viable corneas were transplanted after the epithelium had been removed (Table 1). Histological examination of selected organ cultured non-viable donor rims showed a total absence of cells. Explants from the epithelium-removed group as well as the control group showed extensive cellular outgrowth by 2-3 weeks of organ culture indicating viability.

DISCUSSION

In this experiment, all non-viable chicken to rabbit xenografts were rejected, but the rejection times showed a statistically significant delay when compared to fresh controls. A similar delay could be seen when the epithelium was removed from fresh viable donor corneal xenografts prior to transplantation. Therefore, modification of rabbit corneal xenograft reaction occurs when the donor cornea is rendered non-viable by repeated freeze-thaw injury or when the epithelium is removed from viable donor corneas. However, this modification is manifested by only a modest delay in rejection time and not by elimination of the xenograft response. The most likely reason for this delay is reduction of donor cellularity. This is supported by the results from the epithelium-removed group where the donor cornea was viable as proven by extensive outgrowth of cells in organ culture from the donor rim. Since the delay in rejection time was similar to the non-viable group, this suggests that the effect freeze-thaw injury has on the xenograft response is due to reduction in number of cells, thus reducing the antigenic load.

The xenograft model was chosen because, unlike experimental rabbit corneal allografts, xenografts produce consistent and severe reactions based upon well documented immunologic mechanisms (Elliot & Leibowitz, 1965). The placement of the corneal button is important in this model. A centrally placed intralamellar xenograft may not reject because of its isolation from the afferent immune limbus (Geerats, et al., 1965). In this study we assured immunologic exposure of the xenograft to the host by placing the donor cornea near the limbus and excluding from our data any graft from which the blood vessels from the limbus had not grown to the graft edge. (Less than 1% of grafts excluded were excluded on this basis). Early rejection of our control xenografts confirmed that our experimental design was adequate.

How do we reconcile our experimental results with the conclusions of others? Lorenzetti & Kaufman (1966) noted no significant difference in rejection time between fresh and frozen porcine interlamellar corneal xenografts in rabbits. They assumed that freezing the cornea at $-90°$F for 18-24 hrs before thawing would render the cornea non-viable. No viability tests were performed on these corneas to prove this assumption. In pilot studies done for this experiment, we froze donor corneas at $-70°$C for 18-24 hrs before thawing and found that all of these corneas had extensive cell out-growth after explantation in organ culture, indicating no loss of viability. Even after three freeze-thaw cycles, 35.7% (10/28) of the chicken corneas in this study remained viable as evidenced by cellular outgrowth during organ culture. Although chicken corneas may be more resistant to freeze-thaw damage than porcine corneas, it is probable that the forzen porcine corneal xenografts used by Lorenzetti & Kaufman (1966) were viable and that explains why they observed no delay in rejection time. This points to the importance of determinig the viability of the donor cornea. It is critical to the experimental design and has not been previously reported in other stud-ies.

Maumenee (1960) and Silverstein (1973) state that non-viable corneal tissue is not antigenic. However, they discussed human allografts and pre-sented no experimental data. The results of these animal xenograft experi-ments cannot be extrapolated to the human allograft situation and therefore their conclusions cannot be refuted or supported. The present studies do support the conclusions of Basu & Ormsby (1956) and Kornbleuth, et al. (1962) that frozen experimental allografts were antigenically modified. However, experimental allografts may not be comparable to experimental xenografts. Although Lee & Basu (1973) feel that experimental corneal xenografts and allografts differ only in degree and severity, Silverstein & Khodadoust (1973) feel that allografts and xenografts are not comparable since xenografts may carry species-specific antigens producing antibodies that may mediate xenograft rejections in a manner different from that of allograft rejections. In addition, viability was not determined in either of these studies. For these reasons these studies cannot be compared.

Do these data explain the results previously reported that organ cultured xenografts are immunologically modified (Doughman, et al., 1976)? In that study organ cultured chicken and guinea pig corneas became increasingly hypocellular during organ culture and after three weeks showed a delay in rejection time similar to the non-viable and epithelium-removed group in this study. Therefore, this present study supports (but does not confirm) the view that antigen modification after organ·culture may be due to donor hypocellularity.

REFERENCES

Abbott, M.A. The Failure of lyopholized skin to induce allograft immunity. *Surg. Forum* 20: *297-299* (1969).

Brent, L. Tissue transplantation immunity. *Prog. Allergy* 5: *271-348* (1958).

Burwell, R.G. Studies in transplantation of bone. *J. Bone Jt. Surg. (Brit.)* 45: *386-391* (1963).

Basu, P.K. & Ormsby, H.L. Intralamellar frozen-stored corneal homografts in rabbits. *Am. J. Ophthal.* 42: *71-76* (1956).

Doughman, D.J., Miller, G.E., Mindrup, E.A. & Harris, J.E. The fate of experimental organ-cultured xenografts. *Transplantation* 22: *132-137* (1976).

Elliott, J.H. & Leibowitz, H.M. Corneal immune rings associated with heterograft rejec-tion. *Archs. Ophthal.* 73: *519-527* (1965).

Geerats, W.J., Lederman, J.R., Woo, I. & Guerry, D. In vivo corneal graft reactions after short-term storage. *Am. J. Ophthal.* 60: *28-39* (1965).

Hall, J.M., Smolin, G., Doughman, D.J., Krasnsobroa, H., & Schmitt, M.K. Changes in the antigenic composition of cultured bovine corneas. *Invest. Ophthal.* 14: *295-299* (1975).

Kornbleuth, W., Nelken, E. & Nelken, D. Modified late clouding in experimental corneal grafts. *Am. J. Ophthal.* 54: *76-82* (1962).

Lee, D.S. & Basu, P.K. A comparative study of the corneal graft reaction in allo- and xenograft models. *Can. J. Ophthal.* 8: *444-450* (1973).

Leibowitz, H.M. & Luzzio, A.J. Transplantation antigens in keratoplasty. *Archs. Ophthal.* 83: *215-222* (1970).

Lorenzetti, D.W.C. & Kaufman, H.E. Experimental production of graft reactions with suppression by topical steroids. *Archs. Ophthal.* 76: *274-281* (1966).

Maumenee, A.E. Biological responses to corneal homografts. *Trans. Am. Acad. Ophthal. Otto-lar.* 64: *765-774* (1960).

McPherson, S.D., Drahiem, J.W., Evans, V.J. & Earle, W.R. The viability of fresh and frozen corneas as determined by tissue culture. *Am. J. Ophthal.* 41: *513-519* (1956).

Polack F.M. Histopathological and histochemical alterations in the early stages of corneal graft rejection. *J. exp. Med.* 116: *709-717* (1962).

Silverstein, A.M. & Khodadoust, A.A. Transplantation immunology of the cornea, in corneal graft failure, Ciba Fdn. Symp. 15 (new series), Associated Scientific Publishers, Amsterdam, 1973. pp. *105-125*.

Silverstein, A.M., Russman, A.M. & deLosa, A.S. Survival of donor epithelium in experimental corneal xenograft. *Am. J. Ophthal.* 69: *448-453* (1970).

Summerlin, W.T., Miller, G.E., Harris, J.E. & Good, R.A. The organ-cultured cornea: An in vitro study. *Invest. Ophthal.* 12: *176-180* (1973).

Van Horn, D.L., Doughman, D.J., Harris, J.E., Miller, G.E., Lindstrom, R. & Good, R. A. Ultra-structure of human organ cultured cornea. II. Stroma and epithelium. *Archs. Ophthal.* 93: *275-277* (1975).

Authors' address:
Department of Ophthalmology
Box 493 Mayo, University of Minnesota Hospitals,
University of Minnesota
Minneapolis, Minnesota, 55455
U.S.A.

MODIFICATION OF SULFHYDRYL GROUPS IN THE CORNEAL ENDOTHELIUM WITH ORGANIC MERCURIALS

HENRY F. EDELHAUSER, DIANE L. VAN HORN
& PATRICIA M. MILLER

(Milwaukee, Wisconsin U.S.A.)

ABSTRACT

The effects of blocking SH groups in the corneal endothelium were studied by perfusing the endothelial surfaces of isolated rabbit corneas with the organic mercurials PCMBS and PCMB. PCMBS caused an increase in the rate of corneal swelling due to disruption of the cell membranes. However, the endothelial barrier function remained at low concentrations. These cellular changes can progress from cell swelling to osmotic lysis with either an increase in concentration of PCMBS or perfusion time. The addition of glucose and either cysteine or reduced glutathione prevented corneal swelling and maintained endothelial ultrastructure.

The hydrophobic form of this compound, PCMB, penetrates cell membranes and in low concentrations causes a more pronounced effect on both corneal swelling and endothelial cell ultrastructure. These results suggest that membrane sulfhydryls are intimately involved in maintaining endothelial cell integrity and therefore the ability of the endothelial monolayer to function as both an effective barrier and pump necessary for preserving corneal detergescence and transparency.

INTRODUCTION

Many functions associated with cellular membranes are inhibited by reagents that bind free sulfhydryl groups (Garraban & Rega 1967, Scott et al., 1970, Sutherland et al., 1967, Rothstein, 1970). These studies have indicated that a given class of sulfhydryl groups can be intimately involved as part of a critical membrane protein (enzyme, transport protein, antigen, etc.) or closely associated with the membrane structure. Much information has been accumulated on the role of sulfhydryl groups in red cell membranes (Rothstein, 1971), and distinct 'classes' of sulfhydryl groups have been defined on the basis of their rates of reaction with and accessibility to different sulfhydryl binding reagents.

Little is known about sulfhydryls in the corneal endothelium although Dikstein & Maurice (1972) reported that the addition of reduced glutathione (GSH) to a bicarbonate perfusion media increases the efficiency of the endothelial pump. Further studies in our laboratory (McCarey et al., 1973) have shown that GSH added to glucose, bicarbonate Ringer's solution

This investigation was supported in part by a grant from the National Eye Institute EY-00933, 1-P30-EY-09131 and research funds from the Veteran's Administration.

271

will also maintain endothelial cellular integrity over extended periods of time. Anderson et al. (1974) have shown that GSH prevents depletion of endothelial cellular ATP, and stimulates trans-endothelial fluid transport by its auto-oxidation. Structurally related disulfides such as cysteine and homocysteine can also stimulate the pump.

More recent studies in our laboratory have shown that perfusion with diamide (a thiol-oxidizing agent) results in disruption of the endothelial cell barrier by causing junctional breakdown and/or contraction of microfilaments (Edelhauser, et al., 1976). This effect could be prevented by the addition of glucose to the perfusion medium and reversed by removal of the diamide and perfusion with a glutathione bicarbonate Ringer's solution (GBR).

Two organic mercurials, PCMB (p-chloromercuri-benzoate) and PCMBS (P-chloromercuriphenyl sulfonic acid) have been used extensively in other membrane systems to distinguish sulfhydryls on the outer surface of the membrane from those within the membrane. PCMB is hydrophobic and readily penetrates the cell membrane and attacks cytoplasmic sulfhydryls. PCMBS is hydrophilic and ionizes in aqueous solutions, it then has minimal penetration and interacts with membrane surface SH groups by mercaptide formation.

The purpose of this study was to use PCMB and PCMBS to chemically probe the role of SH groups in the corneal endothelium by determining the effects of mercurial perturbation on corneal endothelial function and structure.

MATERIALS AND METHODS

Paired eyes from albino rabbits (2-3 Kg) were excised and the corneas were mounted in a dual-chambered specular microscope which permits constant perfusion of the endothelium, sequential measurements of corneal thickness, and continuous observation of the mosaic-like pattern of the endothelial monolayer (McCarey et al., 1973). Changes in the endothelial cell pattern and corneal thickness were recorded throughout the perfusion, and swelling rate (μm/hr) was then calculated by regression analysis. A dose response for PCMBS was established by perfusing corneas with five different concentrations of PCMBS (5 and 2.5 x 10^{-4}, 7, 5 and 2.5 x 10^{-5}M) in bicarbonate Ringer's (BR) solution. The paired corneas were perfused with BR. The composition of the bicarbonate Ringer's solution was NaCl (6.521 g/l), KCl (0.358 g/l), CaCl$_2$ (0.115 g/l), MgCl$_2$ (0.159 g/l), NaHCO$_3$ (2.454 g/l) and NaH$_2$PO$_4$ (0.103 g/l).

The effect of exogenous thiol was studied by adding 2.5 x 10^{-3}M cysteine (CYS) or 1 x 10^{-3}M reduced glutathione (GSH) to BR containing 5 x 10^{-4}M PCMBS. The effects of adding 5mM glucose (GLU) to BR either alone or in combination with CYS or GSH containing 5 x 10^{-4}M PCMBS were also studied.

The effects of PCMBS and PCMB were compared by perfusing the corneal endothelium with equal molar concentration (5 x 10^{-4} or 5 x 10^{-5}M in

Table I. Effect of PCMBS on corneal swelling.

Molar Concentration of PCMBS in Bicarbonate Ringer's	Swelling Rate μm/hr
0 (Bicarbonate Ringer's)	13 ± 4*
2.5 × 10⁻⁵ M	18 ± 4
5 × 10⁻⁵ M	23 ± 2
7 × 10⁻⁵ M	31 ± 3
2.5 × 10⁻⁴ M	36 ± 3
5 × 10⁻⁴ M	74 ± 7

* Mean ± SE, swelling rates were calculated by regression analysis of sequential corneal thickness measurement taken over a 2-3 hour perfusion.
N = 3.

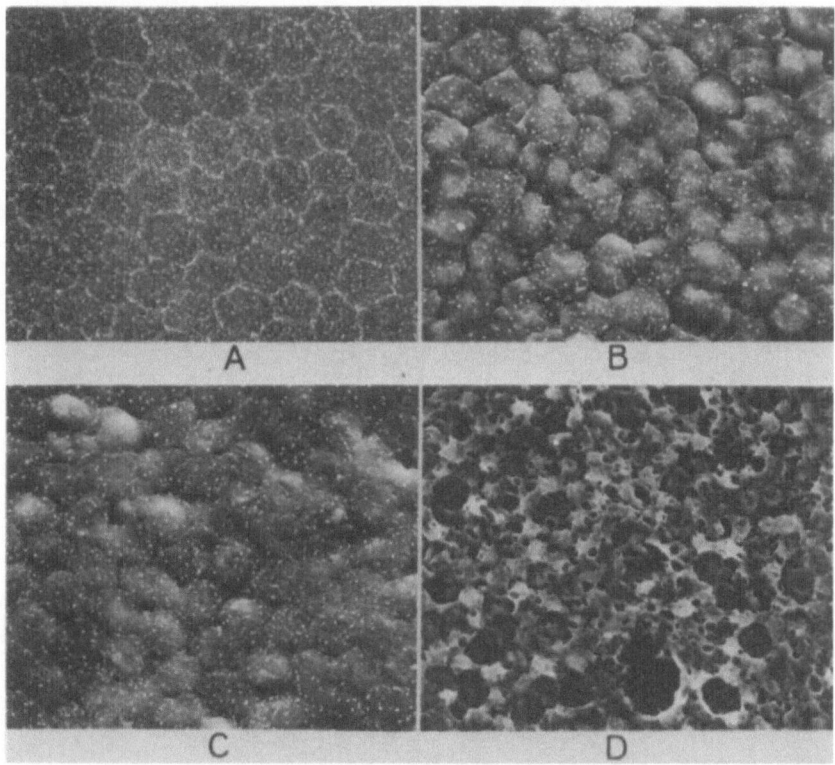

Fig. 1. SEM of corneal endothelial cells perfused for three hours with (A) bicarbonate Ringer's solution (B) 7 × 10⁻⁵ PCMBS, (C) 2.5 × 10⁻⁴ PCMBS and (D) 5 × 10⁻⁴ PCMBS. Cellular swelling is apparent in B and C. Cellular breakdown has occurred in D. (All × 750).

273

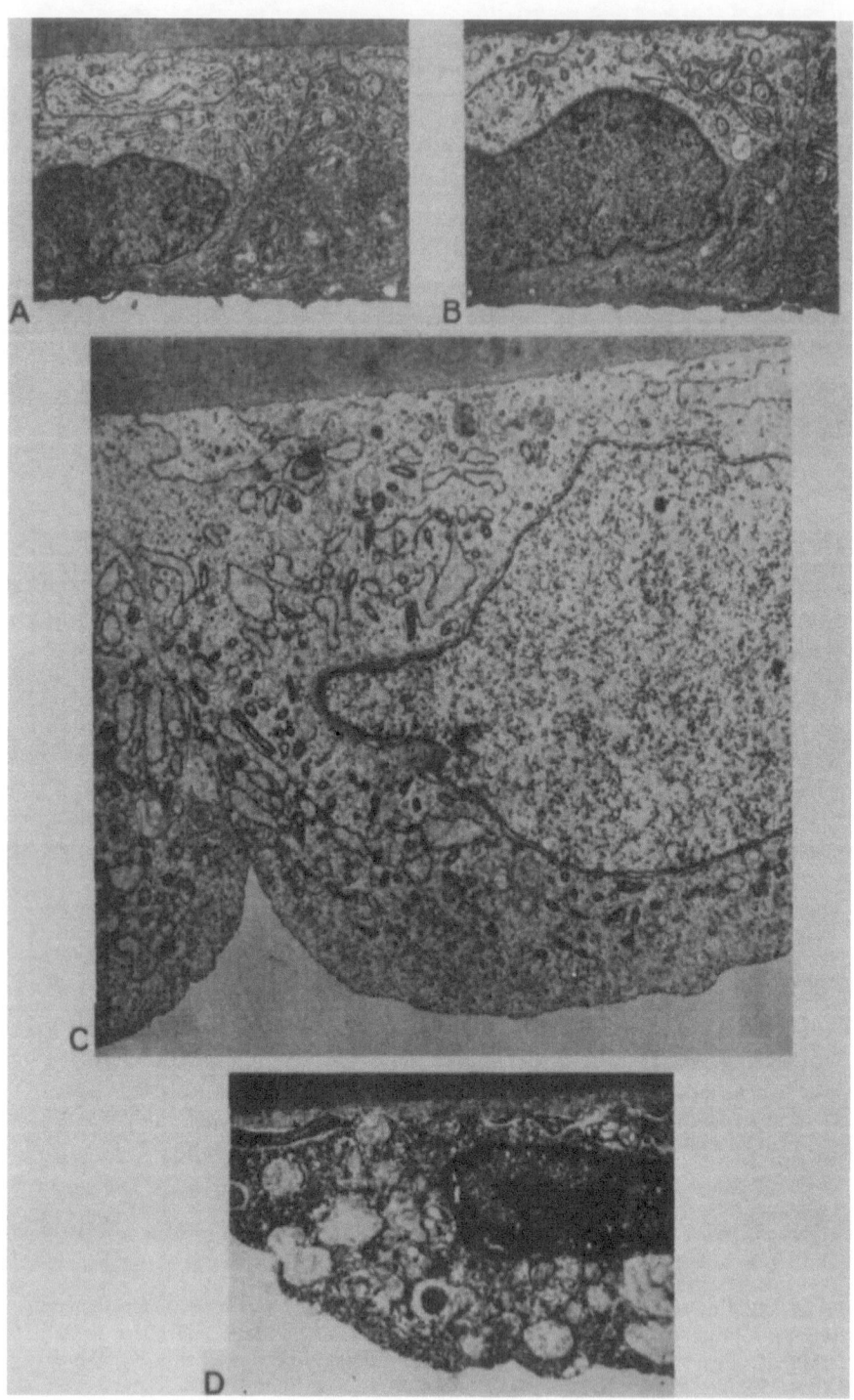

BR) of either PCMBS or PCMB. Both agents were added to BR. However, the low solubility of the PCMB required that it be dissolved in 0.2M NaOH prior to adding it to the BR. The pH of the final PCMB solution was then adjusted to 7.4 with 0.10M HCl.

The corneal endothelia were perfused at a constant rate of 20.6 μl/min. with a Harvard perfusion pump. Both temperature and pressure were monitored and maintained at 37°C and 15 ± 2mmHg respectively. The corneal epithelium in all experiments was intact and covered with medical grade silicone oil (No. 20 CSKS Dow Corning, Midland, Michigan).

At selected times during perfusion the corneas were removed from the specular microscope and fixed for electron microscopy in 2.7% glutaraldehyde in phosphate buffer (pH 7.2, 330 mOsm) for at least eight hours at 4°C. The corneas were then post-fixed in 2% osmium tetroxide and impregnated with a low viscosity epoxy resin. For scanning electron microscopy (SEM), the resin was washed from the endothelial surface of one half of each cornea according to a modified method of Cleveland & Schneider (1969). Small pieces of the other half of each cornea were embedded for transmission electron microscopy (TEM).

RESULTS

Perfusion of rabbit corneal endothelial cells with PCMBS in concentrations varying from 2.5×10^{-5}M to 5×10^{-4}M resulted in a progressive increase in the rate of corneal swelling from 18 to 74 μm/hr (Table I). Scanning and transmission electron microscopy revealed endothelial cell swelling at low concentrations and cell lysis and complete loss of endothelial barrier function at high concentrations (Figs. 1 & 2).

The effect of PCMBS on the corneal endothelium was decreased by the addition of glucose and/or exogenous thiol. The addition of 5mM glucose to a BR + 5×10^{-4}M PCMBS decreased the corneal swelling rate from 74 to 52 μm/hr (Fig. 3) and maintained an intact endothelium (Figs. 4B and 5B) when contrasted to the effect of BR + PCMBS without glucose (Figs. 4A and 5A). When exogenous thiol (cysteine or reduced glutathione) were added the corneas showed no increase in thickness (Figs. 3). There were, however, alterations in the endothelial surface morphology (Fig. 4C and 4E). TEM of these endothelial cells showed condensation of the mitochondria and a dense band of endothelial cell microfilaments at the apical cell borders (Figs. 5C and E). The PCMBS effect on corneal swelling and endothelial structure could be prevented with the further addition of 5mM glucose (Figs. 3, 4D and F and 5D & F).

Fig. 2. TEM of corneal endothelial cells perfused for three hours with (A) Bicarbonate Ringer's, (B) 7×10^{-5}M PCMBS, (C) 2.5×10^{-4}M PCMBS, (D) 5×10^{-4}M PCMBS. Intercellular edema is present in the basal cytoplasm of cells in B. In C the cytoplasm and all organelles except mitochondria are swollen resulting in a cobblestone appearance. In D the posterior plasma membrane of the cell is discontinuous and cellular organelles are difficult to identify. (All X 6700).

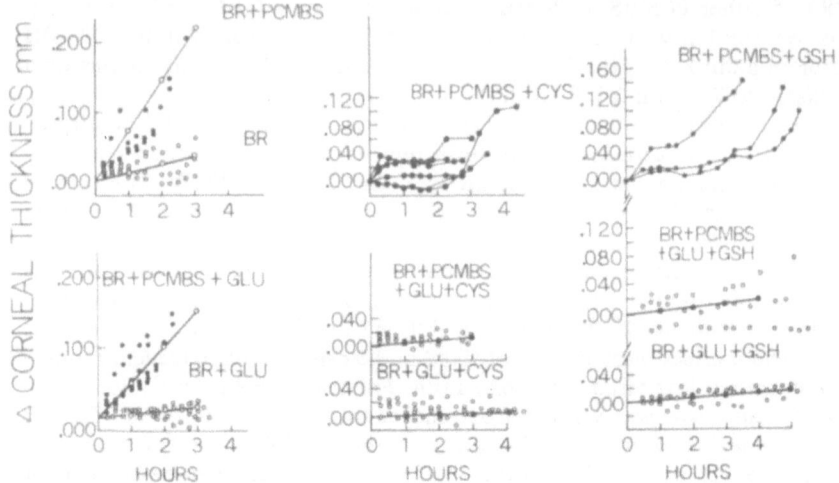

Fig. 3. Changes in corneal thickness with time in corneas perfused with bicarbonate Ringer's solution (BR) alone or in various combinations of 5×10^{-4} M PCMBS, cysteine (CYS), reduced glutathione (GSH) and glucose (GLU). The lines with open circles (left, upper and lower graphs) or solid circles (middle and right lower graphs) are regression lines for an "N" of 3 to 6 perfusions/line.

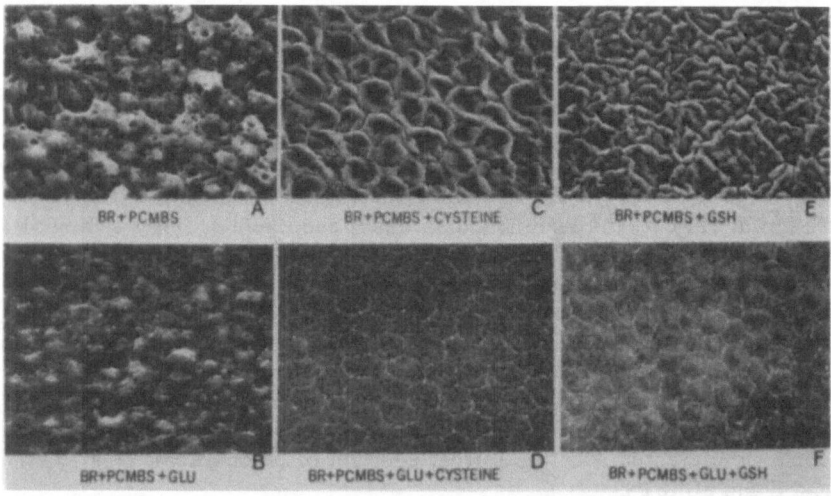

Fig. 4. SEM of corneas perfused with PCMBS in BR alone (A) or in various combinations with cysteine, reduced glutathione and glucose (B-F). (B) Endothelial mosaic-like pattern is obscured but cells are intact in presence of glucose. (C) Mosaic-like pattern is accentuated by irregular contour of posterior surface of endothelial cells in presence of cysteine. (D) Normal endothelial cell morphology is present with glucose and cysteine, (E) Cells have irregular contours with glutathione but are normal in appearance if glucose is also present (F). (All X 400).

276

Corneas perfused with PCMB, the hydrophobic form of PCMBS, increased in thickness at a greater rate than the paired controls perfused with equal molar concentrations of PCMBS (Fig. 6). Morphological alterations were also more severe in corneas perfused with 5×10^{-5} M PCMB compared to those perfused with 5×10^{-5} M PCMBS (Fig. 7).

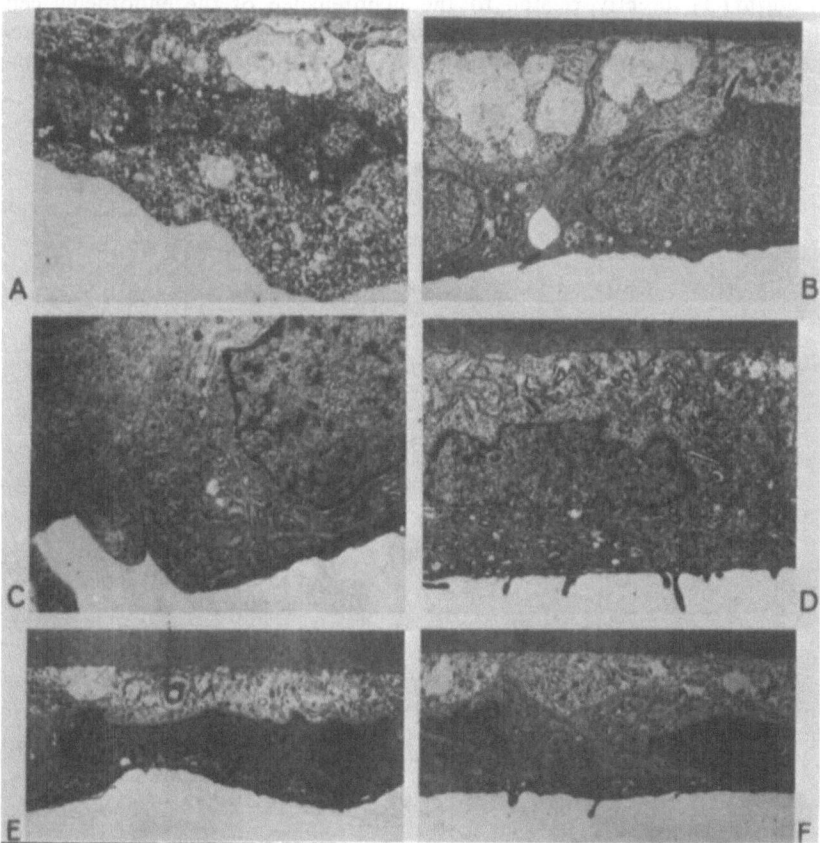

Fig. 5. TEM of endothelium of same corneas illustrated in Fig. 4. (A) Posterior plasma membrane is discontinuous and except for ribosomes and nucleus, subcellular organelles are not readily identifiable. (X 6800). (B) Basal cytoplasmic swelling has occurred in the presence of glucose. (x 8100). (C) Subcellular organelles are normal in appearance but configurational changes have occured in the presence of cysteine (note dense terminal web at the junctional complex). (x 6500). (D) Except for some basal edema, cells appear normal in the presence of glucose and cysteine. (x 7600). (E) Basal cytoplasmic swelling seems to contribute to irregular contour of cells. (x 7724). (F) Except for basal cytoplasmic swelling, cells appear normal in presence of glucose and reduced glutathione. (x 8700).

277

The results of this study show that perturbation of membrane SH groups with PCMBS leads to complete loss of the morphological integrity of the corneal endothelium as well as its function. The response is dose dependent.

Of particular importance is that the endothelial barrier function remains despite the high degree of membrane perturbation and cell swelling with PCMBS (2.5×10^{-4}M). This barrier function (low rate of corneal swelling $36\,\mu$m/hr) is directly related to the maintenance of the endothelial cell junctional complexes (Fig. 2C). In contrast, when the endothelial cell junctional complexes are disrupted by thiol-oxidation of the intracellular gluta-

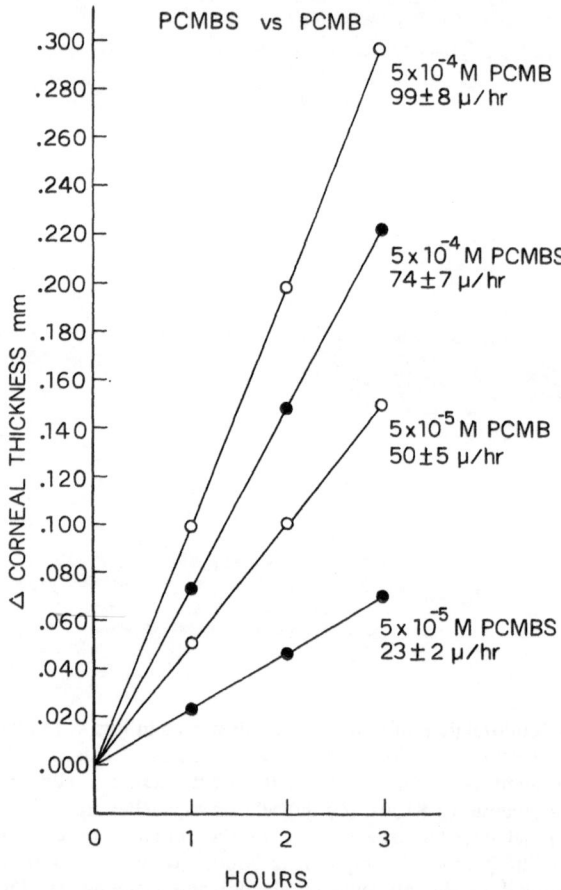

Fig. 6. Increases in corneal thickness with time in corneas perfused with equal molar concentrations of PCMB and PCMBS. The swelling rates (u/hr) are calculated by regression analysis an N-3 for each perfusion.

thione with diamide, loss of endothelial barrier function results leading to marked corneal swelling (Edelhauser et al., 1976). Similarly Sterling (1975) has reported that mercurials do not produce a gross breakdown of ileum brush border membranes or tight junctional integrity. The barrier function, and junctional complexes are only lost in the corneal endothelium by increasing the concentration of PCMBS (5×10^{-4}M) or extending the perfusion time of the lower concentrations.

Ultimately, as increased membrane sulfhydryls are attacked by the PCMBS cation and sugar transport is inhibited which will lead to osmotic cell lysis and complete loss of endothelial barrier function. Cell lysis results from a progressive structural and functional change in the cell from a normal state through the sublethal to a necrotic state. A similar progressive pattern of

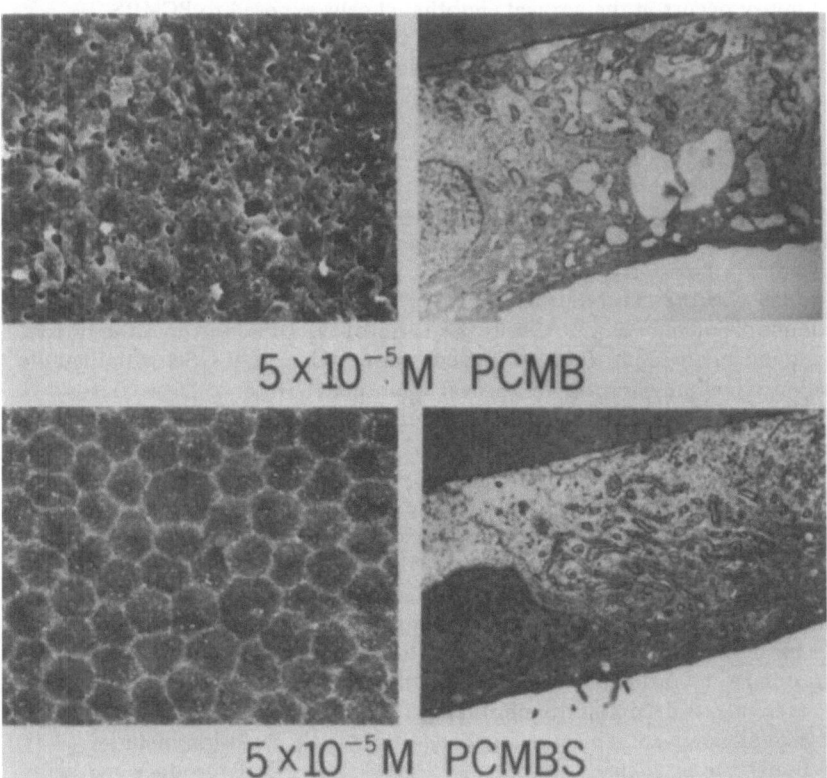

Fig. 7. SEM and TEM comparing morphological alterations after three hours of perfusion with equimolar (but low) concentrations of PCMB and PCMBS. PCMB which penetrates the cell membrane produces cellular vacuolization, and swelling of rough endoplasmic reticulum, nuclei and cytoplasm. PCMBS does little more than produce some basal cytoplasmic swelling and flappiness of junctions.
(SEM both X 600; TEM PCMB = X 5,500 PCMBS = X 11,600).

ultrastructural changes was observed with the use of PCMBS in Ehrlich Ascites tumor cells (Pentila & Trump 1975) and in the isolated kidney tubules of the flounder (Sahaphong & Trump 1971). These authors proposed that SH groups of the membranes are inhibited by mercaptide bonds with PCMBS, resulting in an increase in cell membrane permeability, loss of intracellular K^+, an influx of extracellular Na^+ and water into the cytoplasm and cisternae of the endoplasmic reticulum. This in turn would produce swelling of the cytoplasm, dilation of the endoplasmic reticulum and nuclear envelope (as observed in Fig. 2C). Condensation of the mitochondria (Fig. 2C) would also occur because of the shrinkage of the mitochondrial inner compartments due to loss of ions and water. After prolonged PCMBS treatment the cells undergo further swelling, the mitochondria gradually expand and ultimately cell lysis with high amplitude swelling of mitochondria and fragmentation of membrane systems occurs. A similar pattern of cell injury occurs in the corneal endothelial cells exposed to PCMBS.

Mercaptide bonds formed between PCMBS and membrane SH groups are reversible complexes in other membrane systems. The mercurials can be removed from the protein moiety by the addition of exogenous SH agents such as cysteine or reduced glutathione. In this study, we have compared the effect of the addition of a substrate (glucose) plus the SH agents. Our data show that the addition of either agent markedly decreased corneal swelling and enabled the endothelial cell junctions to remain intact. The addition of both glucose and cysteine or glutathione enabled complete physiological and structural protection of the corneal endothelium from PCMBS. Glucose can be utilized by the endothelium as a substrate for the production of reducing power in the form of NADPH, through the hexose monophosphate shunt (HMS). Indeed, thiol oxidation of GSH with diamide does produce an increase in corneal endothelial HMS activity (Geroski & Edelhauser 1978). It has yet to be determined if PCMBS can increase HMS activity in the corneal endothelium, but it has been shown that PCMB can increase the HMS activity in rat adipocytes (Mukherjee & Lynn 1977). An increased production of NADPH by the endothelium will enable it to withstand oxidative stresses. Because mercaptides form easily reversible complexes, PCMBS can be removed from the membrane proteins by the addition of sulfhydryl-containing agents such as cysteine and reduced glutathione. As in other membrane systems, the removal results in reversal of the inhibitory effect unless the interaction has resulted in irreversible denaturation of the protein (Rothstein 1970). In these studies, the PCMBS effect is reversible and complete endothelial function can be maintained by supplying an energy source and exogenous thiol to the perfusion medium.

Equal molar concentrations of PCMBS and PCMB produce markedly different responses; with the PCMB causing a greater breakdown in the endothelial barrier and greater corneal swelling. This can be attributed to the hydrophobic nature of the PCMB (Van Steverinck et al., 1965) which forms mercaptide bonds not only with surface SH but also with cytoplasmic SH. Once these bonds are formed within the endothelial cells, a pattern of progression of pathophysiologic and ultrastructural changes from the normal steady state through the sublethal states previously described for the high concentration of PCMBS occurs. Our corneal endothelial studies are similar to those of Sahaphong and Trump 1971 who have shown that PCMB can result in an increased rate of mercury induced cell injury, in the red blood cell and in isolated kidney tubules.

REFERENCES

Anderson, E.I., Fischbarg, J. & Spector, A. Disulfide stimulation of fluid transport and effect on ATP level in rabbit corneal endothelium. *Expl. Eye Res.* 19: *1-10*, (1974).

Cleveland, P.H. & Schneider, C.W. A simple method of preserving tissue for scanning electron microscopy. *Vision Res.* 9: *1401-1402*, (1969).

Dikstein, S. & Maurice, D.M. The metabolic basis to the fluid pump in the cornea. *J. Physiol., Lond.* 221: *29-41*, (1972).

Edelhauser, H.F., Van Horn, D.L., Miller, P. & Pederson, H.J. Effect of thiol-oxidation of glutathione with diamide on corneal endothelial function, junctional complexes and microfilaments. *J. Cell Biol.* 68: *567-578*, (1976).

Garrahan, P.J. & Rega, A.F. Cation loading of red blood cells. *J. Physiol., Lond.* 193: *459-466*, (1967).

Geroski, D.H., Edelhauser, H.F. & O'Brien, W.J. Hexose-monophosphate shunt response to diamide in the component layers of the cornea. *Expl. Eye Res.* 26: *611-619*, 1978.

McCarey, B.E., Edelhauser, H.F. & Van Horn, D.L. Functional and structural changes in the corneal endothelium during in vitro perfusion. *Invest. Ophthal.* 12: *410-417*, (1973).

Mukherjee, S.P. & Lynn, B.F. Reduced nicotinamide adenine dinucleotide phosphate oxidase in adipocyte plasma membrane and its activation by insulin. *Archs. Biochem. Biophys.* 184: *69-74*, (1977).

Pentila, A. & Trump, B.F. Studies on the modification of the cellular response to injury III Electron microscopic studies on the protective effect of acidosis on p-chloromercuribenzene sulfonic acid (PCMBS) induced injury of Ehrlich Ascites tumor cells. *Virc. Arch. B.* 18: *17-34*, (1975).

Rothstein, A. Sulfhydryl groups in membrane structure and function, in: *Current Topics in Membrane Transport* (ed: Bonner, F. & Klunzeller, A.) Academic Press, New York, 1970, pp. *135-175*.

Rothstein, A. Sulfhydryl groups in red cell membranes. *Expl. Eye Res.* 11: *329-337*, (1971).

Sahaphong, S. & Trump, B.F. Studies on cellular injury in isolated kidney tunules of the flounder. V. Effects of inhibiting sulfhydryl groups of plasma membrane with organic mercurials PCMB (parachloromercuribenzoate) and PCMBS (parachloromercuribenzene sulfonate). *Am. J. Path.* 63: *277-292*, (1971).

Scott, K.M., Knight, V.A., Settlemire, C.T. & Brierley, G.P. Differential effects of mercurial agents on membrane thiols and on the permeability of heart mitochondrion. *Biochemistry* 9: *714-724* (1970).

Sterling, C.E. Mercurial perturbation of brush border membrane permeability in rabbit ileum. *J. Membr. Bio.* 22: *33-56*, (1975).

Sutherland, R.M., Rothstein, A. & Weed, R.I. Erythrocyte membrane sulfhydryl groups and cation permeability. *Int. Cell. Physiol*: 69: *185-198*, (1967).

Van Steverinck, J., Weed, R.I. & Rothstein, A. Localization of erythrocyte membrane sulfhydryl groups essential for glucose transport. *J. gen. Physiol.* 48: *617*, (1965).

Authors' address:
Department of Physiology
The Medical College of Wisconsin
P.O.Box 26509
Milwaukee, Wisconcin 53226
USA

282

Docum. Ophthal. Proc. Series, Vol. 18

CURRENT CONCEPTS IN THE PHYSIOLOGY OF THE CORNEA

DAVID M. MAURICE

(Stanford, California, U.S.A.)

Since the standard texts (Duke-Elder, 1968; Davson, 1969) were last re-vised, there have been few major advances in our understanding of how the cornea carries out its function, but, rather, earlier concepts have been conso-lidated or modified. This article will review the present status of some of the more important aspects of corneal physiology and problems arising from them, and will deal in turn with the transparency and the mechanics of the tissue and then with its hydration control and nutrition.

TRANSPARENCY

Stroma

It is generally accepted that the clarity of this tissue follows from the ordered arrangement of its collagen fibrils which results in the destructive interference of their scattered light (Maurice, 1957). The strict crystalline order proposed in that paper is no longer considered to be necessary but only a general regularity in which the fibrils are approximately equidistant from each other (Hart & Farrell, 1969; Benedek, 1971; Cox, Farrell, Hart & Langham, 1970; Twersky, 1975) (Fig. 1). There is less agreement about the cause of the clouding that occurs in the edematous, stressed stroma. The mechanism originally suggested was that the fibrils separated from each other and lost their regular arrangement (Maurice, 1957). Benedek (1971) has proposed, on the other hand, that clouding is the result of the formation of fibril-free spaces, or 'lakes', which scatter light because their refractive index differs from the surrounding tissue (Fig. 2), and this has been con-firmed by others (Farrell, McCally & Tatham, 1973). In my laboratory such lakes have not been observed by electron microscopy in swollen corneas (Gallagher & Maurice, 1977), and I still favor the original theory. Evidence from light scattering measurements should be able to resolve the uncertain-ties resulting from the possibility of distortion introduced in preparation for electron microscopy, but such measurements are not yet in accord with one another (Farrell, McCally & Tatham, 1973; Feuk, 1971). A complicating factor is that the greater part of the light scattered by the stroma comes from the nuclei of the keratocytes and other cellular structures (Maurice, 1974).

283

The edema of the epithelium is at least as important as that of the stroma in causing clouding of vision. In the normal state it is optically empty when viewed by the specular microscope, which is a form of high power slit-lamp. The transparency of the epithelial cytoplasm is possibly related to that of the lens, for it is found to contain γ-crystallin (Bours, 1975). It is remarkable also that the nuclei cannot be distinguished in dark field illumination except when the cells are highly edematous.

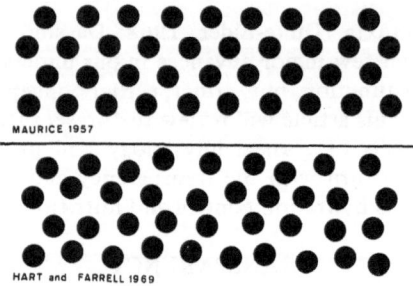

Fig. 1. Illustrating the parade ground regularity of the collagen fibrils originally believed to be necessary for corneal transparency, and the quasi-ordered state that is presently considered to be adequate.

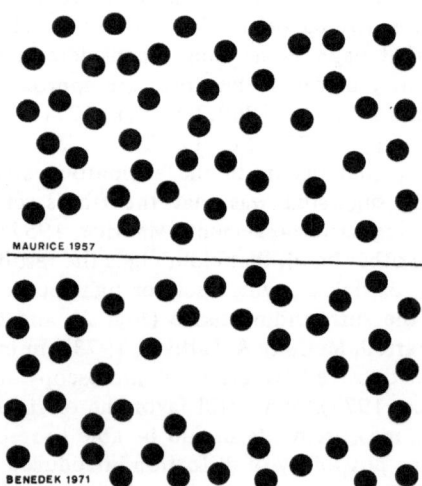

Fig. 2. Illustrating the alternative explanations that have been put forward to account for the cloudiness of the edematous cornea. Above, the random disorder of the fibrils and below, the formation of lakes.

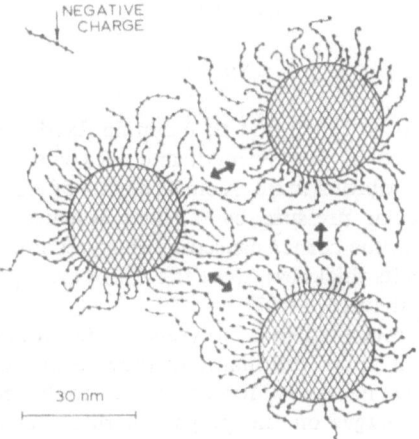

NEGATIVE
CHARGE

30 nm

Fig. 3. Speculative impression of the distribution of polysaccharide in the ground substance leading to the material repulsion of the collagen fibrils. Crosslinking is proposed as one possible way in which the swelling of the stroma is limited.

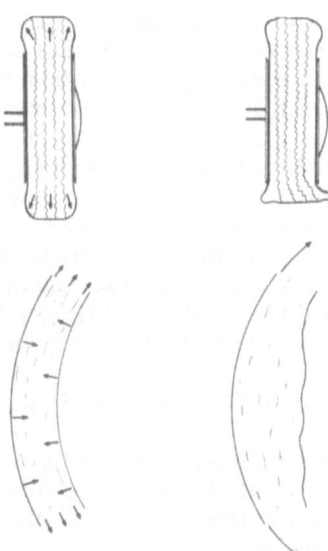

Fig. 4. Illustrating the mechanical firmness imposed by the positive internal pressure in a car tire and the negative internal pressure in the cornea. The structural rigidity is lost with the pressure in the case of a flat or of stromal edema.

285

MECHANICS

Stroma

The eyeball needs to be tough and to maintain fixed dimensions, and these properties are ensured by the strength and inextensibility of the collagen which makes up the fibrous tunic. A small degree of elasticity is provided at the normal intraocular pressure by a slight waviness of the collagenous fibrils. The tension in the cornea caused by this pressure appears to be taken up uniformly across its thickness, since the fibrils are equally extended in all layers (Gallagher & Maurice, 1977).

The fibrils are embedded in a polysaccharide ground substance which serves to brace them apart and maintain their regular order in the normal unswollen state. The necessary forces appear to be connected with the negative electrical charges on the polysaccharide chains (Fig. 3), but the details of the interaction are not fully understood (Hart & Farrell, 1971; Brenner & Parsegian, 1976). In many ways the polysaccharide behaves as if it were a sleeve covering the fibrils which prevents them from coming into contact with one another (Twersky, 1975). The force of expansion of the ground substance manifests itself externally as the swelling pressure of the cornea (Maurice, 1957), which is normally about 60 mm Hg but rapidly rises if the tissue becomes dehydrated or falls if edematous.

In its normal state the force of expansion pushes the structural framework of the tissue against the surface layers and creates a suction within the interstitial fluid (Hedbys, Mishima & Maurice, 1963). Among other things this helps to hold the epithelial cell layer in place (Ytteborg & Dohlman, 1965). When the cornea swells or the IOP rises so that the suction is reversed to a positive fluid pressure, the epithelium tends to be pushed off, leading to bullous keratopathy (Ytteborg & Dohlman, 1965).

The balance of forces may be looked at from the opposite viewpoint, where the suction in the tissue fluid is seen as pulling inwards on the surfaces of the cornea and compressing and packing together the fibrils, thus establishing the order essential for the transparency of the tissue. The compression of the structural framework of the stroma as a result of the fluid suction within it causes it to become compact and firm in the same way that the opposite mechanism leads to structural rigidity in a car tire; an edematous cornea, just as a flat tire, lacks mechanical stability (Fig. 4).

HYDRATION CONTROL

The expansive power of the stroma tends to draw in fluid, and both Davson (1955) and Harris & Nordquist (1955) showed that this fluid was removed by a metabolic process. The thickness of the stroma is considered to be established by a pump-leak process controlled by the superficial cell membranes, particularly the endothelium.

This cell layer is quite permeable to salts and low molecular weight solutes as well as to water; it even permits the slow passage of proteins of moderate size. This permeability allows aqueous humor to be slowly drawn in as a result of the suction in the interstitial fluid. There is little disagreement that a principal function of the endothelial layer is to actively pump this fluid out again and so maintain the suction and with it the transparency of the stroma (Fig. 5). The active movement of fluid can be observed in isolated preparations of the layer (Maurice, 1972), and the rate at which fluid is pumped, 6 μl/cm^2 hr, is relatively fast, for it signifies that in every three minutes the cells are actively transferring more than their own volume of fluid.

The underlying mechanism of the pump is not understood, although some factors influencing its performance have been established and some preliminary attempts have been made to explain its action (Barfort & Maurice, 1974; Fischbarg & Lim, 1974; Hodson, 1974). The depression of pump activity by ouabain (Trenberth & Mishima, 1968; Fischbarg, 1972) and

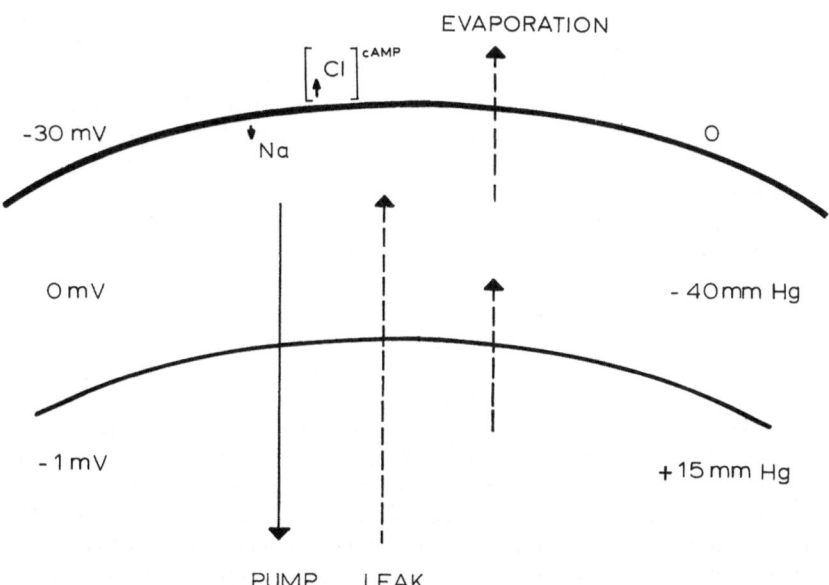

Fig. 5. The electrical potentials, water fluxes and hydrostatic pressures associated with the layers of the rabbit cornea. The length of the arrows roughly corresponds to the magnitude of the water fluxes. Passive fluxes are shown by broken lines. The leak across the endothelium is a result of the imbibition pressure of the stroma, and opening the lids allows evaporation to take place. Active fluxes are shown by full lines. The small water flux across the epithelium may be inward, associated with Na ion transport, or outward, associated with c-AMP stimulated Cl ion transport.

carbonic anhydrase inhibitors (Fischbarg & Lim, 1974) or by the absence of Na^+ and HCO_3^- (Hodson, 1974; Fischbarg, 1972; Hodson, 1971; Dikstein & Maurice, 1972) suggests that these ions are directly or indirectly involved. Recently, Hodson & Miller (1976) and Hull et al. (1977) have presented direct evidence of the existence of a HCO_3^- transport but it is not clear how this is coupled to fluid movement. There is a potential of about 1 mV developed across the endothelial layer, the aqueous humor negative to the stroma, but it is not certain whether this is related to the fluid transport (Barfort & Maurice, 1974; Fischbarg & Lim, 1974; Hodson, 1974).

Progress has been hindered in this field because it has been found very difficult to maintain the isolated perfused cell layer in a functional state for more than a few hours. This appears to conflict with the behavior of isolated cells which will survive in tissue culture and ultimately form a confluent layer that lays down a Descemet's membrane (Perlman & Baum, 1974). The cause of failure may be that so far unidentified metabolites essential to the pump are absent from the medium and are washed away by perfusion.

Epithelium

This layer exhibits a considerable obstruction to the passage of ions, as is shown by its electrical resistance, which, in the rabbit, is around 9000 ohm cm^2 compared to 50 ohm cm^2 for the endothelium. This obstruction, which seems to be located principally in the superficial cells, becomes even greater as the molecular size of the permeant increases. Lipid soluble solutes pass across the layer with much greater facility because they can cross cell membranes.

Ion transport mechanisms have been identified in the epithelium, and these result in an electrical potential of about 30 mV negative to the blood being present in the tear film. One transport mechanism, that of Na^+, was found in the rabbit many years ago; this is directed from the tear film into the cornea and would result in an inward movement of salt and water. Recently an outward transport of Cl^- has also been shown both in the frog (Zadunaisky, 1966) and in the rabbit (Klyce, Neufeld & Zadunaisky, 1973). This activity is not constant like the Na^+ mechanism but is turned on by agents which increase the intracellular level of cyclic AMP (Klyce, Neufeld & Zadunaisky, 1973; Klyce, 1975). Under open circuit conditions, corresponding to the normal state of the open eye, the outward movement of Cl^- ions overwhelms the inward movement of Na^+ and leads to an overall movement of salt from the cornea to the tear film, which carries water with it by osmotic forces. This has been shown directly to result in a large water flow in the frog (Candia, 1976), but in the rabbit it is about 15 times less than that resulting from the endothelial pump (Klyce, 1975). In the latter species very slow water movements into or out of the stroma can be effected by the epithelium according to whether the c-AMP system is stimulated or not. It seems unlikely to the author that this is of any significance in the regulation of the hydration of the mammalian cornea, but it is possible that it could be a control mechanism for the maintenance of the tear film in animals like the rabbit, which blink very infrequently. In this respect it is noteworthy that in man, whose tear film is renewed by frequent blinking, the surface electrical potential is very small (Maurice, 1973; Fischer, Voigt, Liegl & Wiederholt, 1974).

Passive factors

Although the corneal hydration is principally controlled by the active pump located in the endothelium, it can also be affected to a lesser degree by physical factors. Thickening or thinning of the tissue, usually transient in nature, results from the surface application of hypo- or hypertonic solutions. When the eyes are opened, evaporation takes place, which is largely compensated for by the osmotic withdrawal of water from the anterior chamber. A reduction in thickness of a few percent has been recorded both in the rabbit and human cornea as a result (Mishima & Maurice, 1961; Mandell & Fatt, 1965). Normally, evaporation is retarded by the presence of a monomolecular film derived from the meibomian glands, and if the integrity of this film is destroyed, the thinning of the cornea is much more pronounced, resulting in some cases in the formation of dellen (Mishima & Maurice, 1961; Baum, Mishima & Boruchoff, 1968).

Mechanical factors have been suggested as playing a role in the control of hydration (Ehlers, 1967; Mayes & Hodson, 1978). The stroma can be considered as being compressed between the intraocular pressure pushing on the endothelium on one side and the centripetal component of the tension in the outer lamellae on the other side. This effect should be more prominent the more the tension in the cornea is distributed in its anteriormost layer, such as in the very swollen tissue. If the epithelium is absent in this condition, allowing free exchange of fluid across the anterior chamber, the intraocular pressure pushing against the endothelium can limit stromal swelling. When the anterior surface is sealed with an intact epithelium, the relationship becomes complicated (Berkley, 1971; Friedman, 1972).

NUTRITION

The cells in each of the layers of the cornea require the nutrients that are essential to all cells to maintain their basic metabolism and morphological integrity. In addition, the endothelium may require a significant source of energy for its fluid pumping activity, and the epithelium must have access to the metabolites needed for the synthesis of the cells that replace those constantly lost by desquamation.

There are three potential sources of nutrition for the cornea: across the surfaces (from the aqueous humor and tears) or from the blood through the limbus. Substances that enter from the blood can move toward the center of the cornea by diffusion, but they are continuously reduced in concentration by metabolism or by leaking out across the limiting layers. Thus the concentration at the apex of the cornea will be smaller than that at the periphery for substances entering by this route, and calculations based on their known diffusional properties show that molecules smaller in size than proteins will not penetrate far from the limbus in significant proportions (Davson, 1969). Over most of the central areas of the cornea the supply of metabolites, as well as the excretion of waste products, must be across the surfaces of the tissue.

Because the permeability of the endothelium is much greater than that of the epithelium, the major metabolic exchanges will take place with the aqueous humor. Furthermore, mechanisms for the rapid transfer of glucose and some amino-acids across the endothelial cells have been identified (Hale & Maurice, 1969; Scott & Friedenthal, 1973; Riley, 1977). An exception occurs in the case of oxygen and carbon dioxide, which are fat-soluble and can penetrate readily across the epithelium. The greater part of respiration of the cornea takes place across its front surface, and oxygen is directly supplied from the air (Hill & Fatt, 1963; Riley, 1969). When the eye is closed, the conjunctiva takes over as the source of oxygen. The palpebral conjunctiva of the upper lid is specially modified so that there is very little tissue between the capillaries and the surface, thus ensuring an ample gas exchange across the epithelium (Kwan & Fatt, 1971). In fact, this is the only region on the surface of the body where it is possible to accurately monitor the oxygen level in the blood with an external electrode.

ACKNOWLEDGEMENTS

The preparation of this paper was supported by N.I.H. Grant EY 00431.

REFERENCES

Barfort, P. & Maurice, D.M. Electrical potential and fluid transport across the corneal endothelium. *Expl. Eye Res.* 19: *11-19* (1974).

Baum, J.L., Mishima, S. & Boruchoff, A. On the nature of dellen. *Archs. Ophthal.* 79: *657-662* (1968).

Benedek, G.B. Theory of transparency of the eye. *Appl. Opt.* 10: *459-473* (1971).

Berkley, D.A. Influence of intraocular pressure on corneal fluid pressure, tissue stress and thickness. *Expl. Eye Res.* 11: *132-139* (1971).

Bours, J. The pressure of albumin and other serum proteins and crystallins in chick cornea and in corneal endothelium and epithelium. *Expl. Eye Res.* 20: *187-188* (1975).

Brenner, S.L. & Parsegian, V.A. Suggested explanation for the anomalous temperature dependence of the corneal swelling pressure. *Expl. Eye Res.* 22: *95-99* (1976).

Candia, O. A. Fluid and Cl transport by the epithelium of the isolated frog cornea *Fed. Proc.* 35 (3): *703* (1976).

Cox, J.L., Farrell, R.A., Hart, R.W. & Langham, M.E. The transparency of the mammalian cornea. *J. Physiol., Lond.,* 210: *601-616* (1970).

Davson, H. The hydration of the cornea. *Biochem. J.* 59: *24-28* (1955).

Davson, H. The Eye, Vol. 1, 2nd edition, Chapter 7, Academic Press, New York, 1969.

Dikstein, S. & Maurice, D.M. The metabolic basis to the fluid pump in the cornea. *J. Physiol., Lond.,* 221: *29-41* (1972).

Duke-Elder, W.S. System of Ophthalmology, Vol. IV. The Physiology of the Eye and of Vision, C.V. Mosby Co., St. Louis, 1968.

Ehlers, N. Mechanical factors in the maintenance of normal corneal deturgescence. *Acta Ophthal.* 45: *658-672* (1967).

Farrell, R.A., McCally, R.L. & Tatham, P.E.R. Wave-length dependencies of light scattering in normal and cold swollen rabbit corneas and their structural implications. *J. Physiol., Lond.,* 233: *589-612* (1973).

Feuk, T. The wavelength dependence of scattered light intensity in rabbit corneas. *IEEE Trans. bio-med. Eng. BME-18*: *92-96* (1971).

Fischbarg, J. Potential difference and fluid transport across rabbit corneal endothelium. *Biochim. biophys. Acta* 288: *362-366* (1972).

Fischbarg, J. & Lim, J.J. Role of cations, anions and carbonic anhydrase in fluid transport across rabbit corneal endothelium. *J. Physiol.* 241: *647-675* (1974).

Fischer, F., Voigt, G., Liegl, O. & Wiederholt, M. Effect of pH on potential defference and short circuit current in the isolated human cornea. *Pflugers Arch. ges. Physiol.* 349: *119-131* (1974).

Friedman, M.H. A quantitative description of equilibrium and homeostatic thickness regulation in the in vivo cornea. I. Normal cornea. *Biophys. J.* 12: *648-665* (1972).

Gallagher, B. & Maurice, D. Striations of light scattering in the corneal stroma. *J. Ultra. Struct. Res.* 61: *100-114* (1977).

Hale, P.N. & Maurice, D.M. Sugar transport across the corneal endothelium. *Expl. Eye Res.* 8: *205-215* (1969).

Harris, J.E. & Nordquist, L.T. The hydration of the cornea. I: Transport of water from the cornea. *Am. J. Ophthal.* 40: *100-110* (1955).

Hart, R.W. & Farrell, R.A. Light scattering in the cornea. *J. opt. Soc. Am.* 59: *766-774* (1969).

Hart, R.W. & Farrell, R.A. Structural theory of the swelling pressure of corneal stroma in saline. *Bull. math. Biophys.* 33: *165-186.*(1971).

Hedbys, B.O., Mishima, S. & Maurice, D.M. The imbibition pressure of the corneal stroma. *Expl. Eye Res.* 2: *99-111* (1963).

Hill, R.M. & Fatt, I. Oxygen uptake from a reservoir of limited volume by the human cornea in vivo. *Science* 142: *1295-1297* (1963).

Hodson, S. Evidence for a bicarbonate-dependent sodium pump in corneal endothelium. *Expl. Eye Res.* 11: *20-29* (1971).

Hodson, S. The regulation of corneal hydration by a salt pump requiring the presence of sodium and bicarbonate ions. *J. Physiol., Lond.,* 236: *271-302* (1974).

Hodson, S. & Miller, F. The bicarbonate ion pump in the endothelium which regulates the hydration of rabbit cornea. *J. Physiol., Lond.,* 263: *563-573* (1976).

Hull, D.S., Green, K., Boyd, M. & Wynn, H.R. Corneal endothelium bicarbonate transport and the effect of carbonic anhydrase inhibitors on endothelial permeability and fluxes and corneal thickness. *Invest. Ophthal.* 16: *883-892* (1977).

Klyce, S.D., Neufeld, A.H. & Zadunaisky, J.A. The activation of chloride transport by epinephrine and Db cyclic-AMP in the cornea of the rabbit. *Invest. Ophthal.* 12: *127-139* (1973).

Klyce, S.D. Transport of Na, Cl and water by the rabbit corneal epithelium at resting potential. *Am. J. Physiol.* 228: *1446-1452* (1975).

Kwan, M. & Fatt, I. A noninvasive method of continuous arterial oxygen tension estimation from measured palpebral conjunctival oxygen tension. *Anesthesiology* 35: *309-314* (1971).

Mandell, R.B. & Fatt, I. Thinning in the human cornea on awakening. *Nature* 208: *292-293* (1965).

Maurice, D.M. The structure and transparency of the cornea. *J. Physiol., Lond.,* 136: *263-286* (1957).

Maurice, D.M. Nutritional aspects of corneal grafts and prostheses. Corneo-Plastic Surgery (Proceedings of the 2nd International Corneo-Plastic Conference) (ed. Rycroft, P.V.) London, 1967, Pergamon Press, Oxford, 1969, pp.. *197-208.*

Maurice, D.M. The location of the fluid pump in the cornea. *J. Physiol., Lond.,* 221: *43-54* (1972).

Maurice, D.M. Electrical potential and ion transport across the conjuctiva. *Expl. Eye Res.* 15: *527-532* (1973).

Maurice, D.M. A scanning slit optical microscope. *Invest. Ophthal.* 13: *1033-1037* (1974).

Mayes, K.R. & Hodson, S. Some effects of hydrostatic pressure on corneal pressure during specular microscopy. *Expl. Eye Res.* 26: *141-146* (1978).

Mishima, S. & Maurice, D.M. The effect of normal evaporation on the eye. *Expl. Eye Res.* 1: *46-52* (1961).

Perlman, M. & Baum, J.L. The mass culture of rabbit corneal endothelial cells. *Archs. Ophthal.* 92: *235-237* (1974).

Riley, M.V. Glucose and oxygen utilization by the rabbit cornea. *Expl. Eye Res.* 8: *193-200* (1969).

Riley, M.V. A study of the transfer of amino acids across the endothelium of the rabbit cornea. *Expl. Eye Res.* 25: *35-44* (1977).

Scott, W.N. & Friedenthal, D.F. A proposed role for ascorbate in the transport of amino acids and ions in the cornea. *Expl. Eye Res.* 15: *683-692* (1973).

Trenberth, S.M. & Mishima, S. The effect of ouabain on the rabbit corneal endothelium. *Invest. Ophthal.* 7: *44-52* (1968).

Twersky, V. Transparency of pair-correlated, random distributions of small scatterers, with application to the cornea. *J. opt. Soc. Am.* 65: *524-530* (1975).

Ytteborg, J. & Dohlman, C.H. Corneal edema and intraocular pressure. II. Clinical results. *Archs. Ophthal.* 74: *477-484* (1965).

Zadunaisky, J. Active transport of chloride in frog cornea. *Am. J. Physiol.* 221: *506-512* (1966).

Author's address:
Division of Ophthalmology
Stanford University Medical Center
Stanford, California, 94305 U.S.A.

Docum. Ophthal. Proc. Series, Vol. 18

PENETRATING KERATOPLASTY IN THE GUINEA PIG

ELIZABETH A. MINDRUP & WILLIAM B. RATHBUN

(Minneapolis, Minnesota U.S.A.)

ABSTRACT

A procedure is described for penetrating corneal transplantation in guinea pigs in which an 84% success rate was achieved in 74 consecutive allografts. Fourteen of the grafts remained continuously clear for at least 200 days, and two, for over 12 months. In a companion study, topical challenge by skin grafts over a time span of 0 to 250 days following keratoplasty resulted in donor corneal rejection in all cases, two to three weeks following the challenge. Subcutaneous placement of the donor skin produced more variable results, 26% failing to reject the cornea. Skin challenge in isogeneic animals uniformly failed to cause corneal transplant rejection.

INTRODUCTION

The immune response has been generally recognized as being a major cause of corneal opacification following keratoplasty which had been technically successful both clinically and experimentally (Elliot, 1971; Harris & Rathbun, 1972). Virtually all experimental keratoplasty has been restricted to the rabbit, for which very successful procedures have been developed (Khodadoust, 1968). In certain studies, the use of highly inbred strains is extremely desirable. Although such rabbit strains are now no longer generally available, certain highly inbred strains of guinea pigs may yet be obtained. It is the purpose of this communication to report a procedure for penetrating corneal allografts in the guinea pig which has afforded a high rate of success, as well as the subsequent rejection of clear allografts induced by skin transplants applied at various time intervals following successful keratoplasty.

MATERIALS AND METHODS

Animals

Albino and pigmented guinea pigs of mixed breeding as well as animals of the inbred NIH strain 2 (National Institutes of Health, Bethesda, Maryland) weighing 550-800 grams were used in this study. These guinea pigs exhibited

This investigation was supported in part by Public Health Service Grants Nos. EY-00426 and EY-01197 and a grant from the Graduate School of the University of Minnesota.

slightly elliptical corneas whose major axis (horizontal) averaged 7.5 mm, and whose minor axis (vertical) averaged 7.0 mm. The in vivo corneal thickness was 0.2 mm centrally and 0.32 mm near the limbus (measured with a pachometer).

Anesthesia

Following light sedation with ether, the animals received an intraperitoneal injection of sodium pentobarbital, 30 mg/kg body weight. This was supplemented during the surgical procedure by inhalation, for short intervals, of methoxyflurane.

Animal Preparation

The guinea pigs were paired, each animal acting as both a donor and a host during a simultaneous interchange of grafts. The iris was dilated by instillation of a 10% solution of phenylephrine hydrochloride. Retrobulbar injection of 0.1 c.c. of Lidocaine hydrochloride, 1% w/v, served as a nerve block as well as for elevation of the eye. A 5-0 suture was placed through both the upper and lower eye lids about 1.5 mm lateral to the nasal canthus. The eye was proptosed, the eye lids were tucked behind the eye and the suture tied. Following rinsing of the eye with sterile saline, the animals were draped with a Steri-Drape (Minnesota Mining and Manufacturing Co.). The drape was cut out and pressed down around the proptosed eye, in order to keep hair from the operative field and to provide the needed exposure, as well as to stabilize the eye.

Surgical Procedure

The surgical procedure was performed with sterile instruments and clean technique entirely with the aid of a 15 x Stereozoom microscope (Bausch & Lomb, model SVB-73). A 3 mm Castroviejo trephine with 0.3 mm depth was used. The maximal trephine cutting depth was adjusted to prevent anterior chamber penetration, thereby reducing the possibility of lens damage. Entrance was then made with a discission blade.

Following penetration, the eye was immediately flooded with sterile sodium heparin, 1:1000, repeated frequently throughout the procedure to prevent clot formation of the aqueous humor. Excision of the donor corneal button was completed with subminiature corneal scissors while a slight tension was placed upon the button to insure a vertical incision. Care was taken in manipulation of the button, as guinea pig lamellae separate quite easily compared to those of the rabbit. Before excision was complete, a 10-0 monofilament nylon suture was placed in the donor button at a depth just anterior to Descemet's membrane to enable its transfer and also to serve as the first suture. The button was left in its bed while the procedure was repeated on the partner, and then the grafts were exchanged between animals and sutured into place with interrupted 10-0 Ethilon sutures (Ethicon,

Inc.). Four cardinal sutures were placed in the first graft, making certain that the graft remained in place with evenly distributed tension and with good apposition, then the partner's graft was completely secured with eight equally spaced sutures at a depth just anterior to Descemet's membrane before returning to the first graft. Following completion of corneal suturing, the proptosing suture near the medial canthus was removed and the eye was returned to its orbit. A drop of 2% atropine sulfate and some Neosporin ointment were instilled. This procedure can be accomplished by an unassisted operator, and with practice may be completed in approximately one hour.

Postoperative Care

Initially the animals were grossly examined daily, and at least three times a week with the aid of the operating microscope, and treated as needed. Sutures were removed with the aid of the microscope using topical anesthesia (0.5% proparacaine HCl), on the seventh postoperative day. Daily examination was continued for four additonal days and grossly three times weekly thereafter.

Postoperative Course

The mild host edema evident on the first postoperative day peaked in intensity by day three with perilimbal inflammation followed by ingrowth of blood vessels onto the host cornea, especially towards the sutures and graft. In some instances, a few blood vessels reached the wound but were never seen in the graft. The observation of blood vessels in the scar was confirmed by examination of histologic sections, but such blood vessels were never seen in the graft. These vessels subsided quickly after removal of sutures. With time, the scar continued to diminish in size, in some cases forming a fine line barely visible with the unaided eye. At no time was the donor button observed to be cloudy in the postoperative course of a successful graft.

Skin Grafts

Full thickness grafts were cut free hand with scissors from the dorso-lateral thorax, and exchanged between animals. The grafts were elliptical, approximately 2 cm long, with a maximum width of 1.5 cm and were held in place with 4-0 chromic gut sutures. All skin grafts were made on the thorax, being placed either topically or subcutaneously. Following placement on the host, these grafts were observed daily.

RESULTS

Mixed Breeds

Following the initial adaptation of the general transplantation technique to the guinea pig, 62 of 74 (84%) consecutive penetrating grafts were clear, without complications, for four weeks or longer. Fourteen animals having clear grafts were retained for an observation period of at least 200 days and two for at least 12 months. All grafts which were clear during the initial four postoperative weeks remained continuously clear for the duration of the observation period.

The main criterion used for determination of donor cornea viability was a continuous clarity of the graft. As additional proof that continuously clear grafts retained viable donor tissue, graft rejection was induced by skin implants from the corneal donor. Attempts to cause corneal rejection by topical skin grafts were totally successful regardless of the length of time the corneal graft had remained clear (Table I). The average day of rejection following topical skin transplantation was 16 ± 2.3. The observation (Polack, 1962) that the skin transplant must be viable, not subjected to freezing, was confirmed. Immune rings were observed only in the three animals in which corneal and skin grafts were performed simultaneously.

The implantation of donor skin subcutaneously was less successful for induction of corneal graft rejection (Table I). The period required to reject the corneal grafts was longer and more variable, averaging 20 ± 8 days following skin implantation, while 26% (5 animals) failed to reject at all.

Table I. Rejection Induced By Topical and Subcutaneous Skin Transplants

Topical Skin Transplants		Subcutaneous Skin Transplants	
Days clear before *skin transplant*	Day rejected after *skin transplant*	Days clear before *skin transplant*	Day rejected after *skin transplant*
0	12	0	8
0	12	0	13
0	14	13	14
0	14	13	16
27	14	13	19
34	16	13	35
34	16	14	14
44	20	14	14
44	19	16	*
45	20	16	*
100	16	21	28
149	17	21	*
149	16	27	16
153	18	27	30
153	16	30	23
214	18	30	29
250	16	54	16
		54	*
		60	*

* No rejection during an observation period of at least 104 days.

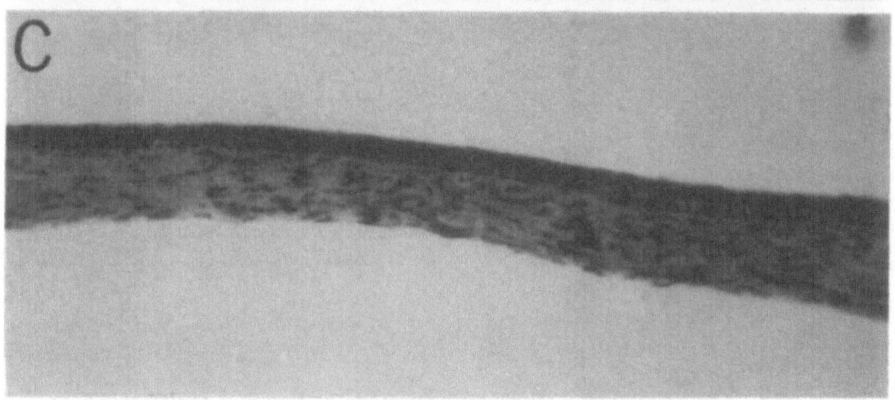

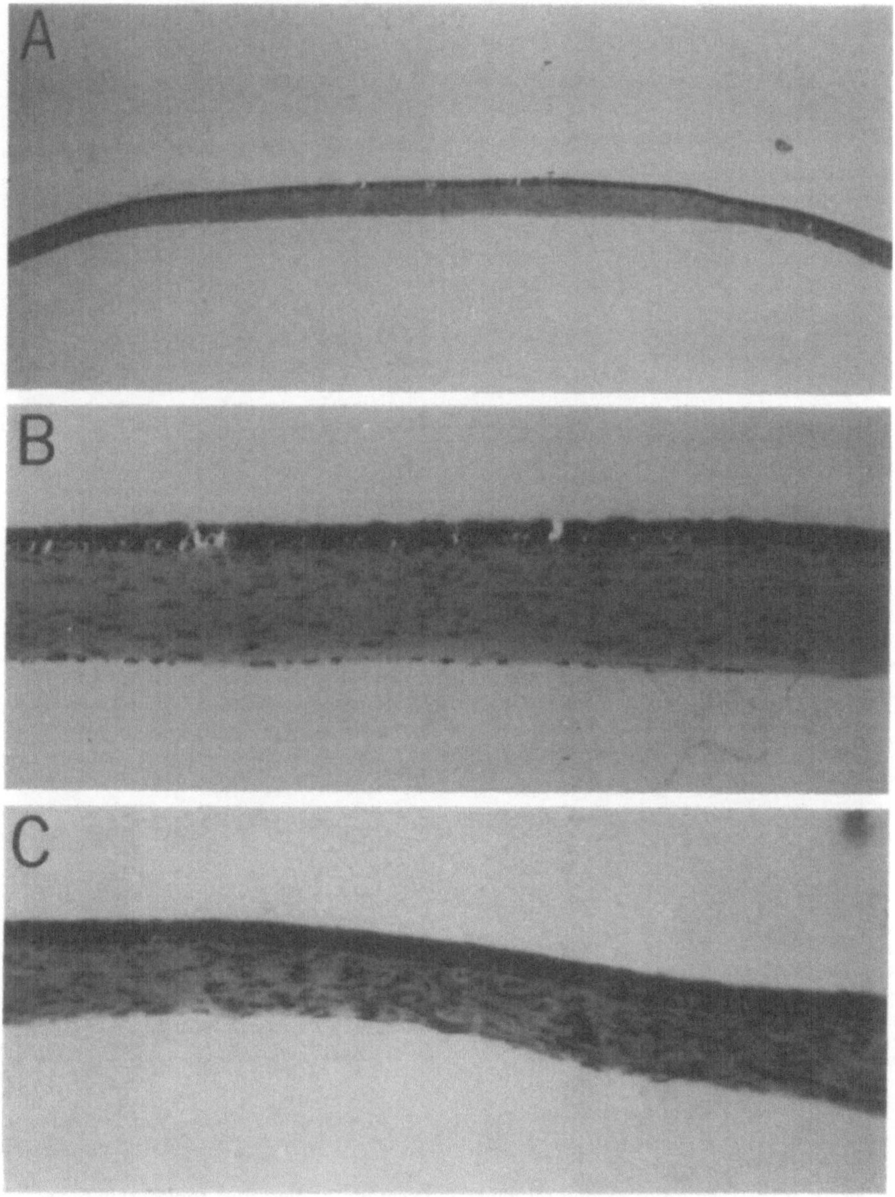

Fig. 1. Cross section of a clear allograft 57 days post surgery.
A. Cross section of entire cornea. Magnification: 2.5 X
B. Center of above cross section. Magnification: 10 X
C. Right scar of above cross section with donor tissue on left, host on right. Magnification: 10 X.

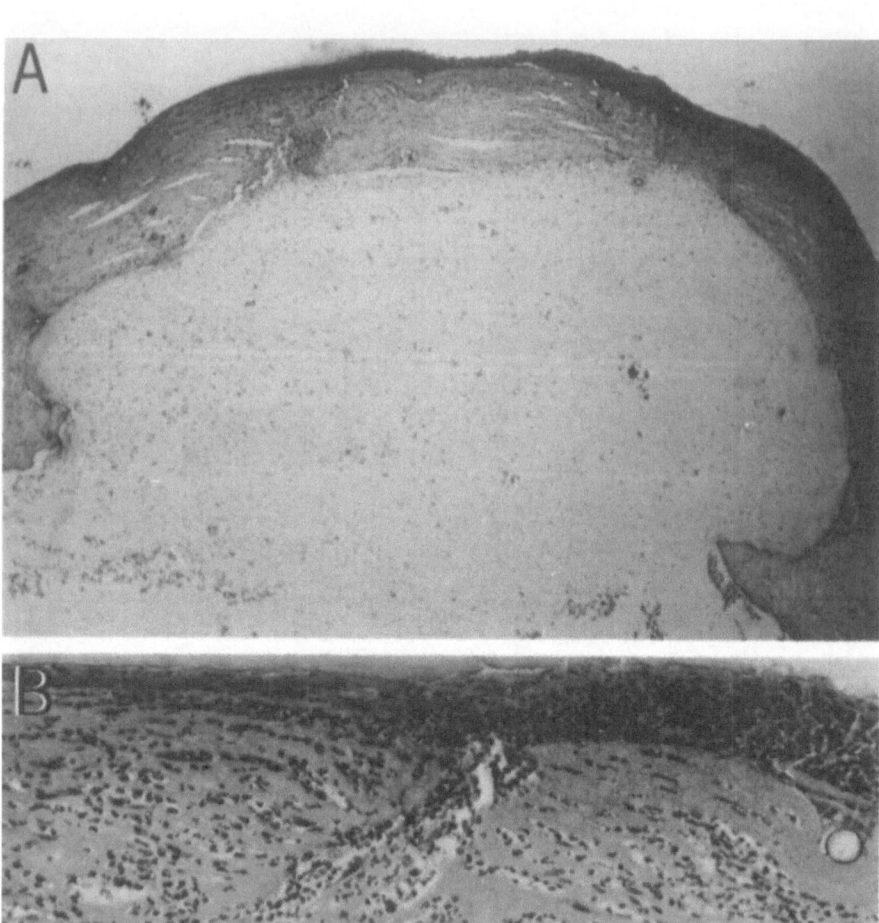

Fig. 2. Cross section of second set allograft rejection 20 days post topical skin transplantation (129 days post keratoplasty).

A. Cross section of entire cornea illustrating deterioration of cornea, and showing sutures still in place. Comparison with Fig. 1 A at same magnification allows estimation of the gross edema. Magnification: 2.5 X.

B. Left corneal wound of above cross section showing invasion of massive quantities of immune cells. Comparison with Fig. 1 C illustrates edema. Magnification: 10 X.

Histologic sections (stained with hemotoxylin and eosin) of long term clear grafts were examined. Among these were ten successful allografts which had remained continuously clear for 6 to 12 months (Fig. 1). These sections uniformly consisted of normal appearing grafts of usual thickness. The endothelium was of normal appearance and extended in a continuous layer to the scar, giving no reason to believe that the endothelium was not derived from the donor.

Histologic sections of rejected corneal grafts contained large numbers of immune rejection cells, polymorphonuclear leukocytes, lymphocytes, and multiple eosinophils throughout the cornea and the graft (Fig. 2). The presence of endothelium was difficult to establish in the later stages of rejection.

The frequently seen pinpoint opacities of the lens were usually isolated and probably due to slight trauma. In the authors' experience, this does not occur in rabbits. These opacities of the lens apparently had no influence on the course of the graft as clear grafts were sometimes obtained in eyes containing totally opaque lenses. Corneal bulging, which did not affect graft clarity, also occurred, but never until at least one month postoperatively. Incidence decreased when sutures were left in longer than the usual period.

Isogeneic Breed

Guinea pigs of the isogeneic NIH strain 2 were used for corneal grafts. Skin was transplanted topically six weeks following the corneal allograft in three pairs of animals, using full-thickness skin grafts. Corneal rejection was not noted in any of these animals after an observation period of over two months following skin transplantation.

DISCUSSION

Khodadoust & Silverstein (1969b), using the rabbit, expored the effects of rejection of individual corneal cell layers. Isolated stromal rejection was grossly observed as a transient clouding of the cornea, after which the cornea returned to a totally normal appearance. Rejection of the donor endothelium, however, resulted in widespread disruption of the donor cell layer in what has to be described as a violent reaction, resulting in development of edema, and clouding of the stroma which persisted for several months.

In this study viable donor endothelium as well as stroma cells were present in all the continuously clear grafts in the guinea pig. When such continuously clear grafts were challenged with donor skin antigens, a very rapid, intense reaction was initiated, clearly resulting in the destruction of the endothelium as revealed by comparison of the histologic sections of these with sections from continuously clear grafts. A completely opaque cornea resulted which never cleared in the ensuing months. In the authors' experience, this rejection reaction was strikingly similar to that observed in the rabbit and described in detail by Khodadoust & Silverstein (1969b). It is evident that such destruction of the endothelium would not have resulted had the donor endothelium been earlier replaced by the host.

This work demonstrates that guinea pig donor cornea can survive longer than six months and then be readily rejected following sensitization to donor skin. This observation is not in accord with early studies using rabbits reported by Maumenee (1951) and O'Gawa, et al. (1966) in which the second set corneal rejection appeared to be highly time dependent with the rate being universely proportional to time. However, Khodadoust & Silverstein (1969a) also using rabbits, observed rejection of corneal epithelium occurring as late as six months following corneal transplantation. Engelstein, et al. (1972) reported that challenge by skin seven to ten weeks following keratoplasty caused rejection of corneal grafts in 14 of 15 rabbits. Data from this latter study allowed the authors to conclude that corneal allografts fail to initiate systemic sensitization due to a block of the afferent limb of the immune system.

The ability of the guinea pig cornea to induce cellular sensitivity was demonstrated by various methods by Ugrinski & Kirkpatrick (1974). Such evidence of delayed sensitivity could not be demonstrated in isogeneic guinea pigs. Both in the present study and in that by Hand & Johnson (1974) exchange of corneal grafts between isogeneic animals followed by challenge by skin failed to cause corneal rejection.

ACKNOWLEDGEMENT

The authors wish to thank Dr. Donald J. Doughman for interpretation of the histologic sections used in this study as well as for review of the manuscript.

REFERENCES

Elliot, J.H. Immune factors in corneal graft rejection. *Invest. Ophthal.* 10: *216-234* (1971).

Engelstein, J.M., Herberman, R.B. & Waltman, S.R. Protection of penetrating corneal allografts from immune rejection. *Am. J. Ophthal.* 74: *311-315* (1972).

Hand, T.G. & Johnson, G.J. A model of primary corneal graft rejection using inbred strains of guinea pigs. *Can. J. Ophthal.* 9: *367-371* (1974).

Harris, J.E. & Rathbun, W.B. Ocular tissues, in transplantation (ed. Najarian, J.S. & Simmons, R.L.) Philadelphia, Lea and Febiger, 1972, p. *613.*

Khodadoust, A.A. Penetrating keratoplasty in the rabbit. *Am. J. Ophthal.* 66: *899-905* (1968).

Khodadoust, A.A. & Silverstein, A.M. The survival and rejection of epithelium in experimental corneal transplants. *Invest. Ophthal.* 8: *169-179* (1969a).

Khodadoust, A.A. & Silverstein, A.M. Transplantation and rejection of individual cell layers of the cornea. *Invest. Ophthal.* 8: *180-195* (1969b).

Maumenee, A.E. The influence of donor-recipient sensitization on corneal grafts. *Am. J. Ophthal. Ser.* 3, 34: *142-152* (1951).

O'Gawa, G.M., Guyton, J.S., Sanders, W.R. Inch, F.A.B. & Ellis, R.C. Behavior of clear penetrating corneal homografts in rabbits. *Am. J. Ophthal. Ser.* 3, 61: *267-273* (1966).

Polack, F.M. Histopathological and histochemical alterations in the early stages of corneal graft rejection. *J. exp. Med.* 116: *709-717* (1962).

Ugrinski, P.S. & Kirkpatrick, C.H. Corneal cellular immunity in the guinea pig. *Am. J. Path.* 74: *365-376* (1974).

Authors' address:
Department of Ophthalmology
Box 376 Mayo Memorial Building
University of Minnesota
Minneapolis, MN 55455 U.S.A.

Docum. Ophthal. Proc. Series, Vol. 18

ASCORBIC ACID, GLUTATHIONE AND LACTATE IN EXPERIMENTAL ULTRAVIOLET KERATITIS

MARTIN REIM, EBERHARD SCHUETTE, GISELA SCHARSICH,
MARIETTA SEIDL & HEINZ G. KESTERNICH

(Aachen, F.R.D.)

ABSTRACT

In rabbits, ultraviolet keratitis was produced by irradiation of one eye with an analytical UV lamp. The glutathione (GSH and GSSG) levels of the cornea epithelium did not change before the epithelium showed visible lesions. At that time, about 10 hours after the irradiation, an increase of the GSH and a decrease of the GSSG levels were observed by enzymatic analyses of the corneal epithelium. During the lag period of the UV keratitis, 30 min. and 3 hours after the irradiation, the ascorbic acid (ASC) levels of the stroma and the epithelium of the cornea were decreased. After 4 hours the lactate levels were also slightly decreased. The lactate/pyruvate ratios did not change. The biochemical lesion of UV light could not be identified by the results of this study. But the early decrease of the ASC in the corneal epithelium and stroma may point to a damage of this tissue by perioxides as postulated by several authors.

INTRODUCTION

The transparent tissues of the eye are not protected from the light by absorbent pigment layers. UV keratitis is the dramatic debridement of the corneal epithelium following UV irradiation. After a lag period of 6-10 hours, the disease begins with the onset of heavy pains, congestion of the conjunctiva and lacrimation.

A corneal erosion is observed and lasts for 24 to 48 hours (Birch-Hirschfeld, 1904). The silent incubation period drew our attention to this disease. According to a hypothesis of Pirie (1946, 1965) it was postulated that the light produced peroxides in the transparent tissues of the eye. These peroxides were supposed to be toxic to cells, attacking primarily all membrane structures.

In the cornea a reduction of the toxic perioxides is possible by means of the glutathione peroxidase (GSHPX) and by direct non-enzymatical oxidation of ascorbic acid. The resulting dehydroascorbic acid as well as the glutathione obtain their reducing potentials from the glutathione reductase and further from the hexose phosphate shunt.

The enzymes involved were demonstrated in the cornea by estimation of their activities (Reim et al., 1971; Reim et al., 1974). The chemical reactions of this metabolic pathway were shown to take place by the determination of the steady state levels of the metabolites involved (Reim et al., 1976).

In rabbits it is possible to produce the UV keratitis in a model experiment (Duke-Elder, 1972). But the energy necessary to produce a UV keratitis in rabbits is larger than in man. Cogan & Kinsey (1946), Kinsey (1948) & Bachem (1956) found a spectral sensitivity of the cornea in the ultraviolet range from 280 to 310 nm and the maximum sensitivity at 288 nm.

METHODS

We used an analytical UV lamp to produce experimental UV keratitis (Original Hanau Fluotest forte, Typ 5261, 210 W, Original Hanau Quarzlampen GmbH, Hanau, Germany; Fig. 1). Rabbits of a grey german wild strain weighing 2,5-3,5 kg were operated on in general anesthesia by i.v. injection of pentobarbital (35 mg/kg). The cornea of one eye was irradiated for 15 min. in a distance of 30 cm. To avoid drying of the corneal surface, it was carefully rinsed with saline (four drops per minute). Then the lids were closed with adhesive tape as long as the animal was kept in general anesthesia. The other eye of the animal served as control. It was kept closed by adhesive tape during the irradiation of the experimental eye.

At different time intervals following the UV irradiation, again under general anesthesia the corneal epithelium was scraped with a blunt hockey knife and immediately brought into liquid nitrogen or directly into perchloric acid. The corneal epithelium was extracted in 0,2 ml and reextracted in 0,1 ml of 0,5 N perchloric acid in a cooled micro glass in glass homogenizer.

The anterior chamber was punctured at the limbus with a 17 gauge needle and 0,2 ml aqueous humour were aspirated and extracted in 0,2 ml of 10% oxalic acid. The stroma was excised at the limbus with scissors and

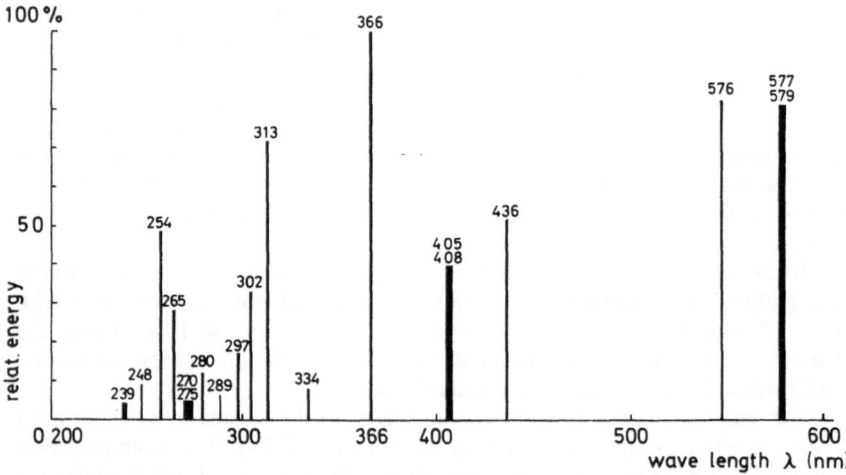

Fig. 1. Relative spectral energy of the UV lamp used in this investigation. (Original Hanau Fluotest forte, Typ 5261, 210 W).

cut into small pieces with scissors or crushed under liquid nitrogen in a mortar. Then the stroma was homogenized in a glass in glass homogenizer using 1,0 and 0,5 ml of 0,5 N perchloric acid and extracted like the epithelium. In each of the extractions the protein precipitate was separated from the homogenate by centrifugation at 2000 g. For the assay of the reduced (GSH) and oxidized (GSSG) glutathione and the lactate, the supernatants were neutralized with 10 N KOH to pH 3,0.

Since the assay of the glutathione was somewhat difficult in single rabbit epithelium we also used isolated bovine eyes. The bovine eyes were obtained freshly from the slaughter house and kept in a moist chamber at room-temperature. The UV irradiation began 30 min. after death of the cattle. The same irradiation conditions were used for the isolated bovine eyes as in rabbits in vivo. The same preparation and extraction methods were used as in rabbit eyes. Only the extraction volumes of 0,5 N perchloric acid were changed to 1,5 ml for corneal epithelium, 3,5 ml for the stroma, and 2,0 ml for the aqueous humour. The reduced and oxidized glutathione were assayed in the combined optic enzymatic test using crystallized glyoxalase I and glutathione reductase as described previously (Reim, et al., 1976). The lactate levels were determined enzymatically according to Hohorst et al. (1959). The ascorbic acid was assayed using the photometric test with 2,6-dichlorophenolindophenol. The method described by Reim & Luthe (1977) was slightly modified by using perchloric acid in the tissue extrac-

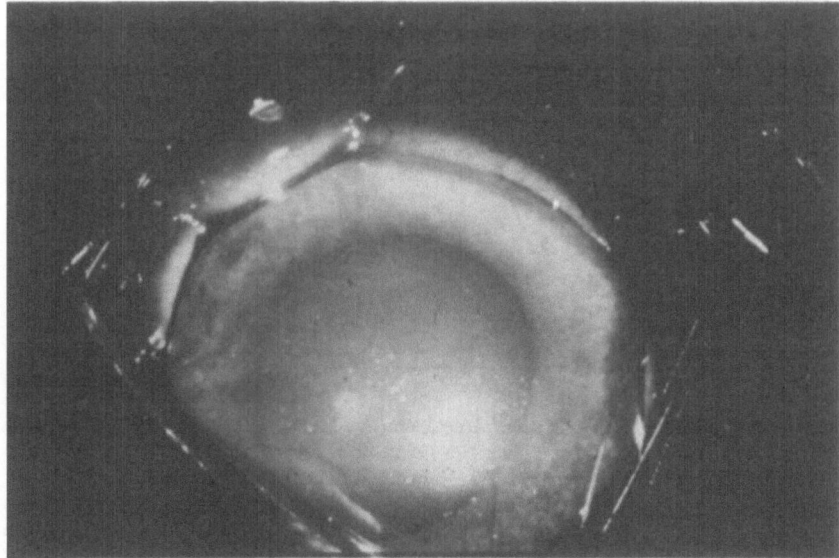

Fig. 2. Rabbit eye 14 hours after UV irradiation. The erosion of the cornea in the irradiated area is stained with fluorescein. The lower part of the cornea, that was covered by the lids, is not damaged.

tions. Analytical controls showed that in tissue extractions the use of perchloric acid gave more reproducible results than oxalic acid. The dye concentration was 0,1 M 2,6-dichlorophenolindophenol. The test was made up with 1,0 ml K, Na, phosphate, 100 mM, pH 6,6 and 0,05 ml 2,6-dichlorophenolindophenol. In a normal cuvette with 1 cm light path the initial extinction was recorded at 600 nm for 3 min. Then 0,05-0,30 ml of the neutralized extract supernatant were added and the final extinction recorded for 3 min. The extinction differences were proportional to the ASC content and calculated by use of a calibration line and defined ascorbic acid solutions. As described previously (Reim & Luthe, 1977) this method proved to be reliable in the corneal layers and in the aqueous humour.

RESULTS

After UV irradiation, the cornea remained normal up to ten hours. Then the exposed area of the corneal epithelium developed punctate keratitis and some time later a superficial defect staining with fluorescein. The conjunctiva was red and swollen. 24 to 48 hours after the UV irradiation the epithe-

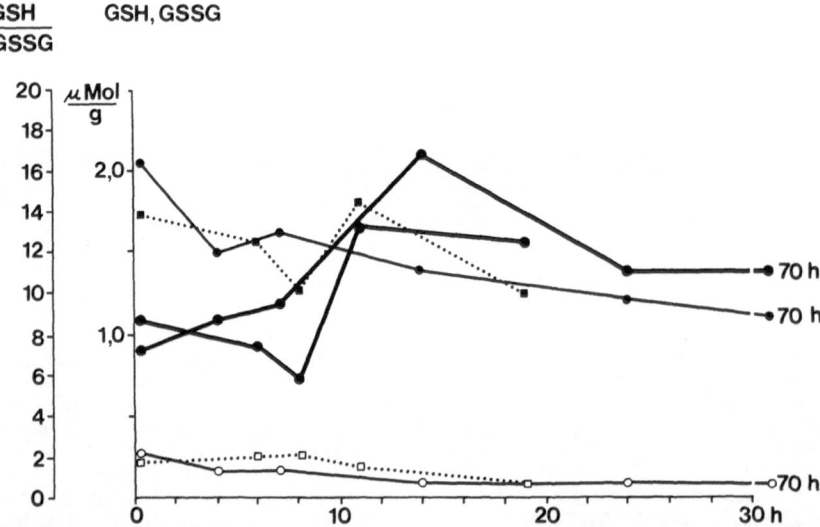

Fig. 3. Glutathione levels in the corneal epithelium of rabbits in vivo and isolated bovine eyes. The first ordinate gives the glutathione levels in μMol/g wet weight. The upper lines and the closed symbols represent the reduced glutathione (GSH). The lower lines with open symbols represent the oxidized glutathione (GSSG). The continuous lines were obtained from rabbit eyes in vivo, and the dotted ones from isolated bovine eyes kept in a moist chamber. The thickly drawn lines represent the ratios of GSH/GSSG the values of which are given in the second ordinate. Each of the symbols represents the mean value of 10 experiments. The standard deviations were calculated and did not exceed 20% of the mean value.

lium was regenerated and looked quite normal (Fig. 2). The results of the glutathione assays were demonstrated in the diagram of Fig. 3. After UV irradiation both forms of the glutathione decreased, the GSH more slowly after the onset of the UV keratitis. Therefore, an increase of the GSH/GSSG ratio was observed between 9 and 11 hours after UV irradiation. No significant change of the glutathione levels was observed during the incubation of the UV keratitis. So the initial lesion of the cornea by UV light did not affect the glutathione.

Fig. 4 shows the results of the ascorbic acid assays. At 30 minutes after the UV irradiation the ASC levels of the corneal epithelium did not change significantly, but the ASC levels of the stroma were statistically significantly reduced. At 3 hours after the UV irradiation also the ASC levels in the epithelium were decreased. These changes were observed although the epithelium looked completely normal at that time.

At 24 hours after the UV irradiation the UV keratitis was fully developed. The decrease of the ASC levels in each of the compartments was surely a consequence of the visible damage to the epithelium.

In the incubation period of the UV keratitis the lactate levels showed only slightly, but not significantly decreased levels (Fig. 5). At later stages

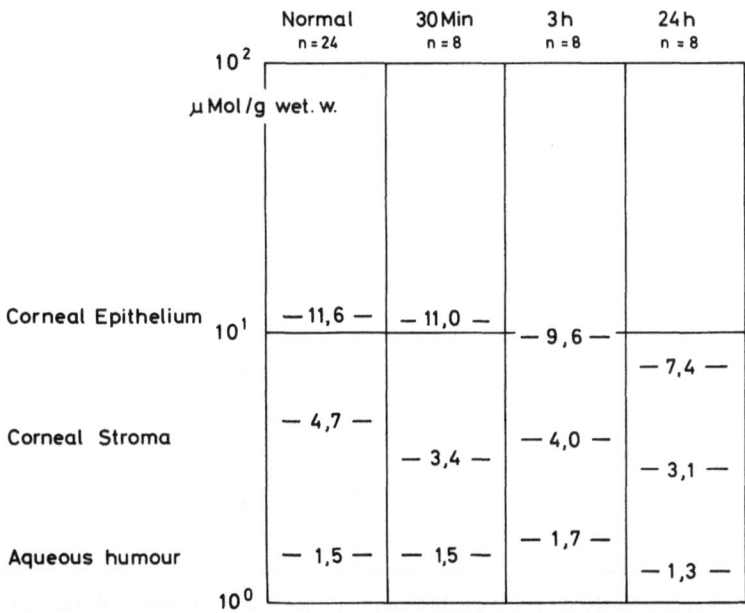

Fig. 4. Ascorbic acid levels after UV irradiation of rabbits. The logarithmic ordinate gives the ascorbic acid levels in the corneal epithelium, stroma and in the aqueous humour (μMol/g wet weight). Each figure in the diagram represents the average of the number of experiments indicated on the top of the columns. The standard deviations of the mean values were calculated and did not exceed 10% of the mean values.

of the disease, the decrease of the lactate levels may be related to the destroyed corneal epithelium, the lactate production of which was certainly reduced. This observation was in correlation to previous results after freezing the corneal epithelium in vivo (Reim et al., 1971).

DISCUSSION

This investigation showed a significant reduction of the ascorbic acid levels in the anterior eye segment, already during the incubation period of the UV keratitis. Therefore, the initially mentioned hypothesis of Pirie (1946) may be correct according to which the light produced peroxides in the eye and oxidized the ascorbic acid. The unexpected observation that the stroma ascorbic acid levels were more and earlier affected than those of the corneal epithelium may be explained by the fact, that the compensation mechanisms of the epithelium were much stronger than in the stroma.

The corneal epithelium has the active hexose phosphate shunt and an

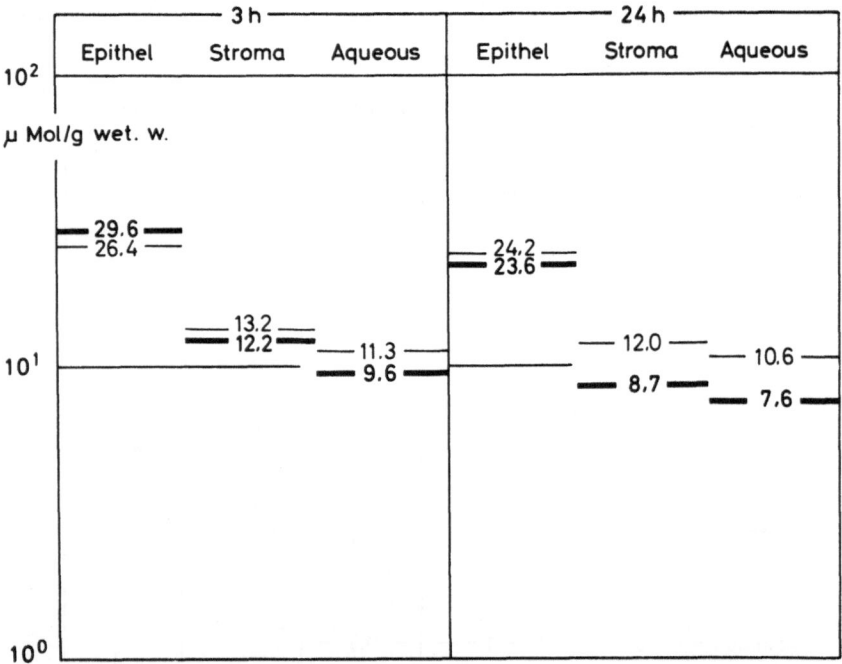

Fig. 5. Lactate levels after UV irradiation of rabbits. The thick lines and figures in the diagram demonstrate the lactate levels of the eyes after UV irradiation. The thin lines and the corresponding figures represent the values of the normal fellow eyes of the same animals. The logarithmic ordinate gives the lactate levels in μMol/g wet weight. Each of the figures represents the average of 8 experiments. The standard deviations of the mean values were calculated and were lower than 10% of the mean values.

efficient glutathione reducing system. These reactions were known to operate well under unfavourable conditions. (Reim & Ashauer, 1975). Therefore, the glutathione levels and the GSH/GSSG ratios too, remained unchanged in the epithelium during the incubation of the UV keratitis.

The well reduced state of the glutathione in the corneal epithelium may have effected a rapid reduction of dehydroascorbic acid possibly formed by the peroxides after UV irradiation.

Apparently, the conditions of the reduction of the dehydroascorbic acid were not so favourable in the stroma of the cornea as in the epithelium, since in the stroma a large proportion of the ascorbic acid was located in the extracellular space and therefore was not in immediate contact to the strictly intracellular reducing system of the glutathione and the hexose phosphate shunt.

The investigation of the glutathione and ascorbic acid levels in the cornea demonstrated that the reducing capacities of the hexose phosphate glutathione system were strong enough to compensate for the irradiation effect leading to UV keratitiso long as as the epithelium is intact. The maximal UV absorption of the cornea between 280 and 310 nm as demonstrated by Cogan & Kinsey (1947) may lead further investigations to substances that show absorption bands in this region.

Kinsey (1948) supposed that the UV irradiation may affect primarily the nucleoproteines. Therefore, the nucleotide levels are presently investigated to search for the primary biochemical lesion of the cornea by UV light.

ACKNOWLEDGEMENTS

This work was supported by the Deutsche Forschungsgemeinschaft 53 Bonn — Bad Godesberg.

The results of this paper were presented at the 18th Meeting of the Association for Eye Research at Bonn, July 1977.

REFERENCES

Bachem, A. Ophthalmic Ultraviolet Action Spectra. *Am. J. Ophthal.* 41: *969-975* (1956).

Birch-Hirschfeld, A. Die wirkung der ultravioletten strahlen auf das auge.*A. v. Graefes Arch. Ophthal.* 58: *469-562* (1904).

Cogan, D.G. & Kinsey, E. Action spectrum of keratitis produced by ultraviolet radiation. *Arch. Ophthal., Chicago*, 35: *670-677* (1946).

Duke-Elder, W.S. Action on the outer eye. Photoophthalmia. System of Ophthalmology, Vol. IXX. Injuries Part II, Chapter (1972) *918-928.*

Hohorst, H.J., Kreutz, F.H. & Dücher, T.H. Über metabolitgehalte und metabolitkonzentrationen in der leber der ratte. *Biochem. Z.* 332: *18-46* (1959).

Kinsey, V.E. Spectral transmission of the eye to ultraviolet radiations. *Arch. Ophthal., Chicago*, 39: *508-513* (1948).

Pirie, A. Ascorbic acid content of the cornea. *Biochem. J.* 40: *96-99* (1946).

Pirie, A. Glutathone peroxidase in lens and source of hydrogen peroxide in aqueous humour. *Biochem. J.* 96: *244-253* (1965).

Reim, M., Ashauer, D. The glutathione of the cornea. *Arch. Ophthal., Paris,* 35: *153-158* (1975).

Reim, M., Beerman, H.R., Luthe, P. & Cattepoel, H. The redox state of the glutathione in the bovine corneal epithelium. *A. v. Graefes Arch. klin. exper. Ophthal.* 201: *143-148* (1976).

Reim, M., Heuvels, B. & Cattepoel, H. Glutathione Peroxidase in Some Ocular Tissues. – *Ophthal. Res.* 6: *228-234* (1974).

Reim, M., Hennigheusen, U., Hildebrandt, D. & Maier, R. Enzyme activities in the cornea epithelium and endothelium of different species. – *Ophthal. Res.* 2: *171-182* (1971).

Reim, M., Boeck, H., Krug, P. & Venske, G. Aqueous humour and cornea stroma metabolite levels under various conditions. *Ophthal. Res.* 3: *241-250* (1972).

Reim, M. & Schmidt, F. Biochemische Veränderungen bei der Vereisung der Hornhaut in vivo. Ein beitrag zur Kältetherapie. *Klin. Mbl. Augenheilk.* 150: *96-103* (1967).

Reim, M., Lipp, U. & Venske, G.: Biochemical changes in the cornea after cryotherapy. Proc. XXI. Int. Congr. Ophthal., Mexico 1970; Excerpta Medical Amsterdam 1971, *550-554.*

Reim, M. & Luthe, P., Compartmentation of redox metabolites in the anterior eye segment? – *A. v. Graefes Arch. klin. exper. Ophthal.* 204: *135-140* (1977).

Author's address:
Prof. Dr. med. M. Reim
Vorstand der Abteilung für Augenheilkunde
der Medizinischen Fakultät der RWTH
Goethestraße 27-29
5100 Aachen
Germany

OCULAR FINDINGS IN ADOLESCENT AND ADULT CYSTINOSIS

HANS-EBERHARD VÖLCKER, ERIK HARMS, GERHARD WEISS & GOTTFRIED O.H. NAUMANN

(Tübingen, Heidelberg, F.R.G.)

ABSTRACT

Report on two patients with non-infantile cystinosis. In both cases the ophthalmologist first made the diagnosis.
1. A 12 year old boy with normal visual function suffered from photophobia and showed the typical corneal and conjunctival deposits of crystine crystals. A conjunctival biopsy and skin fibroblast culture studies confirmed the diagnosis. Electroretinography was normal.
2. A 24 year old male suffered from renal disease starting at the age of 9 years. The diagnosis was made by the ophthalmologist because of the typical conjunctival and corneal cystine crystals. Skin fibroblast cultures confirmed the diagnosis biochemically.

All patients with renal disease of unknown etiology should be seen by an ophthalmologist.

INTRODUCTION

Cystinosis results from an autosomal recessive metabolic disease, probably due to an unknown enzyme deficiency. Crystalline cystine is deposited in lysosomes of reticulo-endothelial cells of liver, lymph nodes, bone marrow, kidney and eye. *Infantile cystinosis*, the most common type, is characterized by renal tubular disfunction (generalized aminoaciduria, glucosuria and phosphaturia), rachitic dwarfism and progressive glomerular damage of the kidney within the first years of life leading to death from uremia before puberty (Bickel et al., 1952). *Adolescent* cystinosis shows the first symptoms in late childhood, the progressive glomerular damage of the kidneys occurs later. The patients therefore may survive to the third decade. So far it has not been ascertained that this is a genetically different disease. Perhaps adolescent cystinosis represents only a particularly slow and protracted course of the same entity as infantile cystinosis. Adult cystinosis is a rare entity, quite distinct however from infantile and adolescent cystinosis. There is no renal damage at all.

Since Bürki (1941) deposits of cystine crystals in cornea and conjunctiva have been frequently reported in infantile cystinosis; later also in other ocular tissues: choroid, retina, optic nerve (Ullerich, 1951; Cogan et al., 1956; Cogan, 1966; Wong et al., 1967; Bickel et al., 1968; Kenyon & Sensenbrenner, 1974; Sanderson et al., 1974; Cogan & Kuwabara, 1960).

The typical conjunctival and corneal findings associated with photophobia frequently lead to clinical diagnosis.

In contrast to this there have been only sporadic observations of cystinosis after childhood and in adults. The purpose of this report is to document two patients of 12 and 24 years where the ophthalmologist first made the clinical diagnosis of cystinosis. Histologic findings of the conjunctiva and determination of the cystine-content in skin fibroblast cultures confirmed the entity.

PATIENTS AND METHODS OF INVESTIGATION

During the summer of 1975 two patients aged 12 and 24 years were seen because of visual deterioration and photophobia. A clinical diagnosis of cystinosis was made.

I. *A conjunctival biopsy* was obtained from the 12 year old boy (R.K.) and studied with two methods:

Conjunctival stroma was placed on a slide and studied with polarized light. Another piece of conjunctiva immediately after biopsy was placed in 2-Methylbutane (C_5H_{12}) frozen by fluid nitrogen to about $-100°C$. Sections by a cryotom measured about $10\,\mu$. Unstained sections were placed in Glycerin-Gelatine and studied with the phase contrast microscope.

II. *Cystine determination in skin fibroblast cultures:* The diagnosis was biochemically established by determination of free non-protein bound cystine in skin fibroblast cultures. A skin biopsy from the upper arm was obtained for primary culture in cover slip technique. Culture medium was HAM's F10 supplemented with 20% fetal calf serum, 100 IU penicillin-G/ml and 0,1 mg streptomycin sulphate per ml. Further passages of the primary cell line were performed in the same culture medium supplemented with 10% fetal calf serum.

Cystine-content of monolayer cultures of the 6th-10th passage were determined by automatic aminoacid analysis (Schneider et al., 1967). The column-chromatographic separation was performed via 0,6 x 32 cm Durrum-DC-6A in an aminoacid analyzer of the type BioCal BC 201 (LKB, Gräfelfing, Germany).

CASE REPORTS

Case No. 1 (R.K.) born August 9th, 1963
Ocular findings: This 12 year old boy consulted us because of photophobia. Visual acuity was OU: 1,0; intraocular pressure measured OU: 16 mm Hg. The motility of the globe was unremarkable. The tarsal and bulbar conjunctiva showed numerous confluent glistening crystals within its stroma. These crystals were particularly dense at the limbus and around vessels (Fig. 1). Biopsy from the fornix showed colorless birefringent rectangular, hexagonal or polygonal crystals both extra- and intracellularily (Fig. 2). There was no inflammatory reaction. The cornea showed profuse deposition of crystals within the *stroma* in all its layers at the limbus; the corneal

center showed a decrease in the density of crystals from the anterior to the posterior layers (Fig. 3). Corneal epithelium, iris, lens and fundus did not reveal pathologic changes. The visual field was normal; electroretinography did not show any abnormalities.

Diagnosis: 'Cystinosis' of cornea and conjunctiva
Systemic findings: Family history was unremarkable. At the age of 6 years (1969) this boy developed scarlet fever and was treated with sulfonamides. At this time a moderate albuminuria was noted and interpreted as a part of a 'membranous glomerulonephritis'. There was no erythrocyturia and blood pressure was normal. 1972 a renal biopsy showed 'normal parenchymal structures'. *The diagnosis of cystinosis was first introduced by the ophthalmologist in summer of 1975.* Regular check-ups by the internist up to 1978 showed only moderate proteinuria, amino-acid determination in blood and urine were normal and there was no hyperaminoaciduria. Only after the diagnosis of cystinosis was made by us in 1975 were cystine crystals found in bone marrow.

Cystine determination in fibroblast tissue cultures was 13,7; 5,9; and 7,3 nMol half-cystine/mg protein (determinations from 3 cultures). Cystine determination in a 3 year older sister revealed 0,56 nMol half-cystine/mg protein. This suggests a heterozygosty.
Diagnosis: 'Adult cystinosis'

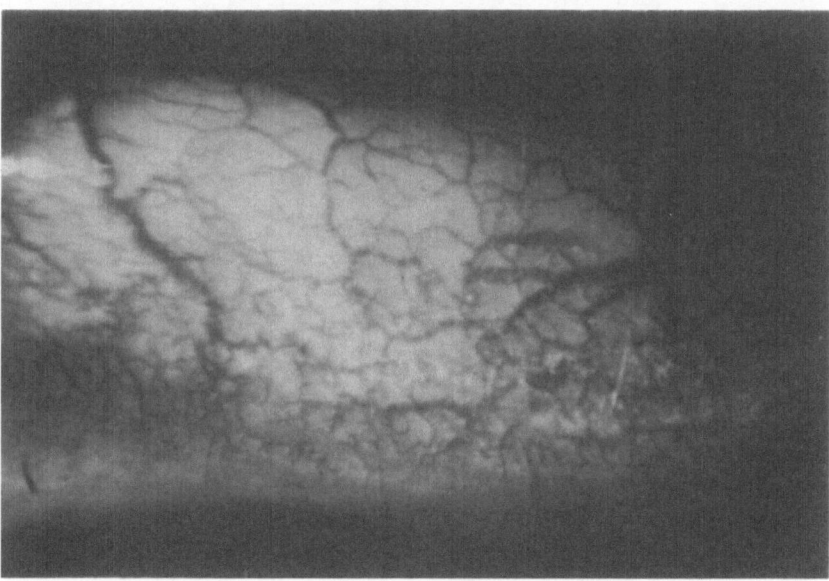

Fig. 1. Tarsal conjunctiva with numerous glistening crystals particularly dense around the vessels.

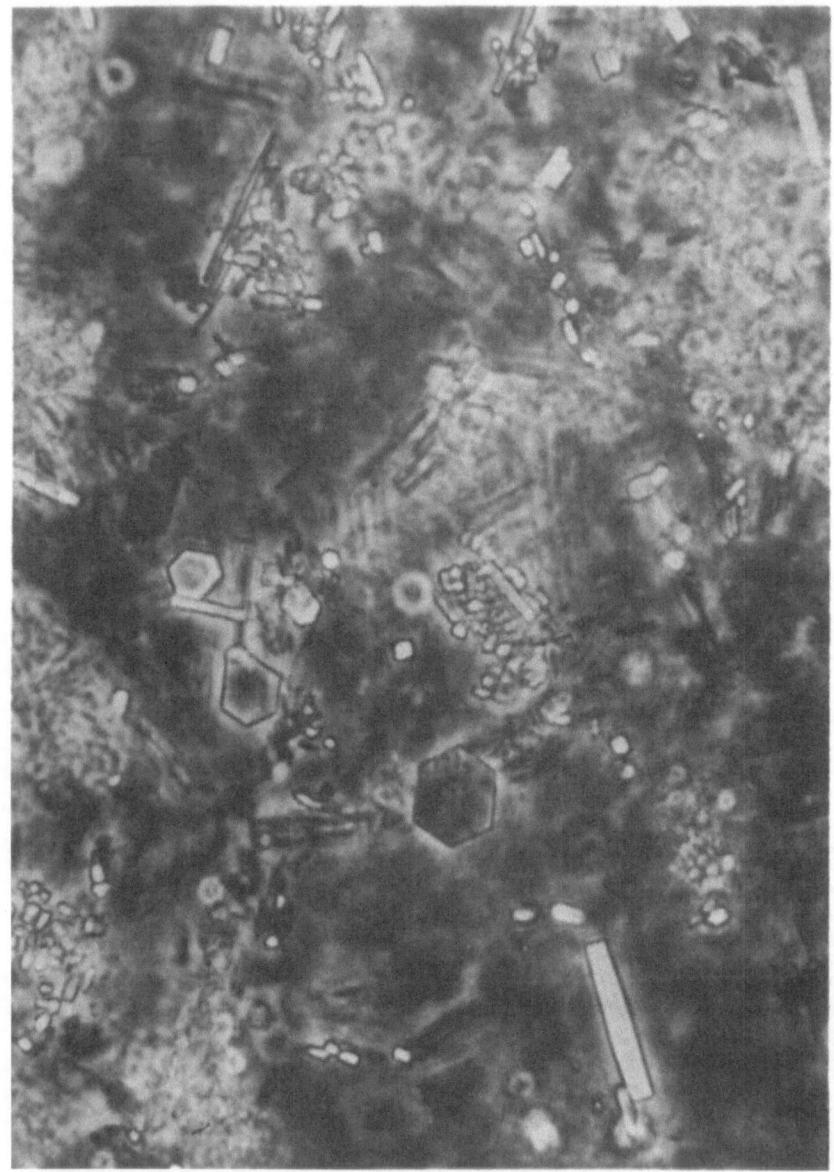

Fig. 2. Phase contrast microscopic picture of the conjunctival biopsy (see Fig. 1): typical colorless birefringent rectangular, hexagonal and polygonal cystine crystals (unstained frozen sections 1:180).

314

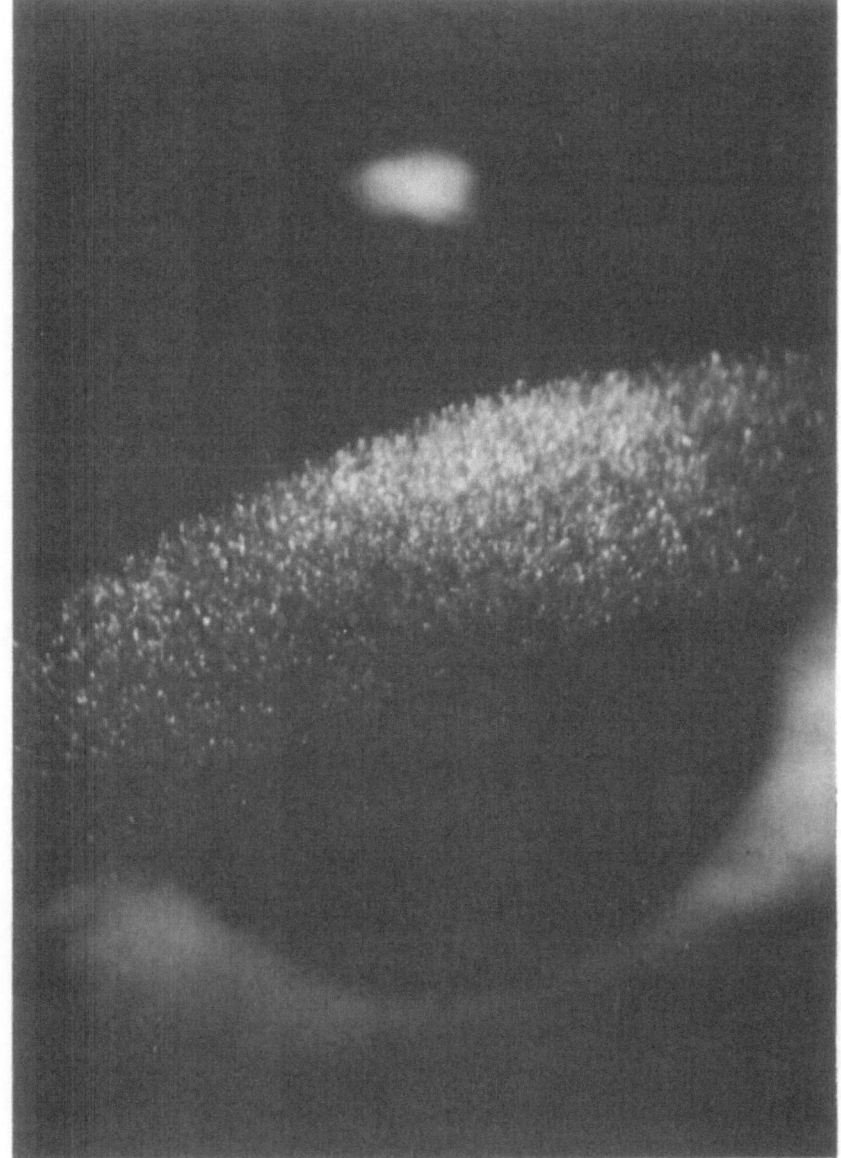

Fig. 3. Slit lamp picture of the cornea: profuse deposition of cystine crystals within the stroma.

Case No. 2 (G.St.) Born November 20th, 1951

Ocular findings: This 24 year old male consulted us because of deterioration of vision but did not complain of photophobia. Visual acuity was OD: 0,7; OS: 0,6; intraocular pressure OU: 14 mm Hg. The conjunctiva again revealed numerous minute crystalline deposits in the tarsal and bulbar conjunctiva with marked condensation of these crystalline deposits around vessels. The corneal stroma showed numerous crystalline deposits with increasing density towards the periphery. At the limbus all corneal layers were effected; the central portions showed a decrease of the crystal density from the anterior to the posterior layers. The corneal epithelium was unremarkable. Anterior chamber and iris did not reveal any abnormalities. The lens showed granular opacities of the anterior and posterior cortex and fine opacities of the posterior subcapsular area (cataracta complicata). The fundus did not show any abnormalities in the macular area or periphery.

Systemic findings: Family history was unremarkable. This boy developed normally until he was found to have marked proteinuria at the age of 9 years (1960). A diagnosis of 'nephrosis' was made. The proteinuria decreased after therapy with corticosteroids. In 1969 hospitalization was necessary because of polyuria (1900 ml daily). A renal biopsy was interpreted as 'advanced chronic glomerulo-nephritis'. The serum creatinine level was 3,9 mg%, urea nitrogen 33 mg% and creatinine-clearance 32 ml/min. In 1969 a uremia developed with urea N-values of 118 mg%, creatinine 11,6 mg% and uremic gastritis. Ever since there have been repeated peritonealdialysis and hemodialysis. A renal transplant in 1973 failed. Since then the patient is regularly treated in a dialysis center. The *diagnosis of cystinosis was first suggested by an ophthalmologist in summer of 1975.* Determination of cystine in skin fibroblast cultures revealed pathologic findings of 2,64; 3,22 and 5,22 nMol half-cystine/mg protein.

Diagnosis: 'Adolescent cystinosis'

DISCUSSION

The ophthalmologist can make the diagnosis of benign or adult forms of cystinosis, where renal tubular or glomerular defects are missing. Since the first description of 'adult cystinosis' (Cogan, 1957) — a possible case of cystinosis from Bürki & Rohner (1955) was later described as 'multiple myeloma with paraprotein-deposits (Cogan, 1958) — further cases have been described: Lietmann et al., 1966 (3 cases between the age of 37 and 48 years); Schneider et al., 1968 (3 cases between the age of 37 to 53 years); Brubaker et al., (1970) (2 cases between the age of 11 to 16 years) and Kraus & Lutz, (1971) (1 case at the age of 46 years). In all these cases there were no renal symptoms and no retinal participation, as seen in infantile cystinosis (Francois et al., 1972; Read et al., 1973; Wong et al., 1967; & Schneider et al., 1974). In most of the above mentioned cases cystine could be found, as in our patient, in bone marrow.

The cystine-content in fibroblast cultures, as described by Brubaker et al., (1970) and Schneider et al., (1968) in their adult cystinosis patients, showed the same values as in our patients. Schneider et al., (1968) state that the free cystine content of leukocytes and fibroblasts in adult cystinosis patients averages 30 to 50 times higher than in controls. They are between the values of patients with heterozygotic or homozygotic infantile cystinosis.

Cystine content of fibroblast tissue cultures varies according to the culture medium even with the same cell line remarkably. Therefore any attempt to classify these various types of cystinosis according to the cystine content of fibroblasts would require standardization of the culture media. Our case No. 1 appears to be one of the youngest patients with adult cystinosis — only Brubaker's (1952) case of 11 years was younger. At this stage one can not rule out whether within the second decade an aminoaciduria may occur. If this should happen a reclassification as adolescent cystinosis would be necessary.

All patients classified as 'adolescent' cystinosis (Goldman et al., 1971; Zimmerman, et al., 1974) showed at the time of diagnosis both the characteristic ocular findings and renal damage as Fanconi-Syndrome. (Patients of Goldman at the age of 10 and 11, patient of Zimmerman at the age of 13 years). Therefore we have no doubts that both symptoms and course of our patient no. 2 belong to this category of adolescent cystinosis. The nature of the lens changes found cannot be interpreted with certainly. Most likely they represent complications of the pre-uremic condition of the patient — however from a theoretical point of view the influence of cystinosis cannot be ruled out with certainty.

The interpretation of the minimal proteinuria of our patient 1 is of interest. As it has remained stationary for more than 6 years, this could represent a consequence of scarlet fever because the aminoacid content in the urine has been normal and as there have been no renal symptoms.

Table I. Cystinosis: Differential diagnosis according to clinical findings.

Symptomatology	Infantile	Adolescent	Adult
General:			
Age of manifestation	early childhood	2nd decade	undetermined
Life expectancy	childhood	undetermined	normal
Ocular findings: corneal and conjunctival			
deposits	+	+	+
retinopathy	+	−	−
Renal:			
Glomerular and tubular insufficiency (FANCONI-syndrome)	1. decade generalized	1. to 2. decade generalized	missing

According to Goldman et al., (1971) the most important clinical findings of infantile, adolescent and adult forms of cystinosis reveal that all show corneal and conjunctival changes while retinal findings so far have only been observed in infantile cystinosis (Tab. I).

Structure and localization of the cystine crystals in the conjunctival biopsy are identical to those of cystinosis (Schulman et al., 1970; Kraus, 1971). In cases of doubt conjunctival biopsy is technically simple, safe and permits biochemical differentiation from paraproteinous crystal deposits (Wong et al., 1970). Another method of identification of cystine crystals is x-ray refraction (Bickel & Smellie, 1952; Frazier & Wong, 1968).

Electroretinographic studies in our patient with adult cystinosis did not reveal any abnormalities. This does however not rule out deposits within the retinal pigment epithelium as described by Wong et al. (1970). The ophthalmologist has the key to the clinical diagnosis of cystinosis particularly in its adolescent and adult from. If visual decrease due to the corneal deposits should become severe corneal grafting would appear to be no problem.

In view of the difficulty of the clinical diagnosis by the pediatrician and nephrologist, all patients with renal disease of uncertain etiology should be seen by an ophthalmologist to rule out early cystinosis.

REFERENCES

Bickel, H., Baar, H.S., Astley, R.D., Douglas, A.A., Finck, E., Harris, H., Harvey, C.C., Hickmans, E.M., Philpott, M.G., Smallwood, W.C., Smellie, J.M. & Teall, C.G. Cystine storage disease with aminoaciduria und dwarfism (Lignac-Fanconi) disease. *Acta Paediat.* 42 (Supp 90) (1952).

Bickel, H., Jaeger, W., Wollensak, J., Teller, W. & Kraus, E. Augenveränderungen bei hereditären stoffwechselerkrankungen im kindesalter. *Ber. deutsch. ophthal. Ges.* 69: *16-24* (1968).

Bickel, H. & Smellie, J.M. Cystine storage disease with aminoaciduria. *Lancet* 262: *1023-1095* (1952).

Brubaker, R.F., Wong, V.G., Schulman, J.D. & Seegmiller, J.E. Benign cystinosis. *Am. J. Med.* 49: *546-550* (1970).

Bürki, E. & Rohner, M. Ein seltener fall von kristalliner hornhautdegeneration. *Ophthalmologica* 129: *211-217* (1955).

Bürki, E. Über die Cystinkrankheit im Kleinkindesalter unter besonderer berücksichtigung des augenbefundes. *Ophthalmologica* 101: *257-272* (1941).

Cogan, D.G., Kuwabara, T., Kinoshita, J. & Sheehan, L. Cystinosis in an adult. *J.A.M.A.* 164: *394-396* (1957).

Cogan, D.G. & Kuwabara, T. Ocular pathology of cystinosis. *AMA Arch. Ophthal.* 63: *51-57* (1960).

Cogan, D.G., Kuwabara, T., Kinoshita, J. & Sudarsky, D. Ocular manifestations of systematic cystinosis. *AMA Arch. Ophthal.* 55: *36-41* (1956).

Cogan, D.G. Ocular correlates of inborn metabolic defects. *Canad. Med. Assoc. J.* 95: *1055-1065* (1966).

Cogan, D.G., Kuwabara, T. & Hurlbut, C.S. Further observations on cystinosis in the adult. *J.A.M.A.* 166: *1725-1726* (1958).

Francois, J., Hanssens, M., Coppieters, R. & Evens, L. Cystinosis. *Am. J. Ophthal.* 73: *643-650* (1972).

Frazier, P.D. & Wong, V.G. Cystinosis. *Am. Arch. Ophthal.* 80: *87-91* (1968).

Goldman, H., Scriver, C.R., Aaron, K., Delvin, E. & Canlas, Z. Adolescent cystinosis: comparisons with infantile and adult Form *Pediatrics* 47: *979-988* (1971).

Kenyon, K.R. & Sensenbrenner, J.A. Electron microscopy of cornea and conjunctiva in childhood cystinosis *Am. J. Ophthal.* 78: *68-76* (1974).

Kraus, E. & Lutz, P. Ocular cystine deposits in an adult *Am. Arch. Ophthal.* 85: *690-694* (1971).

Lietman, P.S., Frazier, P.D., Wong, V.G., Shotton, D. & Seegmiller, J.E. Adult cystinosis — benign disorders. *Am. J. Med.* 40: *511-517* (1966).

Read, J., Goldberg, M.F., Fishman, G. & Rosenthal, I. Nephropathic cystinosis. *Am. J. Ophthal.* 76: *791-796* (1973).

Sanderson, P.O., Kuwabara, T., Stark, W.J., Wong, V.G. & Collins, E.M. Cystinosis. A clinical, histopathologic and ultrastructural study. *Am. Arch. Ophthal.* 91: *270-274* (1974).

Schneider, J.A., Verroust, F.M., Kroll, W.A., Garvin, A.J., Horger, E.O., Wong, V.G., Spear, G.S., Jacobson, C., Pellett, O.L. & Becker, F.L.A. Prenatal diagnosis of cystinosis, *New Engl. J. Med.* 290: *878-882* (1974).

Schneider, J.A., Wong, V.G., Bradley, K. & Seegmiller, J.E. Biochemical Comparisons of the adult and childhood forms of cystinosis. *New Engl. J. Med.* 279: *1253-1257* (1968).

Schneider, J.A., Rosenbloom, F.M., Bradley, K. & Seegmiller, J.E. Increased free-cystine content of fibroblasts cultured from patients with cystinosis. *Biochem. Biophys. Res. Commun.* 29: *527-531* (1967).

Schulman, J.D., Wong, V.G., Olson, W.H. & Seegmiller, J.E. Lysosomal site of crystalline deposits in cystinosis as shown by ferritin uptake. *Arch. Path.* 90: *259-264* (1970).

Ullerich, K. Über Augenveränderungen bei der cystinkrankheit. *Ber. deutsch. ophthal. Ges.* 57: *306-309* (1951).

Wong, V.G., Lietman, P.S. & Seegmiller, J.E. Alterations of pigment epithelium in cystinosis. *Am. Arch. Ophthal.* 77: *361-369* (1967).

Wong, V.G., Schulman, J.D. & Seegmiller, J.E. Conjunctival biopsy for the biochemical diagnosis of cystinosis. *Am. J. Ophthal.* 70: *278-281* (1970).

Wong, V.G., Kuwabara, T., Brubaker, R., Olson, W., Schulman, J. & Seegmiller, J.E. Intralysosomal cystine crystals in cystinosis. *Invest. Ophthal.* 9: *83-88* (1970).

Zimmerman, T.J., Hood, I. & Gasset, A.R. 'Adolescent' cystinosis. *Am. Arch. Ophthal.* 92: *265-268* (1974).

Docum. Ophthal. Proc. Series, Vol. 18

IN VITRO CORTICOSTEROID SENSITIVITY IN PATIENTS WITH FUCHS' DYSTROPHY

STEPHEN R. WALTMAN & PAUL F. PALMBERG &
BERNARD BECKER

(St. Louis, Missouri, U.S.A.)

ABSTRACT

Of 16 patients with Fuchs' corneal dystrophy who were classified prospectively and in masked fashion by an in vitro assay of corticosteroid responsiveness (using their lymphocytes), only 2 (13%) were found to be markedly responsive. Both developed clinically significant elevations of intraocular pressure in the eyes subjected to topical corticosteroids postkeratoplasty and required anti-glaucomatous therapy for more than three months postoperatively. Of the 10 other patients undergoing keratoplasty, one developed a clinically significant pressure elevation in one eye but not in his fellow eye.

Since peripheral anterior synechias were present in the affected eye and not in the contralateral eye that received the same postoperative corticosteroid therapy, cortico-steroid-induced pressure elevation seemed unlikely in this patient.

These preliminary results suggested that in vitro corticosteroid testing prior to keratoplasty might be helpful in identifying those patients who will develope cortico-steroid-induced intraocular pressure elevation.

INTRODUCTION

The postoperative management of patients who undergo penetrating kerato-plasty or combined procedures for Fuchs' corneal dystrophy is not infre-quently complicated by glaucoma. Such glaucoma may be pre-existing, in-duced by postoperative corticosteroids, or due to peripheral anterior syne-chias.

It is estimated that 10-15% of patients with Fuchs' dystrophy have an associated open-angle glaucoma prior to surgery (Kolker & Hetherington, 1976). It is not known whether this is primary open-angle glaucoma or involvement of the trabecular meshwork endothelium by the same disease process that occurs in the corneal endothelium. It is also possible that those patients with Fuchs' dystrophy who consult an ophthalmologist have higher intraocular pressures and symptomatic epithelial edema. If the glaucoma is primary open-angle glaucoma, one would anticipate that postoperative corti-costeroids would exacerbate it (Becker & Mills, 1963; Armaly, 1963).

Even if there is no relationship between primary open-angle glaucoma

Supported in part by grant EY-01167 from the National Eye Institute, Bethesda, Maryland.

and Fuchs' dystrophy, one can anticipate that some preoperatively normotensive patients will develop elevated intraocular pressures while on long-term topical corticosteroid therapy (Becker, 1971); to prevent graft rejection.

It is useful clinically to know, therefore, which patients will develop corticosteroid-induced pressure elevation or exacerbation of existing glaucoma. Preoperative topical corticosteroid testing in eyes with compromised corneas is complicated by altered drug penetration in eyes with epithelial edema, difficulties in measuring pressures, and increased the risk of corneal infection. Fortunately, an in vitro assay of corticosteroid responsiveness (using the patients' lymphocytes) is available that correlates well with the ocular corticosteroid response (Bigger et al., 1975). Patients with primary open-angle glaucoma are particularly responsive (Bigger et al., 1975; Foon et al., 1977).

We report a group of patients with Fuchs' dystrophy classified as to *in vitro* responsiveness to corticosteroid in which intraocular pressures after penetrating keratoplasty were followed.

SUBJECTS AND METHODS

Sixteen patients with Fuchs' corneal dystrophy without prior ocular surgery were studied. All had clinically advanced disease with corneal thickening, epithelial edema, and reduction of visual acuity to less than 20/100. Many also had cataracts. All patients had preoperative intraocular pressures below 20 mm Hg by applanation and Mackay-Marg tonometry. They all had deep anterior chambers, and where visible the cup/disc ratio never exceeded 0.3 by color. There were 13 females and 3 males, and all but one were over the age of 60 years. Twelve patients underwent penetrating keratoplasty, four of these bilaterally. Eleven of the operations were combined keratoplasty and cataract extractions. The remaining four patients have not yet undergone keratoplasty. In vitro testing was done prior to any ocular surgery, and the results were not revealed to the surgeon until after completion of six months postoperative follow up.

The technique of in vitro assay of corticosteroid response and data analysis has been described previously (Bigger et al., 1975). The method was adapted in the present study to a microtiter plate system (Foon et al., 1977). The concentrations of prednisolone-21-phosphate required to inhibit tritiated thymidine uptake by 50% (half inhibition concentration, or I_{50} value) in phytohemagglutinin-P stimulated lymphocytes were determined concurrently for 16 patients with Fuchs' dystrophy, a control group of 17 ocular normotensive patients, and 7 patients with known primary open-angle glaucoma.

RESULTS

In the lymphocyte assay, lower I_{50} values signified greater sensitivity to corticosteroids. The mean I_{50} value of the control group was 165 ± 14 (SE) ng/ml, significantly (p < 0.001) higher than the result for the primary open-angle glaucoma patients, 78 ± 9. The mean I_{50} value for the Fuchs' dystrophy patients was 134 ± 14 (SE) ng/ml, also significantly greater than that of the glaucoma patients (p < 0.01), but not differing significantly from the control group.

Designating a level of 103 ng/ml or less as indicating marked in vitro corticosteroid responsiveness, all seven primary open-angle glaucoma patients, but just two of the 17 controls, and two of the 16 Fuchs' dystrophy patients fell into this category. Thus the distribution of responses of the Fuchs' dystrophy patients resembled that of the control patients, but differed significantly (Chi-square p < 0.01) from the glaucoma patients.

Intraocular pressure was monitored immediately postoperatively and at follow up in all patients. No eye had an intraocular pressure elevation immediately following surgery of greater than 45 mm Hg despite the fact that 11 had combined keratoplasty and cataract extraction. There were no wound leaks and no flat chambers. All grafts remained clear six months postoperatively.

Three patients have required topical medication for elevated intraocular pressures for more than three months after surgery. Two of these were designated preoperatively as markedly responsive to corticosteroids by the in vitro assay. The first patient had an I_{50} value of 51 ng/ml. He developed an intraocular pressure over 30 mm Hg, which led to minimal but definite graft edema. His visual field and optic cup remained entirely normal, and the intraocular pressure was normalized with topical pilocarpine, with clearing of the corneal edema. The second patient had an I_{50} value of 21 ng/ml. She developed extensive cupping with marked field loss in the operated eye, and when maximum medical therapy failed to bring her pressure below 35 mm Hg, cyclocryotherapy was required. Although both patients had their corticosteroids reduced to a low concentration of prednisolone (0.12%) every day or every other day, resolution of the elevated intraocular pressure did not occur. In addition, gonioscopy was somewhat difficult in these patients, and they may have had multiple small peripheral anterior synechias.

The third patient, who had an average in vitro corticosteroid response, underwent bilateral keratoplasties without intraoperative complication. One eye has developed extensive cupping and field loss with pressures that are

Table 1. Prednisolone Phosphate Inhibition of Lymphocyte Transformation in Fuchs' Corneal Dystrophy.

	Number patients	Mean I_{50} (ng/ml)	Standard error
Fuchs'	16	134	14
Normals	17	165	14
Primary open-angle glaucoma	7	78	9

35-40 mm Hg without glaucoma therapy. The pressure was later brought under medical control. The other eye maintains normal intraocular pressure despite the similar use of corticosteroids. Although this patient maintained deep anterior chambers postoperatively, gonioscopy reveals an asymmetry, with more synechias in the eye with the elevated pressure.

DISCUSSION

Of the 16 patients with Fuchs' corneal dystrophy who were classified by in vitro corticosteroid responsiveness, only 2 (13%) had the marked responsiveness characteristic of primary open-angle glaucoma and of ocular normotensive persons known to be highly responsive to topical steroids. Both developed clinically significant elevations of intraocular pressure (> 30 mm Hg) that required topical medication for more than three months postoperatively. Although their glaucoma may have been induced by corticosteroids, reduction in steroid dosage did not lead to pressure reduction. Of the 10 other Fuchs' dystrophy patients who underwent keratoplasty (with or without cataract extraction), only one developed a clinically significant pressure elevation. In that case extensive synechia formation was noted, and the contralateral eye, which was similarly operated upon and received the same postoperative corticosteroid therapy, did not develop pressure elevation. Thus, corticosteroid-induced pressure elevation seemed unlikely in this patient.

Our results suggest that in vitro corticosteroid testing prior to keratoplasty may be helpful in identifying those patients who will be susceptible to corticosteroid-induced intraocular pressure elevations. A much greater number of patients must be studied in order to assess the utility of such testing.

REFERENCES

Armaly, M.F. Effect of corticosteroids on intraocular pressure and fluid dynamics, II. The effect of dexamethasone in the glaucomatous eye. *Archs. Ophthal.* 70: *492* (1963).

Becker, B. & Mills, D.W. Corticosteroids and intraocular pressure. *Archs. Ophthal.* 70: *500* (1963).

Becker, B. Diabetes mellitus and primary open-angle glaucoma. *Am. J. Ophthal.* 71: *1* (1971).

Bigger, J.F., Palmberg, P.F. & Zink, H.A. In vitro corticosteroid response: Correlation with primary open-angle glaucoma and ocular corticosteroid sensitivity. *Am. J. Ophthal.* 79: *92* (1975).

Foon, K.A., Yuen, K., Ballintine, E.J. & Rosenstreich, D.L. Analysis of the systemic corticosteroid sensitivity of patients with primary open-angle glaucoma. *Am. J. Ophthal.* 83: *167* (1977).

Kolker, A.E. & Hetherington, J. Becker-Shaffer's Diagnosis and therapy of the Glaucomas, 4th edition, Mosby, St. Louis, 1976, p. *265*.

Authors' address:
Department of Ophthalmology
Washington University
School of Medicine
660 South Euclid
St. Louis, Missouri 63110
USA

Docum. Ophthal. Proc. Series, Vol. 18

STIMULATION OF MITOSIS AND HYPERTROPHY OF CORNEAL STROMAL CELLS BY MESODERMAL GROWTH FACTOR. INFLUENCE OF ENDOTHELIUM AND EPITHELIUM

VIRGINIA WEIMAR & KENNETH HARAGUCHI

(Portland, Oregon, U.S.A.)

ABSTRACT

Rabbit corneal buttons, with and without epithelial and/or endothelial layers, were incubated in organ culture in the presence and absence of mesodermal growth factor (MGF). MGF stimulated cell hypertrophy, fibroblast growth, and mitosis of corneal stromal cells. In buttons with both epithelial and endothelial layers present, the greatest stimulation with growth factor was found near the wound edge. Removal of either the epithelium or the endothelium produced, in the presence of growth factor, cell growth throughout the button. Growth factor stimulated and sustained corneal fibroblast growth in the absence of epithelium.

INTRODUCTION

Regenerating corneal epithelium, growing over denuded stroma, stimulates underlying keratocytes to transform into fibroblasts. In the absence of epithelium, fibroblast formation in a healing corneal wound is decreased and does not reach a normal rate until the epithelium has grown across the anterior surface of the incision (Dunnington & Weimar, 1958). The tensile strength of healing central wounds is markedly decreased in the absence of epithelium (Gasset & Dohlman, 1968). These results suggest that growing epithelium may liberate a factor stimulating the growth of fibroblasts in wound repair.

In our search for naturally occurring biological compounds which might initiate the growth of corneal fibroblasts in wound healing, we have isolated, from the mouse submaxillary gland, a factor which stimulates the growth of corneal fibroblasts in tissue culture (Haraguchi & Weimar, 1978), in organ culture (Weimar & Haraguchi, 1975), and in rabbit corneas *in vivo* (Rich, Weimar, Squires & Haraguchi, 1978). The purpose of this investigation was (1) to determine the effect of the epithelium and the endothelium on the penetration of this growth factor into the stroma, and (2) to determine if this growth factor stimulates growth of corneal fibroblasts in the absence of the corneal epithelium.

MATERIALS AND METHODS

Corneas: Young adult New Zealand white rabbits (about 2 kg) were used for all experiments. Rabbits were sacrificed by air injection into an ear vein,

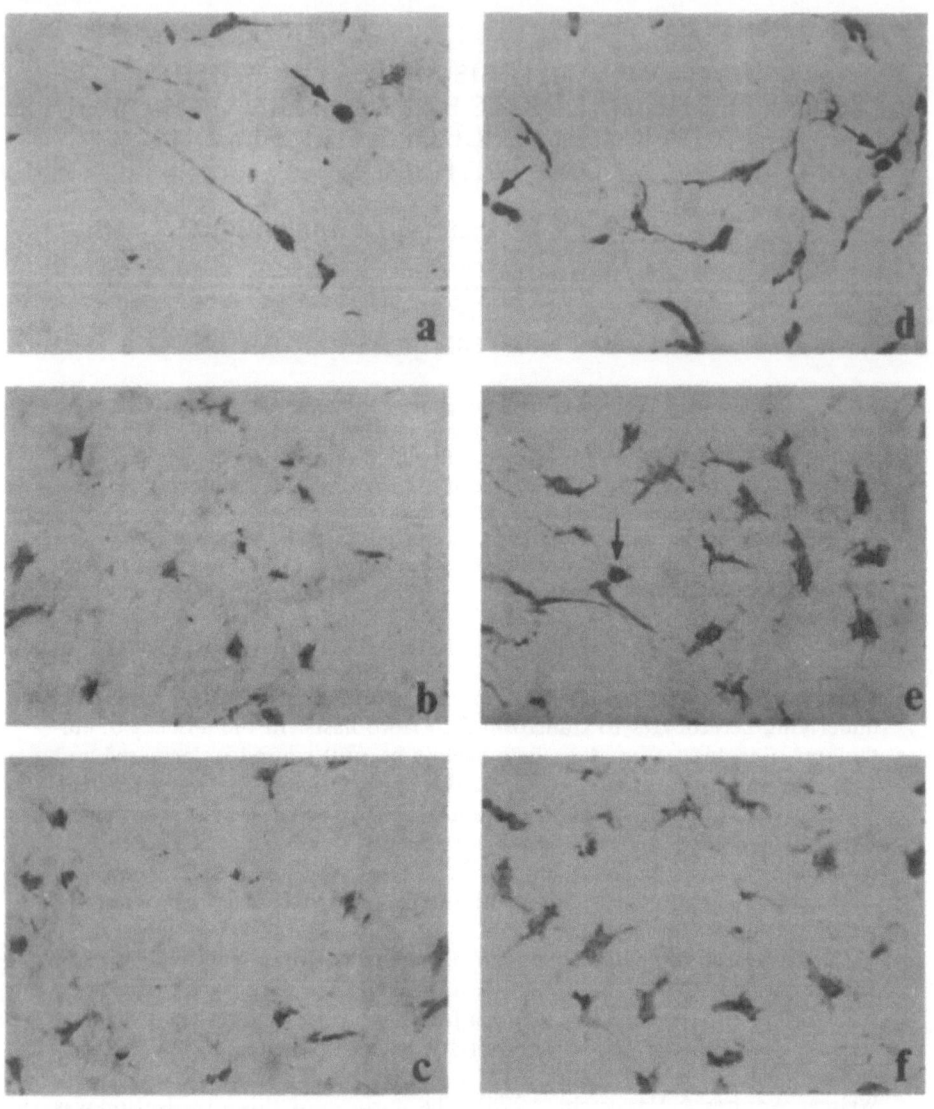

Fig. 1. Epithelial and endothelial layers present. Each microscopic field, left to right, is 355 micrometers. Arrows indicate mitotic figures. (a, b, c): Tangential sections of wound edge (a) and two successive microscopic fields (b and c) from wound edge of *control* corneas after 48 hours of culture. X 180. (d, e, f): Tangential sections of wound edge (d) and two successive microscopic fields (e and f) from wound edge of *MGF-treated* corneas after 48 hours of culture. X 180.

and the eyes enucleated and rinsed in Ringer's solution. Corneas were dissected with a 2-3 mm scleral rim for handling, and the iris and lens excised. Corneal buttons were cut from the endothelial side with an 8 mm trephine. Epithelium was removed with a motor-driven brush (Weimar, 1971) after enucleation of the eye and before dissection of the globe. For removal of the endothelium, the corneoscleral preparation was inverted on the end of a test tube and the endothelium removed with the motor-driven brush.

Organ cultures: Corneal buttons were transferred with a loop to sterile organ culture medium for 20 minutes and then transferred to 10 ml of organ culture medium in 50 ml Belco tissue culture flasks and incubated at 34°C in a New Brunswick air-CO_2 Gyrotory incubator. The platform rotation speed was adjusted to move the buttons very slowly, but continuously, around the flask. The composition of the organ culture medium was as follows: Eagle's minimum essential medium (Earle's base) containing phenol red and supplemented with glutamine, 2 mM/l; Eagle's non-essential amino acids, each 0.1 mM/l; penicillin, 100 units/ml; streptomycin, 100 μg/ml; fungizone, 0.25 μg/ml; $FeSO_4.7H_2O$, 0.426 mg/l; $CuSO_4.5H_2O$, 0.238 mg/l; $ZnSO_4.7H_2O$, 0.143 mg/l; $MnCl_2.4H_2O$, 0.053 mg/l; $CoCl_2.6H_2O$, 0.105 mg/l; and $(NH_4)_6Mo_7O_{24}.4H_2O$, 0.114 mg/l.

Histology: At the end of the incubation period the corneal buttons were fixed in Carnoy's overnight, rehydrated by passage through absolute alcohol, 95% alcohol, 70% alcohol, and water for 1 hour each, and then frozen. Serial sections were cut tangential to the surface of the cornea, stained lightly with Giemsa, and mounted in Permount.

Growth factor: The growth factor was obtained from murine submaxillary glands after the method of Taylor, Cohen & Mitchell (1970). Their procedure was modified in our laboratory by the addition of 10^{-3} M Benzamidine hydrochloride. The crude mesodermal growth factor was further isolated by reverse-flow recycling Sephadex G-100 column chromatography (5.0 x 100 cm). The growth factor fraction was allowed to recycle for two complete cycles prior to its collection on the third pass. The semi-purified growth factor was subsequently desalted by dialysis, lyophilized, and stored as a powder in a Revco freezer at − 80°C until ready for use.

RESULTS

Wound edge: Corneal buttons were cultured for 48 hours in the presence of 20 μg/ml of partially purified MGF. The growth factor was omitted from the control cultures. Some stimulation of fibroblast growth and cell hypertrophy occurred at the wound edge (Fig. 1a) of control buttons and extended from 350-450 micrometers from the wound edge (Fig. 1b). Occasionally a mitotic figure was found (Fig. 1a). In the presence of growth factor, however, a much broader band (750-1000 micrometers) of growth stimulation occurred (Fig. 1d, e, f). Numerous mitotic figures, spindle-shaped fibroblasts, and enlarged cells are clearly evident in growth factor-treated buttons (Fig. 1d, e). The progressive decrease of these effects away from the wound edge is shown in Figure 1: (d) 0-355 micrometers from the wound edge; (e) 355-710 micrometers from wound edge; (f) 710-1065 micrometers from wound edge.

Away from wound edge: To determine the effects of growth factor in the presence and absence of epithelium, endothelium, or both, the effect of growth factor was evaluated in the center of 8 mm corneal buttons in serial sections cut tangentially from the anterior to the posterior surface of the cornea. Photographs were taken at the center of the sections at standard distances from the anterior to the posterior surface of the cornea: (1) at the anterior surface of the stroma just under the epithelium, (2) half the distance from the anterior to the posterior surface of the button, and (3) two-thirds the distance from the anterior to the posterior surface of the button. Figure 2 shows these areas in normal buttons in the absence (a, b, and c) and presence (d, e, and f) of growth factor. Cell hypertrophy is clearly evident in the posterior half of the growth factor-treated buttons. (Compare Fig. 2b and c, with e and f.) The growth stimulation observed, however, is slight when compared with that observed near the wound edge in growth factor-treated buttons (Fig. 1d, e).

If either the endothelial or the epithelial layer was removed, growth factor stimulated fibroblast growth and cell hypertrophy throughout the button (not shown). Maximal stimulation of fibroblast growth, cell hypertrophy and mitosis occurred in corneal buttons treated with growth factor in the absence of both epithelium and endothelium (Fig. 3d, e, f).

DISCUSSION

The results indicate that in the presence of both endothelial and epithelial layers, stimulation of corneal fibroblasts growth by growth factor occurs primarily inward from the cut edge of the button (Fig. 1d, e, f). The growth factor used in these experiments is a polypeptide with a molecular weight of about 26,000 (Haraguchi & Weimar, 1978). It is well established that both the endothelial and epithelial layers of the cornea form relatively impermeable barriers to polar compounds. Horseradish peroxidase, a protein with a molecular weight of about 40,000, has been demonstrated to enter the

328

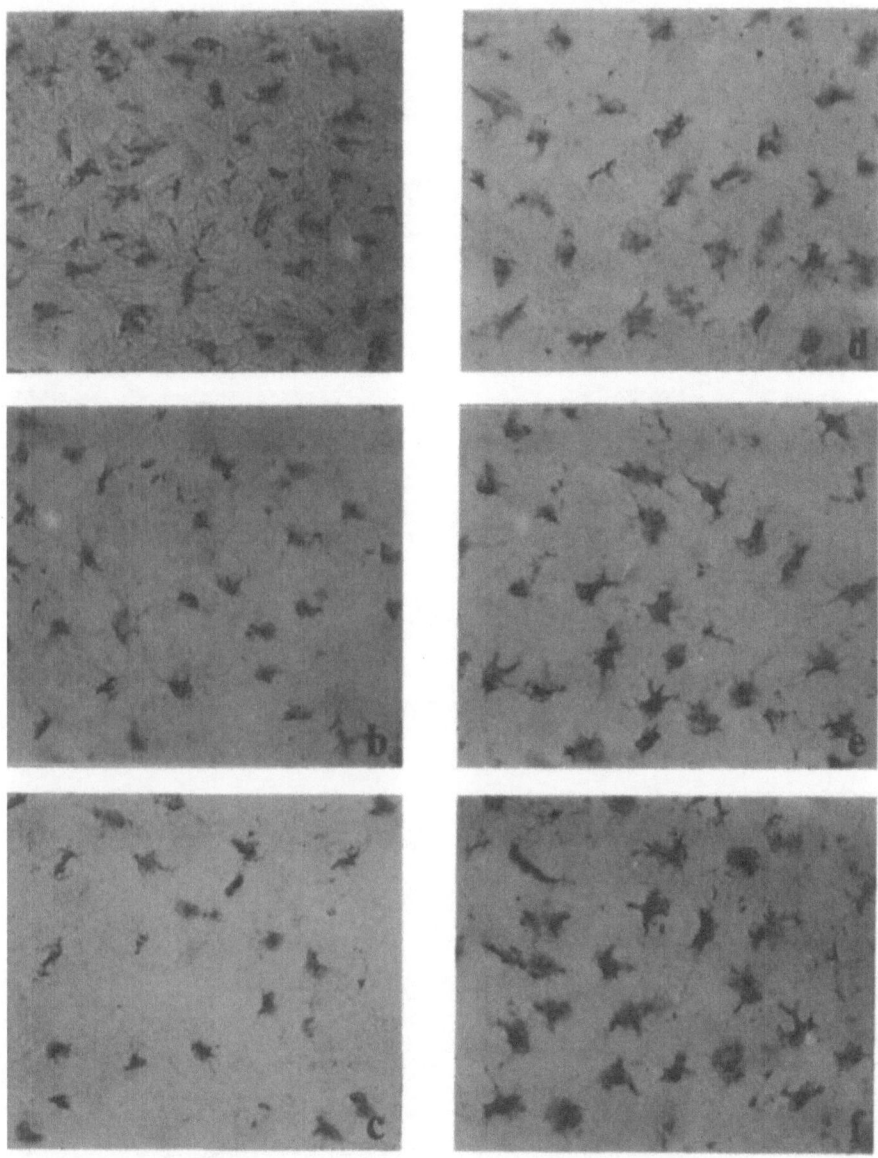

Fig. 2. Epithelial and endothelial layers present (a, b, c): Tangential sections of center of *control* corneal button under epithelium (a), halfway through button (b), and two-thirds of distance from anterior to posterior surface of button (c), after 48 hours of culture. x 180. (d, e, f): Tangential sections of center of *MGF-treated* corneal button under epithelium (d), halfway through button (e), and two-thirds of distance from anterior to posterior surface of button (f) after 48 hours of culture. X 180.

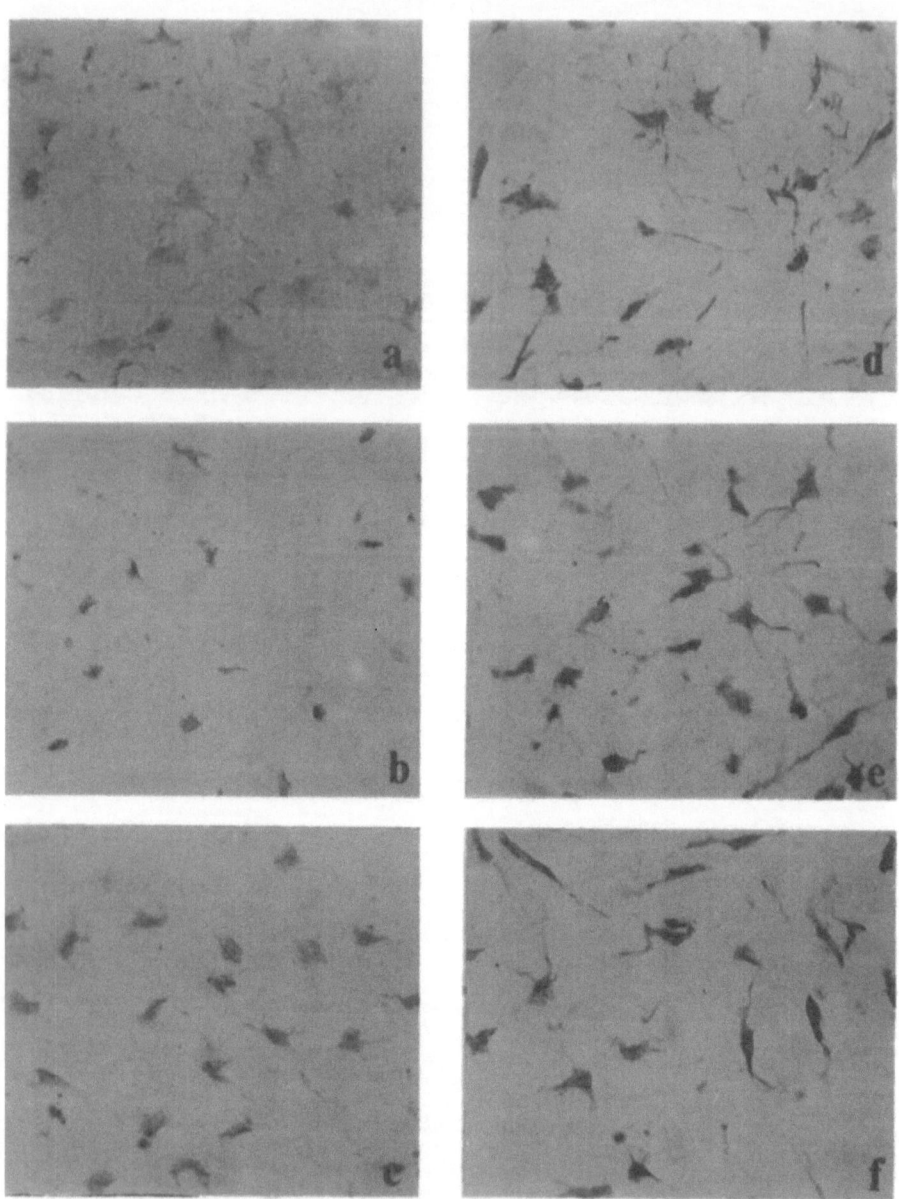

Fig. 3. Epithelial and endothelial layers removed. (a, b, c): Tangential sections of center of *control* button near anterior surface of cornea (a), halfway through button (b), and two-thirds of distance from anterior to posterior surface of button (c), after 48 hours of culture. ✕ 180. (d, e, f): Tangential sections of center of *MGF-treated* corneas near anterior surface of button (d), halfway through button (e), and two-thirds of distance from anterior to posterior surface of button (e), after 48 hours of culture. ✕ 180.

intercellular spaces of the endothelium (Kaye, Sibley & Hoefle, 1973). Some penetration of the endothelium by growth factor must have occurred as indicated by increasing hypertrophy in the cells in the posterior half of the stroma when both endothelium and epithelium were present (Fig. 2e, f).

The results further indicate that growth factor stimulates and supports fibroblast growth in the absence of epithelium (Fig. 3d, e, f). Recently it has been proposed that a new class of polypeptide hormones which have been isolated from the mouse submaxillary gland and from bovine pituitary may represent a group of growth hormones which normally regulate cell growth *in vivo* (Rudland, Gospodarowicz & Seifert, 1974). The growth factor used in our experiments might, for example, be a 'wound hormone.'

REFERENCES

Dunnington, J.H. & Weimar, V. Influence of the epithelium on the healing of corneal incisions. *Am. J. Ophthal.* 45 (Part II): *89-95* (1958).

Gasset, A.R. & Dohlman, C.H. The tensile strength of corneal wounds. *Archs. Ophthal.* 79: *595-602* (1968).

Haraguchi, K.H. & Weimar, V. Corneal connective tissue cell growth factor: Its isolation and purification. (Manuscript in preparation.)

Kaye, G.I., Sibley, R.C. & Hoefle, F.B. Recent studies on the nature and function of the corneal endothelial barrier. *Expl. Eye Res.* 15: *585-613* (1973).

Rich, L.F., Weimar, V., Squires, E.L. & Haraguchi, K. Stimulation of corneal wound healing responses by mesodermal growth factor. ARVO Abstracts, 1978 p. *200*.

Rudland, P.S., Gospodarowicz, D. & Seifert, W. Activation of guanyl cyclase and intracellular cyclic GMP by fibroblast growth factor. *Nature* 250: *741-742* and *773-774* (1974).

Taylor, J.M., Cohen, S. & Mitchell, W.M. Epidermal growth factor: high and low molecular weight forms. *Proc. Natn. Acad. Sci. U.S.A.* 67: *164-171* (1970).

Weimar, V. Neutral red uptake by corneal epithelial cells and by injury-activated corneal stromal cells. I. A comparison of the effects of various metabolic inhibitors and lysosome labilizing and stabilizing agents. *Expl. Eye Res.* 11: *57-69* (1971).

Weimar, V.L. & Haraguchi, K.H. A potent new mesodermal growth factor from mouse submaxillary gland. A quantitative, comparative study with previously described submaxillary gland growth factors. *Physl. Chem.* 7: *7-21* (1975).

Authors' address:
Department of Ophthalmology
University of Oregon Health Sciences Center
3181 S.W. Sam Jackson Park Road
Portland, Oregon 97201, USA

Docum. Ophthal. Proc. Series, Vol. 18

ENZYMATIC ACTIVITIES FOUND IN HUMAN TEARS

JANET A. ANDERSON & IRVING H. LEOPOLD

(Irvine, California, U.S.A.)

ABSTRACT

Many active proteins including enzymes have been observed in human tears. Some of these proteins, including the enzymes lysozyme and amylase, are secreted by the lacrimal gland. Other enzymes found in tears are lysosomal in origin and the tissue source is not yet known. Desquamating epithelial cells of the cornea and conjunctiva are another source of enzymes found in tears. One of the major functions of tear proteins including the enzyme lysozyme appears to be protection of the eye from microorganisms. Other enzyme activities of the tears are probably important in breaking down the cellular debris of microorganisms and desquamating epithelial cells and assisting in the turnover of tear components.

Tears are produced by a number of glands in and surrounding the eye. Basic tear flow is constantly maintained by basic secretors such as the Meibomian glands, the conjunctival goblet cells and the accessory glands of Krause and Wolfring (Jones, 1973). The main lacrimal gland and the accessory palpebral gland are reflex secretors and provide a changing amount of tears — none at all during sleep (Jones, 1973). Reflex secretion in humans can be stimulated by emotions, light, chemicals and irritation of the eye. Tears are made up of water, salts, lipids, free amino acids, glucose, urea and a number of protein-aceous compounds (Iwata, 1973). The high molecular weight components of the tears have been identified by various electrophoretic methods (Smolens et al., 1949; Liotet & Reveilleau, 1965; McEwen et al., 1958). The major components are albumins which make up about 30% of the protein in a normal eye and lysozyme which makes up another 30% of the protein (Liotet & Reveilleau, 1965). The remaining proteins form electrophoretic patterns similar to the serum globulins (McEwen et al., 1958). These fractions contain a number of immunoglobulins, with IgA as the predominant species. IgG is also present while IgM and IgE have occasionally been detected (Allansmith, 1973). These fractions also contain the tear glycoproteins and mucins (McEwen et al., 1958). Although the major components of the tear film have been identified, many minor components are still being found. The interrelationships and the functional roles of all components are currently under investigation in a number of laboratories.

In this review, the enzyme and related protein activities that are found in tears, their possible physiological roles and their use in the diagnosis of disease will be discussed.

Lysozyme is the major enzyme in tears. Its source, activity and physiological role have been the object of intensive research since first described by Fleming (1922). Lysozyme obtained from egg white has been most widely studied but the enzyme is present in many plant and animal tissues. In humans it is found in tears, saliva, nasal mucus, leucocytes and cartilage (Ridley, 1928). Tear lysozyme is similar to egg white lysozyme in size and charge but differs in amino acid content (Bondavida et al., 1967) and in its antigenic properties (Smolens et al., 1949; Bonavida et al., 1967). It has about three times the specific activity of egg white lysozyme (Bonavida et al., 1967) and is produced by the main lacrimal gland (Table 1) (Allen et al., 1972; Covey et al., 1971). Lysozyme concentration in normal tears does not vary with changes in tear flow (Sapse et al., 1968; Haeringen & Glasius, 1974; Mackie & Seal, 1974b). However, after excessive tearing of several hours, there is a decrease in lysozyme concentration (Ridley, 1928). There is no diurnal variation (Pietsch & Pearlman, 1973), although individual variation over longer periods of time (one week to one year) have been reported (Reagan, 1950). Concentration does decrease with age, starting at 10 years (Mackie & Seal, 1976; Pietsch & Pearlman, 1973).

The lysis and killing of bacteria is believed to be the physiological function of lysozyme in tears. The level of activity in tears is sufficient to kill pathogenic bacteria such as staphylococci, streptococci, pneumococci, cholera, gonococcus and meningococcus (Ridley, 1928). Some reports have suggested that the enzyme is also effective against viruses (Ferrari et al., 1959).

Reduction of lysozymal activity has been observed in various ocular disease states, e.g., conjunctivitis (Liotet & Reveilleau, 1965; Ridley, 1928; Reagan, 1950; Gammal & Mostafa, 1971), corneal ulcer (Ridley, 1928; Regan, 1950; Gammal & Mostafa, 1971), lacrimal gland inflammation (Regan, 1950; Gammal & Mostafa, 1971), and herpes keratitis (Eylan et al., 1977) but the results are variable. One group of authors has reported increased levels of lysozyme in conjunctivitis (Janke et al., 1973). The reduced activity observed may be due to the increased tearing associated with these infections (Regan, 1950; Gammal & Mostafa, 1971). None of the reduced levels are sufficiently consistent to be of diagnosistic value. However, in keratoconjunctivitis sicca, lysozymal levels are consistently and significantly lower than in normal tears (Mackie & Seal, 1976; Regan, 1950; Bijsterveld, 1969). The reduction in lysozyme concentration can be used as a diagnostic aid in this disease (Bijsterveld, 1969). Lowered lysozyme levels have also been observed in patients taking practolol, a drug with which ocular toxicity is associated following long-term use (Mackie & Seal, 1975). Since the concentration of lysozyme apparently decreases before any other signs of ocular toxicity appear, measurement of enzyme activity could be used to detect toxicity of this drug and other drugs which have toxic ocular effects (Mackie & Seal, 1975). The measurement of lysozymal activity in tears is a simple procedure in which the breakdown of micrococcus lysodeikticus is monitored either on agar plates (Bonavida & Sapse, 1968) or in a spectrophotometer (Ronen et al., 1975). Measurement of lysis using the spectrophotometric method is a more accurate determination of tear lysozyme activity than the agar technique. There are several other factors in tears which have bacteriocidal or bacteriostatic properties. These activities can be confused with that of lysozyme on the agar plate test. Among these is a heat labile substance of low molecular weight (10,000) which inhibits the growth of a wide range of conjunctival bacteria including some pathogens against which lysozyme is ineffective (Friedland, 1972).

Lactoferrin is an iron-binding tear protein with bacteriostatic properties (Masson et al., 1966). It has a molecular weight of 80-85,000 (Oram & Reiter, 1968) and is secreted by the lacrimal gland (Table 1 Franklin et al., 1973). This protein is found in a variety of external secretions (Masson & Heremans, 1966) including tears where it makes up 2-3% of the total protein content (Masson et al., 1966). As its name indicates, it was first found in milk. Its distribution parallels that of lysozyme suggesting some interaction or complementary functions of these proteins (Masson et al., 1969). Its bacteriostatic properties are enhanced by a number of metal ions except iron. The presence of iron reduces the bacteriostatic activity (Oram & Reiter, 1968).

Another major protein constituent of the tears is one which is not found in other body fluids but which has been found in tears of the several mammalian species tested (Bonavida et al., 1969). It is, therefore, considered to be a specific tear protein. The most acidic protein in tears, it migrates faster toward the anode in acrylamide gel electrophoresis than serum albumin (Bonavida et al., 1969). It is secreted by the lacrimal gland (Table 1 Bonavida et al., 1969). This protein interacts with lysozyme, enhancing its bacteriocidal properties (Josephson & Wald, 1969). No other function for it is presently known.

The main lacrimal gland also synthesizes and secretes amylase (Table 1) (Haeringen & Glasius, 1974b; Haeringen et al., 1975). The isoenzyme patterns and pH activity curves of tear amylase differ from those of salivary amylase and urinary amylase showing separate synthesis of the enzymes found in these three fluids (Haeringen et al., 1975). Tear activities of amylase show considerable variation during lacrimation and also from person to person (Haeringen & Glasius, 1974b). This variation is probably due to the

Table 1. Enzymes and Other Proteins Secreted by the Main Lacrimal Gland.

Lysozyme
Lactoferrin
Specific Tear Protein
Amylase
IgA
Hexokinase
Glutamate-pyruvate transaminase

References: (Allen et al, 1972; Covey et al, 1971; Franklin et al, 1973; Bonavida et al, 1969; Haeringen et al, 1975; Haeringen & Glasius, 1976).

335

mode of secretion of amylase from secretory granules discharged into the acini of the lacrimal gland (Haeringen & Glasius, 1974b). No differences in amylase concentrations have been shown to correlate with sex or ocular disease (Liotet, 1967a). Maximum activity appears in tears of people from 40 to 60 years of age (Liotet, 1967a). The enzyme requires Ca^{++} for activity and is inhibited by EDTA (Haeringen et al., 1975). The physiological role of the enzyme is not known. It has been suggested that the enzyme provides glucose for the metabolism of the corneal epithelial cells (Liotet, 1967a) or it provides a substrate for the formation of mucous material by epithelial cells (Pei & Rhodin, 1971).

Enzymes from the epithelial cells of the conjunctiva and cornea are also found in the tears (Haeringen & Glasius, 1976). The most active of these enzymes is lactate dehydrogenase (Haeringen & Glasius, 1974a). Its concentration in tear samples collected by different methods correlates with the concentrations of the enzymes shown in Table 2 suggesting that these enzymes come from the same source (Haeringen & Glasius, 1974b; Haeringen & Glasius, 1976). The concentrations of these enzymes are high in tears collected with filter paper strips and low in tears collected by glass capillary (Haeringen & Glasius, 1976). Collection of tears by paper strips is irritating to the epithelial surface and this irritation probably releases these enzymes from desquamated epithelial cells. These studies indicate that another source of material found in tears is the epithelial cells of the conjunctiva and cornea. They also suggest that the measurement of lactate dehydrogenase concentration in tears collected by capillary tube would be a sufficient indication for epithelial damage of the eye (Haeringen & Glasius, 1976).

Several lysosomal enzyme activities have been observed in the tears (Table 3). These enzyme activities and their absence are important in several inborn metabolic disorders. The levels in tears are sufficiently high to allow assays for activity for diagnostic purposes.

Table 2. Enzymes from Epithelial Cells of Conjunctiva and Cornea.

Glycolytic Enzymes:
   Lactate dehydrogenase, pyruvate kinase, aldolase

Tricarboxylic Acid Cycle Enzymes:
   Malate dehydrogenase, isocitrate dehydrogenase

Others:
   Glucose-6-phosphate dehydrogenase, sorbitol dehydrogenase, glutamate dehydrogenase, glutamate-oxalate transaminase

Comparison of the enzyme concentrations in tears collected by different methods indicates that these enzymes appear in the tear fluid from the breakdown of epithelial cells.

Reference (Haeringen & Glasius, 1976).

336

In Tay-Sachs Disease the inherited metabolic lesion is the absence of activity of β hexosaminadase A, one of two forms of the hexosaminidase. In tear samples, as in serum samples, hexosaminidase A activities of patient, carrier and normal are clearly different (Carmody et al., 1973; Singer et al., 1973). Heterozygotes cannot be clearly distinguished in assays of saliva samples. The tear enzyme concentrations are 6 to 10 times greater than the serum concentrations (Singer et al., 1973). The ratios of A & B activity change in serum during pregnancy which may lead to false diagnosis, using serum, but the ratios in tears remain constant during pregnancy (Carmody et al., 1973). This method of diagnosis for Tay-Sachs patients and carriers has the further advantages of ease of collection, using filter paper strips, and stability of the enzyme in these strips at room temperature (Singer et al., 1973).

In Fabry disease the metabolic lesion is in the enzyme α galactosidase A. There are also two forms of this enzyme – A & B. The A activity is thermolabile. Tears are collected on filter paper strips and assayed for total galactosidase activity, and after heating for galactosidase B activity (Del Monte et al., 1974; Johnson et al., 1975). The difference is the galactosidase A activity. The affected individuals, carriers and normals can be quite easily distinguished by this method of assay (Del Monte et al., 1974; Johnson et al., 1975). Fucosidosis and mannosidosis are inherited metabolic disorders of lysosomal enzymes which can also be detected by the study of tears (Libert et al., 1976; Van Hoof, 1976). The heterozygous carriers cannot be distinguished in fucosidosis but can be differentiated in mannosidosis (Van Hoof, 1976). The assays are useful in diagnosing these unusual diseases. Samples are easily taken and the enzymes are stable at room temperature (Libert et al., 1976; Van Hoof, 1976).

The presence of lysosomal enzyme activities in tears brings up the question of the source of these enzymes. From their studies of tear enzyme activities using different collection methods, Haeringen & Glasius (1976) concluded that these enzymes come from both the breakdown of epithelial cells and from the lacrimal gland. Active secretion of lysosomes has been observed in some cell types (Davies & Allison, 1976). Whether or not the release from the lacrimal gland is of this nature is not presently known although the high concentration of these enzymes in the tears (Singer et al., 1973) suggests that their presence there is not just a result of cell degradation.

Table 3. Lysosomal Enzymes Found in Tears.

β hexosaminidase
α galactosidase
α fucosidase
α mannosidase

References: (Carmody et al, 1973; Singer et al, 1973; Del Monte et al, 1974; Johnson et al, 1975; Libert et al, 1976; Van Hoof, 1976).

Among the many hydrolases present in lysosomes are proteolytic enzymes. No proteolytic activity has yet been observed in human tears but there is an inhibitor of proteolytic activity present in tears (Kueppers, 1971). This inhibitor has been shown to be active against trypsin, at neutral pH (Kueppers, 1971). In our laboratory, we have found that there is also inhibition of the proteolytic activity of papain present in tears. Proteolytic enzymes active at neutral pH have been isolated from lysosomes, one of which, Cathepsin B, is similar to papain in its activity and cofactor requirements (LoSpalluto et al., 1970; Snellman, 1969). The presence of the inhibitors of proteolytic activity in tears and the presence of other lysosomal enzymes in tears both suggest that proteolytic activity may also be found in tears.

Other enzyme activities that have been detected in tears are hexokinase (Table 1) (Haeringen & Glasius, 1976), glutamate-pyruvate transaminase (Table 1) (Haeringen & Glasius, 1976), serine deaminase (Kahan & Erdei, 1972), alkaline and acid phosphatases (Liotet, 1967).

Human tears contain many different proteins. One of the main functions of these proteins is protection of the eye from microorganisms. Presently, there are four known proteins in the tears with bacteriocidal or bacteriostatic effects: lysozyme, lactoferrin, the specific tear protein, and the immunoglobulins which are also antimicrobial agents. All of these proteins, including IgA, the major immunoglobulin of the tears, are secreted by the main lacrimal gland (Allen et al., 1972; Covey et al., 1971; Franklin et al., 1973. Bonavida et al., 1969; Haeringen et al., 1975). The other protein activities of the tears probably have to do with good housekeeping — removing cellular debris of microorganisms and of the desquamating epithelial cells and assisting in the turnover of the components of the tears. Amylase may act to provide substrate for glycoprotein production (Pei & Rhodin, 1971). The lysosomal enzymes probably act to break down the cellular debris of microorganisms and of the desquamating epithelial cells. These enzymes may also act in the breakdown of the tear components which have fulfilled their functions. The enzymes of the glycolytic and tricarboxylic pathways are apparently not regular constituents of the tears but appear from the degrading corneal and conjunctival epithelial cells (Haeringen & Glasius, 1976).

REFERENCES

Allansmith, Mathea. Immunology of tears in International Ophthalmology Clinics, Vol. 13 (ed. Holly, F.J. & Lemp, M.A.), Little, Brown & Co., Boston, 1973, pp. 47-72.

Allen, M., Wright, P. & Reid, L. The human lacrimal gland, a histochemical and organ culture study of the secretory cells. Archs. Ophthal., 88: 493-497 (1972).

Bijsterveld, D.P. van Diagnostic tests in the sicca syndrome. Archs. Ophthal., 82: 10-14 (1969).

Bonavida, B. & Sapse, A.T. Human tear lysozyme II quantitative determination with standard schirmer strips. Am. J. Ophthal., 66: 70-76 (1968).

Bonavida, B., Sapse, A.T. & Sercarz, E.E. Human tear lysozyme. I purification, physiocochemical and immunochemical characterization. J. Lab. Med., 70: 951-962 (1967).

338

Bonavida, B., Sapse, A.T. & Secarz, E.E. Specific tear prealbumin: A unique lachrymal protein absent from serum and other secretions, *Nature,* 221. *375-376* (1969).

Carmody, P.J., Rattazzi, M.D. & Davidson, R.G. Tay-Sachs Disease: The use of tears for the detection of heterozygates, *New Engl. J. Med.* 289: *1072-1074* (1973).

Covey, W., Perillie, P. & Finch, S.C. The origin of tear lysozyme. *Proc. Soc. exp. Biol. Med.,* 137: *1362-1363* (1971).

Davies, P. & Allison, A.C. The Secretion of lysosomal enzymes, in Frontiers of Biology, Vol. 45. (ed. Dingle, J.T. & Dean, R.T.), North-Holland Publishing Co., Amsterdam, 1976, pp. *61-93.*

DelMonte, M.D., Johnson, D.L., Cotlier, E., Krivil, W. & Desnick, R.J. Diagnosis of Fabry's disease by tear α-Galactosidase. A. *New Engl. J. Med.,* 290: *57-58* (1974).

Eylan, E., Ronen, D., Romano, A. & Smetana, O. Lysozyme tear level in patients with herpes simplex virus infection. *Invest. Ophthal.,* 16: *850-853* (1977).

Ferrari, R., Callerio, C. & Podio, G. Antiviral activity of lysozyme. *Nature.* 183: *548* (1959).

Fleming, A. On a remarkable bacteriolytic element found in tissues and secretions. *Proc. R. Soc.,* London, ser. B 93: *306* (1922).

Franklin, R.M., Kenyon, K.R. & Tomasi Jr., T.B. Immunohistologic studies of human lacrimal gland: localization of immunoglobulins, secretory component and lactoferrin. *J. Immun.,* 110: *984-992* (1973).

Friedland, B.R., Anderson, D.R. & Forster, R.K. Non-lysozyme antibacterial factor in human tears. *Am. J. Ophthal.,* 74: *52-59* (1972).

Gammal, M.Y. el & Mostafa, M.S.E. Estimation of tears lysozyme in some eye diseases. *Bull. Soc. Ophthal. Egypte,* 64: *285-297* (1971).

Haeringen, N.J. van, Ensink, F. & Gasius, E. Amylase in human tear fluid: origin and characteristics, compared with salivary and urinary amylases. *Expl. Eye Res.,* 21: *395-403* (1975).

Haeringen, N.J. van & Glasius, E. Lactate dehydrogenase in tear fluid. *Expl. Eye Res.,* 18: *345-349* (1974a).

Haeringen, N.J. van & Glasius, E. Enzymatic studies in lacrimal secretion. *Expl. Eye Res.,* 19: *134-139* (1974b).

Haeringen, N.J. van & Glasius, E. The origin of some enzymes in tear fluid, determined by comparative investigation with two collection methods. *Expl. Eye Res.,* 22: *267-272* (1976).

Iwata, Shuzo Chemistry of aqueous phase, in International Ophthalmology Clinics (ed. Holly, F.J. & Lemp, M.A.) Vol. 13, Little, Brown & Co., Boston, 1973, pp. *29-46.*

Janke, W., Langmaack, H. & Tiburtuis, H. Bestimmung der lysozymalen aktivität der tränenflüssigkeit mit klinisch anwendbarer Methode. *Klin. Mbl. Augenheilk.,* 163: *366-369* (1973).

Johnson, D.L., DelMonte, M.A., Cotlier, E. & Desnick, R.J. Fabry disease: diagnosis by α-galactosidase activities in tears. *Clinica Chim. Acta,* 63: *81-90* (1975).

Jones, L.T. Anatomy of the tear system, in International Ophthalmology Clinics, Vol. 13 (ed. Holly, F.J. & Lemp, M.A.) Little,Brown & Co., Boston, 1973, pp. *3-32.*

Josephson, A.S. & Wald, A. Enhancement of lysozyme activity by anodal tear protein. *Proc. Soc. exp. Biol. Med.* 131: *677-679* (1969).

Kahan, I.L. & Erdei, Z. On the keto acid content of tears. *Ophthalmologica,* 164: *71-77* (1972).

Kueppers, F. Proteinase inhibitor in human tears. *Biochim. Biophys. Acta,* 229: *845-4849* (1971).

Libert, J., Van Hoof, F. & Tondeur, M. Fucosidosis: ultrastructural study of conjunctiva and skin and enzyme analysis of tears. *Invest. Ophthal.,* 15: *626-639* (1976).

Liotet, S. Pouvoir Amylasique des larmes humaines. *Annls. Oculist.* 200: *526-534* (1967a).

Liotet, S. Étude de L'Activite´transaminasique et de l'activité phosphatasique des larmes humaines. *Annls. Oculist.* 12: *1258-1272* (1967b).

Liotet, S. & Reveilleau, J. Étude des larmes humaines par électrophorese et par immo-électrophorese. *Annls. Oculist.* 198: *12-24* (1965).

LoSpalluto, J.J., Fehr, K. & Ziff, M. Degradation of immunoglobulins by intracellular proteases in the range of neutral pH. *J. Immun.* 105: *886-897* (1970).

Mackie, I.A. & Seal, D.V. Tear fluid lysozyme concentration: guide to practolol toxicity. *Br. med. J.* 4(5999): *732* (1975).

Mackie, I.A. & Seal, D.V. Quantitative tear lysozyme assay in units of activity per microlitre. *Br. J. Ophthal.* 60: *70-74* (1976).

Masson, P.L. & Heremans, J.F. Studies on lactoferrin, the iron-binding protein of secretions, in Protides of the Biological Fluids, Vol. 14, (ed. Peeters, H.) Elsevier Publishing Co, Amsterdam, 1966, pp. *115-124.*

Masson, P.L., Heremans, J.F. & Dive, C. An iron-binding protein common to many external secretions. *Clinica Chim. Acta* 14: *735-739* (1966).

Masson, P.L., Heremans, J.F. & Schonne, E. Lactoferrin, an iron-binding protein in neutrophylic leukocytes. *J. exp. Med.* 130: *643-656* (1969).

McEwen, W.K., Kimura, S.J. & Feeney, M.L. Filter paper electophoresis of tears III human tears and their high molecular weight components. *Am. J. Ophthal.* 45: *67-70* (1958).

Oram, J.D. & Reiter, B. Inhibition of bacteria by lactoferrin and other iron-chelating agents. *Biochim. Biophys. Acta,* 170: *351-365* (1968).

Pei, Y.F. & Rhodin, J.A.S. Electronmicroscopic study of the mouse corneal epithelium. *Invest. Ophthal.* 10: *811-825* (1971).

Pietsch, R.L. & Pearlman, M.E. Human tear lysozyme variables. *Archs. Ophthal.,* 90: *94-96* (1973).

Regan, E. The lysozyme content of tears. *Am. J. Ophthal.,* 33: *600-605* (1950).

Ridley, F. Lysozyme: an antibacterial body present in great concentration in tears and its relation to infection of the human eye. *Proc. R. Soc. Med.,* 21: *1495-1506* (1928).

Ronen, D., Eylan, E. Romano, A., Stein, R. & Modan, M. A spectrophotometric method for quantitative determination of lysozyme in human tears: Description and evaluation of the method and screening of 60 healthy subjects. *Invest. Ophthal.,* 14: *479-484* (1975).

Sapse, A.T., Bonavida, B., Stone Jr., W. & Secarz, E.E. Human tear lysozyme III preliminary study on lysozyme levels in subjects with smog eye irritation. *Am. J. Ophthal.,* 66: *76-80* (1968).

Singer, J.D., Cotlier, E. & Krimmer, R. Hexosaminidase A in Tears and saliva for rapid identification of Tay-Sachs disease and its carriers. *Lancet,* 2: *1116-1119* (1973).

Smolens, J., Leopold, I.H. & Parker, J. Studies of human tears, *Am. J. Ophthal.,* 32: *153-160* (1949).

Snellman, O. Cathepsin, B., The lysosomal thiol proteinase of calf liver, *Biochem. J.,* 114: *673-678* (1969).

Van Hoof, F. Fucusidase and mannosidase in tears, in discussion of Cotlier, E. Identification of homozygotes and heterozygotes by chemical analysis of tears in the eye, in Birth Defects: Original Article Series, Vol. 12, No. 3, The Eye and inborn errors of metabolism (eds. Bergsma, D., Bron, A.J. & Cotlier, E.) Alan R. Liss, Inc., New York, 1976, pp. *111-114.*

Authors' address:
Department of Ophthalmology
California College of Medicine
University of California
Irvine, California 92717, USA

Docum. Ophthal. Proc. Series, Vol. 18

POSSIBLE ADVERSE EFFECTS FROM TOPICAL OCULAR ANESTHETICS

F.T. FRAUNFELDER & J.D. SHARP & B.E. SILVER

(Little Rock, Arkansas U.S.A.)

ABSTRACT

Topical ocular local anesthetics only in rare instances give rise to significant adverse reactions if only a few drops of the medication are given. However, adverse effects do occur that require immediate medical management. Patients with apprehensive type personalities may be the most susceptible to 'emotionally' related adverse responses. The possibility of the oculocardiac reflex and emotional factors playing a role in a significant adverse 'drug' reaction needs to be considered in each case. Irregardless, medical management after the reaction is essential. There is no indication for long-term use of topical ocular local anesthetics since secondary ocular complications are inevitable.

The National Registry of Drug-Induced Ocular Side Effects was established in July, 1976, under the auspices of the Federal Food and Drug Administration and the American Academy of Ophthalmology. Since then, there have been 36 reports by ophthalmologists to the registry of adverse effects probably related to the application of topical ocular local anesthetics. These cases included 15 allergic reactions, 8 cases of syncopy, 6 with significant keratitis, 5 with convulsions, and 2 cases of possible anaphylactic shock.

ALLERGIC REACTIONS

The largest group in our series was allergic reactions. A response of this type consists of epithelial stippling, slight stromal edema, conjunctival hyperemia, chemosis, lacrimation, and lid edema. It is usually accompanied by pruritus. More severe allergic reactions rarely occur, and include angioneurotic edema, urticaria, dermatitis, asthmatic breathing, and anaphylactic shock.

In general, most allergic reactions seldom cause further problems once recognized and the exciting agent is discontinued. Severe allergic reactions are more often seen in patients with an allergic history, in the debilitated, or in pediatric or geriatric age groups. However, one can seldom predict which patients will exhibit a significant adverse response. Theoretically, an allergic

This study was supported by Contract No. 223-76-3018 from the Food and Drug Administration.

reaction cannot develop unless there has been previous exposure to the drug. Cross-allergy occurs when a reaction develops from anesthetics of the same chemical structure. It is not uncommon to see minimal ocular or periocular allergic reactions to procaine, but it is unusual to see them with proparacaine. The amino benzoic acid compounds (tetracaine, benoxinate) are more prone to cause allergic sensitivity reactions than other local anesthetics, and cross sensitivity between members of this group often is observed. There is seldom cross-allergic responses with proparacaine, however, which is also a benzoic ester, though chemically distinct. Dibucaine, a quinoline derivative, may produce an allergic reaction, but does not cross react with other local anesthetics.

SYNCOPE

Occasionally, the topical ocular administration of a local anesthetic will result in a vasopressor reaction consisting of bradycardia, nausea, syncope, and even cardiac arrest. The oculocardiac reflex, activated by pressure on the eyeball or by traction on the extraocular muscles, can elicit this response, and may be responsible for many of these reactions. The reflex is dependent upon trigeminal sensory stimulation with the efferent limb being the vagus nerve to the heart. It is possible to get a cardiac standstill in normal, unanesthetized subjects by pressure on the eyeball. This rapidly wanes when ocular pressure is released (Pontinen, 1966). The reaction can, therefore, follow any ocular manipulation when applying a drop, and can be enhanced by the ocular massage sometimes advocated to aid distribution of the anesthetic. Once the anesthesia has taken effect, the reflex should be diminished since anesthesia inhibits somewhat the initiation of the reflex arc.

Because abnormal reactions, such as the vasovagal response, may occur without apparent cause, or more rapidly than seems likely from a pharmacologic effect, psychogenic factors should be considered. Occasionally, patients will become apprehensive enough to either faint or display some of the subjective signs common to toxic local anesthetic and vasopressor reactions. These include pallor, nausea, diaphoresis, and a fall in blood pressure leading to neurogenic syncope. A psychological origin should be suspected. For example, we received the case of a 31-year-old male who lost consciousness upon the instillation of topical ocular benoxinate. The fact that he fainted on a previous date when blood was drawn leads one to suspect an over-anxious state rather than that of a drug reaction. Incidental reactions such as this are often most difficult to distinguish from a toxic drug effect. They usually occur when the patient is in the upright position. Thus, they are more common in outpatient practice, where topical local anesthesia is used with frequency for minor procedures. Cerebral hypoxia with loss of consciousness, and even tremors and convulsions, may occur before the patient can be placed in the horizontal position (Gordh, 1969).

Realizing that certain individuals are more prone to anxiety and subsequent reactions than others, it may be indicated in rare instances to administer a presurgical sedative. Barbiturates are also given as prophylaxis against genuine toxic reactions. Their value in this regard is doubtful; the minimal lethal dose of local anesthetics in some laboratory animals is increased four-fold after barbiturates (Bryant, 1969). The barbiturates depress the cortex and may obscure early warning signs of a toxic reaction, as well as deepening central nervous system depression which follows cortical stimulation.

KERATITIS

Immediate local reactions following topically applied anesthetics usually include only a stinging sensation which subsides as the anesthesia takes effect. As this occurs, however, the blink reflex is inhibited which may lead to abnormal drying of the cornea. Also, due to the patient's lack of appreciation of corneal exposure, foreign bodies or corneal abrasions may go unnoticed.

Local anesthetics generally have toxic effects directly on the corneal epithelium. They are protoplasmic poisons which can cause tissue death due to chemical changes or dehydration. They depress respiration and glycolysis, increase permeability, and induce sensitization reactions (Epstein & Paton, 1963). Repeated application may seriously delay or prevent regeneration of the epithelium. The dramatic relief of discomfort provided by the topical anesthetics may, in the treatment of cases such as ultraviolet light-induced keratitis, encourage overusage of these drugs. Reapplication of the anesthetic provides only temporary relief of discomfort, and as instillations are made at shorter intervals to achieve the desired effect, chronic ulceration of the cornea becomes more likely. Initially there will be corneal epithelial and stromal edema with folds in Descemet's membrane. The central corneal epithelium may be absent and iritis may be present. Ultimately, a stromal opacity or corneal perforation can occur. There is experimental evidence which demonstrates that the 'caine' drugs are toxic at the cellular level to both corneal fibroblasts and epithelial cells. These drugs have been shown to inhibit corneal epithelial cell metabolism (Herman, Moses & Friedenwald, 1942), miotic activity (Marr, et al., 1957), and migration. Fibroblasts and epithelial cells, which have been exposed to 'caine' drugs, have demonstrated impaired microfilament and microtubular systems within the cells (Burns, et al., 1977). Numerous clinical reports of significant and devastating ocular damage due to prolonged local anesthetic use have been reported (Burns, 1977; Epstein & Paton, 1968; Willis & Laibson, 1970).

Four cases of a dense yellow ring in the corneal stroma following chronic misuse (6 days to 8 weeks) of topical ocular local anesthetics were reported in paramedical personnel (Burns, 1977). The local anesthetics implicated were tetracaine (Pontocaine), benoxinate (Dorsacaine), and proparacaine (Ophthaine). The clinical picture of these patients suggested an allergic reaction; however, no immunologic hyperactivity to local anesthetics could be found. Experimental data suggest a local toxic effect from local anesthetics, and possibly corneal epithelium damage with a secondary stromal reaction. To date, these responses have, in most part, been reversible with discontinuation of the drug.

CONVULSIONS

In ordinary practice, the dosage of topical local anesthetics sufficient to cause a toxic central nervous system reaction are rarely reached. This is because a toxic dose is rarely given. However, of the cases in which a severe systemic reaction to a local anesthetic has occurred, almost all were due to an overdose. Blood levels are a function of the total dose and not of the concentration of the solution. Absorption of some drugs from mucosal membranes (conjunctiva, cornea, nasal mucosa) is so efficient and rapid that even topical application can produce a relatively high blood level of these drugs. To achieve this with proparacaine, however, would require at least 15 drops in each eye. In the 5 cases reported to the Registry, each had only a few drops. The patients developed marked apprehension, anxiety, loquaciousness, dizziness, incoherent speech, diaphoresis, disorientation, and muscular twitching. The skin became pale, diaphoretic, and respiration increased in rate and depth before convulsions occurred. While this is highly suggestive of sudden cortical stimulation due to drug effect, this seems to be unlikely at these low dosages other than as an idiosyncratic or emotional response.

Central nervous system depression may follow or accompany the stage of cortical stimulation. The depression of the cardiovascular centers in the medulla and myocardial hypoxia result in peripheral vascular collapse, producing cyanosis and profuse perspiration. Because cardiac conduction and contractility is inhibited, cardiac arrest may ensue.

POSSIBLE ANAPHYLACTIC SHOCK

Occasionally, individuals exhibit a hypersensitive or idiosyncratic response such as with syncope which occurs from a minimal dose of the drug. These reactions range from an allergic dermatitis, a typical asthmatic, or a toxic reaction of a usual pattern, to a fatal anaphylactic reaction. In acute anaphylactic shock, the predominating feature is an almost immediate circulatory collapse, with pallor and coma. The occasional occurrence of shock and collapse following the topical administration of cocaine is well known, and has been reported following the use of many of the synthetic anesthetics. There need not be any previous exposure to the drug. This reaction is probably due to sudden release of an excessive amount of histamines. This is indeed a rare event. Both cases reported to the Registry recovered without sequel after administration of oxygen and intravenous epinephrine. Some of these reactions may be difficult to distinguish from a severe vasovagal motor response.

REFERENCES

Bryant, J.A. Local and topical anesthetics in ophthalmology. *Surv. Ophthal.* 13(5): *263-283* (1969).

Burns, R.P., Chronic toxicity of local anesthetics on the cornea, in Symposium on Ocular Therapy (eds. Leopold, I.H. & Burns, R.P.) New York, John Wiley & Sons, 1977, pp. *31-44.*

Burns, R.P. Toxicity of local anesthetics on the eye. Presented at the Symposium on Drug-Induced Ocular Side Effects and Ocular Toxicology, September 8-10, 1977, Little Rock, Arkansas.

Epstein, D.L. & Paton, D. Keratitis from misuse of corneal anesthetics. *New Engl. J. Med.* 279(8): *396-399* (1968).

Gordh, T. Complications and their treatment, in Illustrated Handbook in Local Anesthesia, (ed. Eriksson, E.) Year Book Medical Publishers, Inc., Chicago, 1969, pp. *14-17.*

Herman, H., Moses, S.G. & Friedenwald, J.S. Influence of pontocaine hydrochloride and chlorobutanol on respiration and glycolysis of cornea. *Archs. Ophthal.* 28: *652-660* (1942).

Marr, W.G., et al. Effect of topical anesthetics on regeneration of corneal epithelium. *Am. J. Ophthal.* 43: *606-610* (1957).

Pontinen, P.J. The importance of the oculocardiac reflex during ocular surgery. *Acta. Ophthal.* 86 (suppl), 1966.

Willis, W.E. & Laibson, P.R. Corneal complications of topical anesthetic abuse. *Can. J. Ophthalmol.* 5: *239-243* (1970).

Authors' address:
Department of Ophthalmology
University of Oregon Health Science Center
Portland, Oregon 97034 U.S.A.

345

Docum. Ophthal. Proc. Series, Vol. 18

LATTICE DEGENERATION IN THE BLACK AFRICAN

WILLIAM H. KNOBLOCH*

(Minneapolis, Minnesota U.S.A.)

ABSTRACT

Infrequency of retinal detachment in black people has been noted. A survey of the incidence of lattice degeneration in the African was performed. A highly significant difference, 0.6% in black people as compared to 7.1% in Caucasians, was found. The possible relationship of this low incidence of lattice degeneration to the infrequency of retinal detachment was discussed.

INTRODUCTION

Because of reports of the decrease in incidence of retinal detachment among black people (Brown & Thomas, 1965; Michaelson, 1965), Av-Shalom and others surveyed 257 Africans in Tanzania and Liberia for vitreoretinal disease that might be associated with retinal detachment. (Av-Shalom, et al., 1967). They were impressed with the infrequency of vitreous syneresis and myopia in those examined. Lattice degeneration was present in 1.8% of their subjects.

Lattice degeneration occurs with a well documented incidence of about 7% in Caucasians (Straatsma, 1962; Byer, 1965). Studies by Dumas & Schepens, (1966) and Straatsma & Allen, (1962) showed an association of lattice degeneration with retinal detachment in 30% of their patients. Autosomal dominant inheritance of lattice degeneration has already been shown (Everett, 1968; Lewkonia, et al., 1973). This would make lattice degeneration the most commonly inherited retinal lesion that is often a precursor of retinal detachment. If a low incidence of lattice degeneration is confirmed in black people then a possible explanation for the decrease in number of retinal detachment patients can be postulated.

When the opportunity to survey a large number of black Africans for retinal disease presented itself, this study to specifically determine the incidence of the lattice degeneration was undertaken.

---

* This study was carried out while the author was on a sabbatical leave at Dodoma, Tanzania.

SUBJECTS AND METHODS

A total of 500 black individuals were surveyed for retinal disease. All were from central Tanzania and represented 27 different Bantu tribes. Seventy-seven percent of those surveyed were from the Mgogo tribe located near Dodoma, Tanzania. Patients, relatives and visitors from the General Medical Hospitals at Mvumi and Kilimatinde were the primary source of subjects. Excluded were Eye Clinic patients or those with eye complaints. If the media were opaque enough to preclude a good view of the retina, these were also excluded. Non-Bantu African people such as Masai, East Indian or Arabic people were not included.

Of the 500 people examined 326 were female and 174 were male. The youngest was 16 and the oldest was 73. The majority of the subjects were from the younger age groups as shown in Table I. This is important in that Byer (1965) has shown that the incidence of lattice degeneration is higher in the second to third decades.

Pupils of subjects examined were dilated with 10% Phenylephrine Hydrochloride and 1% Cyclopentolate Hydrochlorate each given three times at five minute intervals. The peripheral retina was examined with the binocular indirect ophthalmoscope and scleral indentation. The direct ophthalmoscope was also used for greater magnification and for examining the more posterior lesions. Retinal drawings were made of all eyes with fundus pathology and fundus photographs were taken of significant lesions. Slit lamp examinations and refractive error measurements were not made.

The broad definition of lattice degeneration was used. Included were circumferentially arranged lesions usually located pre-equatorial with sharply demarcated borders. A variable degree of excavation was usually apparent over its roughened surface. Although circumscribed areas of thinning and retinal holes are frequently seen in lattice degeneration, their presence was not required for consideration. Pigmentation and white line arborization occasionally found in lattice degeneration were also not a requisite to be included.

Table 1. Subjects by age groups.

Ages	Number
16-25	188
26-35	183
36-45	62
46-55	29
56-65	28
66-75	10
Total	500

Lattice degeneration was present in three subjects, 25, 30 and 34 years of age. All were bilateral and symmetrical with the superior temporal quadrants involved in two, and the inferior temporal quadrants in one. White branching lines were not evident and pigmentation was minimal. Round holes were present in one subject and cystic areas were noted in the other two. No flap tears were present and there were no associated retinal detachments.

Table II lists in order of frequency other vitreoretinal findings in the study. The very high incidence of chorioretinitis in 10.4% was impressive. Over half of these showed widespread diffuse areas of involvement with chorioretinal stipling, atrophy of the pigment epithelium, vitreous veils and debris, vascular attenuation and sheathing and tractional distortion of the vessels with glial tissue occasionally obscuring the optic nerve. Optic atrophy was frequently associated. The inflammatory response in all appeared inactive. The distortion of the vascular patterns and the 'old' appearance of the chorioretinitis gave the impression that the inflammation had occurred early in life. The other half of the individuals with chorioretinitis had either localized peripapillary scars or small scattered old inflammatory foci. Two patients had lesions typical of toxoplasmosis.

There were five individuals with optic atrophy without other evidence of chorioretinal disease. One was bilateral and the other four unilateral. The etiology was not evident from examination or history.

The three patients with macular degeneration were 60, 67 and 68 years of age. All had 'dry' type of senile macular degeneration with irregular areas

Table 2. Vitreoretinal Lesions as found in survey of 500 black African people

Lesions	Number of Subjects	% Affected
Chorioretinitis	52	10.4
Persistent Hyaloid Remnants	43	8.6
Optic Atrophy	5	1.0
Retinoschisis	4	0.8
Myelinated Nerve Fibers	4	0.8
Lattice Degeneration	3	0.6
Macular Degeneration	3	0.6
Asteroid Hyalosis	3	0.6
Glaucomatous Excavation	2	0.4
Retinal Hemorrhages	2	0.4
Grouped Pigmentation	2	0.4
Melanocytoma	1	0.2
Pigment Epithelium Hypertrophy	1	0.2
Oblique Optic Nerve	1	0.2
Paving Stone Degeneration	1	0.2
Marchesani Syndrome	1	0.2

of atrophy of the pigment epithelium and choriocapillaris with scattered pigment clumping. Disciform scarring was not present.

Four individuals had bilateral retinoschisis. In three the areas were confined to the inferior temporal quadrants and in one to the superior temporal quadrant. All were shallow and anterior to the equator. There were no associated retinal breaks or retinal detachments.

An interesting non-pathological finding in 42 subjects was the hyaloid artery remnants in the vitreous or Bergmeister's papillae at the optic nerve. Some of the epipapillary veils associated with the hyaloid remnants almost obscured the disc in several individuals.

DISCUSSION

In a well documented series of 1,300 patients, Byer found 92 patients (7.1%) with lattice degeneration. In this study of 500 Africans, three (0.6%) had lattice degeneration. This difference is highly significant (Table III). The low incidence of lattice degeneration in the African most likely reflects the low gene prevalence for lattice degeneration when compared to the Caucasian. To determine the relationship of the decreased incidence of lattice degeneration to the infrequency of retinal detachment in black people, a more careful study of the type of retinal detachment found in the African will be needed.

Hilton & Richards (1970) reporting a study of retinal detachment in the American Indian, found an incidence of occurrence of retinal detachment of one in 19,000 individuals per year. This corresponds closely with previous prevalence studies by others (Stein, et al., 1972; Suckling & Hay, 1968). The important finding, however, was that 78% of those detached had retinal dialysis, an infrequent cause of detachment in the Caucasian. Accordingly a careful survey of detachment in the African may reveal similar etiological variations.

It would be difficult to accept the low incidence of retinal detachment to be due entirely to the infrequency of lattice degeneration. As lattice degeneration is etiologically linked to only 30% of retinal detachments in

Table 3. Comparison of the Incidence of Lattice degeneration in Caucasians and black Africans.

Race	Lattice Degeneration	Not Affected	Total Studied	% Affected
Caucasian (Byer)	92	1.208	1,300	7.08
Black Africans	3	497	500	0.60
TOTALS	95	1,705	1,800	

$x^2 = 30.3$ 1 d/f $P < .00001$

350

the Caucasian it would appear likely that other factors are present. Certainly the findings of a low incidence of myopia and vitreous syneresis reported by Av-Shalom (1967a, 1967b) is a likely cause. At this point, racial differences in inheritance of degenerative vitreoretinal disease that preceeds retinal detachment seems evident. Further study to determine these differences may shed light on the whole problem of genetic susceptability to retinal detachment.

REFERENCES

Av-Shalom, A., Berson, D., Blumenthal, M., Gombos, G.M., Landau, L. & Zauberman, H. Prevalence of myopia in africans. *Am. J. Ophthal.* 63: *1728-1731* (1967).

Av-Shalom, A., Berson, D., Gombos, G.M., Landau, L., Michaelson, I.C. & Zauberman, H. The vitreo-retinopathy associated with retinal detachment among africans. *Am. J. Ophthal.* 64: *387-391* (1967).

Av-Shalom, A., Berson, D., Gombos, G.M., Michaelson, I.C. & Zauberman, H. Some comments on the incidence of idiopathic retinal detachment among africans. *Am. J. Ophthal.* 64: *384-386* (1967).

Brown, P.R. & Thomas, R.P. The low incidence of primary retinal detachment in the negro. *Am. J. Ophthal.* 60: *109-110* (1965).

Byer, N.E. Clinical study of lattice degeneration of the retina. *Trans Am. Acad. Ophthal. Otolar.* 69: *1064-1081* (1965).

Dumas, J. & Schepens, C.L. Chorioretinal lesions predisposing to retinal breaks. *Am. J. Ophthal.* 61: *620* (1966).

Everett, W.G. Study Of A family with lattice degeneration and retinal detachment. *Am. J. Ophthal.* 65: *229-232* (1968).

Hilton, G.F. & Richards, W.W. Retinal detachment in american indians. *Am. J. Ophthal.* 70: *981-983* (1970).

Lewkonia, I., Davies, M.S. & Salmon, J.D. Lattice degeneration in a family. *Br.J. Ophthal.* 57: *566-571* (1973).

Michaelson, I.C. Ophthalmology in developing countries. *Am. J. Ophthal.* 59: *409-412* (1965).

Stein, R., Feller-Ofry, V. & Romano, A. The effect of treatment in the prevention of retinal detachment. *Israel J. Med. Sci.* 8.2: *1429-1430* (1972).

Straatsma, B.R. & Allen, R.A. Lattice degeneration of the retina. *Trans. Am. Acad. Ophthal. Otolar.* 66: *600-613* (1962).

Suckling, R.D. & Hay, J.R. A regional survey of retinal detachment. *Trans Ophthal. Soc. N. Z.* 20: *69-74* (1968).

Author's address
William H. Knobloch, M.D.
Department of Ophthalmology
University of Minnesota Medical School
Minneapolis, Minnesota 55455
U.S.A.

Docum. Ophthal. Proc. Series, Vol. 18

THE ADRENERGIC EFFECTS ON CYCLIC AMP AND TENSION OF THE SPHINCTER PUPILLAE OF THE RABBIT

MANABU MOCHIZUKI & SAIICHI MISHIMA

(Tokyo, Japan)

ABSTRACT

Using sphincter pupillae muscle pairs dissected from both eyes of albino rabbits after instillation of an 0.5 percent indomethacin oil-drop, it was found that the cyclic AMP level of the muscle was increased with isoprenaline and epinephrine but not with phenylephrine. The effects of isoprenaline were dose-dependent and the ED_{50} was calculated to be 4.47×10^{-8} mol l^{-1}. Isoprenaline effect was inhibited by pretreatment with propranolol but not with phenoxybenzamine.

Muscle strips obtained without prior topical indomethacin were incubated, and drug effects on the isometric tension were studied. The muscle contraction induced with carbachol was reduced in a dose-dependent manner with isoprenaline; the ED_{50} was $(4.78 \pm 0.56) \times 10^{-8}$ mol l^{-1}. The isoprenaline effects were completely suppressed with propranolol. The maximum relaxation occurred with 10^{-5} mol l^{-1} of isoprenaline which also induced the maximum increase in the cyclic AMP level.

It was concluded that both responses of the sphincter muscle were due to beta-adrenergic stimulation, and a possible relation of these responses was discussed.

INTRODUCTION

It is generally accepted that the action of the beta-adrenergic agonists is mediated by intracellular cyclic adenosine 3′, 5′-monophosphate (cyclic AMP) (Robison et al., 1968). Smooth muscle relaxation induced by these drugs is thought to be dependent on their efficacy to increase the intracellural level of cyclic AMP (Robison et al., 1968; Bärl, 1974), and this has been shown in several smooth muscles, e.g. the guinea pig trachea (Moore et al., 1967), the rat uterus (Dobbs & Robison, 1968), the rabbit colon (Andersson & Nilsson, 1972) and the taenia caecum of guinea pig (Kawasaki et al., 1969; Takayanagi et al., 1972; Inatomi et al., 1974).

The sphincter pupillae muscle of rabbits has beta-adrenergic receptors (Sachsl & Heath, 1940; van Alphen et al., 1965), stimulation of which results in relaxation of the muscle. It is possible that this relaxation is also dependent on the increase of the intracellular cyclic AMP, but no experimental proof is yet available. This paper reports the effects of adrenergic agonists and blockers on the cyclic AMP of the sphincter pupillae muscle of rabbits, on the tension relaxation of the muscle and also the correlation of these effects.

353

MATERIALS AND METHODS

1. Drugs

The following drugs were used: l-isoproterenol HCl (isoprenaline) obtained from Kaken Chemical Co., l-epinephrine bitartrate (epinephrine), l-phenylephrine HCl (phenylephrine), dl-propranolol HCl (propranolol) obtained from Sigma Chemical Co., and phenoxybenzamine HCl (PBA) obtained from Tokyo Kasei Ind..

2. Isolation of the sphincter muscle strip

Adult albino rabbits of both sexes, weighing 2.2-3.5 kg, were killed with an overdose of pentobarbital sodium. The whole cornea was removed in situ and a short incision was made on the iris about 1 mm from the pupillary margin and parallel to it. Two 6-0 silk sutures were placed through the incision and the pupil margin was cut in between the sutures. The incision was extended along the pupil margin and a 1 mm-wide strip was isolated. Histological examination confirmed that the preparation contained all sphincter muscles and few dilator muscles.

3. Incubation of the sphincter muscle strip

The isolated sphincter muscle strip was incubated in an organ bath containing 10 ml of Krebs-Ringers' physiologic solution as reported previously (Ohara, 1977). The solution had the following composition: (m mol 1^{-1}); NaCl, 118.05; KCl, 4.69; $CaCl_2 . 2H_2O$, 2.51; $MgCl_2 . 6H_2O$, 0.54; $NaH_2PO_4 . H_2O$, 1.01; glucose, 11.10 and $NaHCO_3$, 25.01. The bath was kept at $37°C$ and continuously gassed with a mixture of 95 percent O_2 and 5 percent CO_2 to maintain the pH at 7.4.

4. Cyclic AMP study

Instillation to both eyes of an 0.5 percent indomethacin oil-drop was carried out 3, 2, 1 and 0.5 hours prior to the sacrifice of the rabbits. A pair of sphincter muscle strips was used, one for drug effects and the other for the control. They were suspended in the organ bath with a glass weight, weighing 100 mg in water, attached to one end. The incubation medium contained 1 m mol 1^{-1} of amynophyllline (Eisai Pharm. Co.).

After preliminary incubation, the adrenergic agonists were given to the medium at various final concentrations, and the strip was incubated for a further 5 minutes. In another series of experiments, the muscles were incubated for 15 minutes in the medium containing the adrenergic blockers and then the agonists were given as above.

Immediately after the incubation, the muscles were frozen in liquid nitrogen and were subjected to cyclic AMP assay. The frozen muscle strips were homogenized in 1 ml of cold 6 percent trichloroacetic acid and the homogenate was centrifuged at 1,500 g for 15 minutes at 4°C. The supernatant was extracted with 3 volumes of water-saturated ether and the procedure was repeated 3 times. The remaining supernatant was dried at 60°C using nitrogen gas and stored at $-20°C$ until use. The sample was dissolved in 1 ml of 50 m mol 1^{-1} sodium acetate buffer at pH 6.2; an aliquot of 200 μl was subjected to the radio-immunoassay technique described by Steiner et al. (1969) and modified by Sato et al. (1976), using cyclic AMP assay kit (Mitsui Toatsu Chemical). For the statistical processing of the results, the paired t-test was used.

To test the recovery of this method, 50 picomoles of cyclic sodium AMP (Sigma Chemical Co.) and 200 μg of bovine albumin (Daiichi Chemical Co.) were mixed in a glass homogenizer and the homogenate was subjected to the above method of assay. The recovery rate was 87.5 ± 3.1 (mean ± S.E.) percent in 10 trials.

The precipitate of the homogenate was used to measure protein content by the method of Lowry et al. (1951).

5. The drug effects on muscle tension

The sphincter muscle strip was isolated without prior use of indomethacin oil-drop. It was incubated in the medium without amynophylline, the lower end fixed to a glass hook in the organ bath and the upper end attached to a force-displacement transducer (SB-1T-H, Nihon Koden), which was connected to a strain amplifier (6M51, Sanei Instrument) and a recorder (Kasset TO2NS-H, Toshin Electric). To achieve a stable condition of the muscle strip, i.e. appropriate length and responsiveness, a preliminary incubation was carried out with a load of light tension for 30-60 minutes, during which period the medium was changed at a regular interval of 10 minutes. A half-maximum dose of carbachol, 10^{-6} mol 1^{-1}, was given to confirm that the strip showed stable contraction lasting for 10 minutes. About 15 minutes after washing 4 times with the physiologic solution, carbachol was given at the above dose, and the dose-response studies were performed with

Table 1. The effects of the adrenergic agonists on the cyclic AMP of the sphincter muscles.

	No. of experiments	cyclic AMP (mean ± S.E.) pmol / mg protein	
		control	treated
isoprenaline	4	48.9 ± 4.7	154.7 ± 9.5**
epinephrine	4	42.0 ± 7.3	63.9 ± 4.5*
phenylephrine	4	41.7 ± 3.9	38.7 ± 5.6

* P < 0.01
** P < 0.001

cumulative doses of isoprenaline. Subsequently, the muscle strip was washed as above and similar studies were repeated with prior application of 3×10^{-6} mol 1^{-1} propranolol.

RESULTS

1. The level of cyclic AMP in the sphincter muscle

To find the most adequate time for the preliminary incubation, the muscle strip was incubated for 15, 30, 45, 60, 90 and 120 minutes, using 5 muscle strips for each time interval. The lowest average and the least variation of the cyclic AMP level were obtained with 30 minutes incubation; this was chosen as the preliminary incubation time in the following experiments. The cyclic AMP level of 50 control muscle strips averaged 49.6 ± 2.2 (mean ± S.E.) pmol per mg protein. Five pairs of the sphincter muscles were incubated as above and the cyclic AMP level was 49.3 ± 3.5 and 50.1 ± 3.8 pmol per mg protein in the strip prepared first and in the strip subsequently isolated; the difference was not significant.

The effects of isoprenaline, epinephrine and phenylephrine at doses of 10^{-6} mol 1^{-1} are shown in Table 1. With isoprenaline and epinephrine, the cyclic AMP level was significantly higher than that of the control strips; the difference was more pronounced with the former than with the latter. The effects of adrenergic blockers are shown in Table 2. Application of propranolol or PBA, 3×10^{-6} mol$_1$$1^{-1}$, did not alter the cyclic AMP level from that of the control. The pretreatment with propranolol almost completely sup-

Table 2. The influence of the adrenergic blockers on the cyclic AMP and the isoprenaline effects.

	No. of experiments	cyclic AMP (mean ± S.E.) pmol / mg protein
control	4	65.7 ± 10.9
propranolol**	4	71.7 ± 10.2
isoprenaline*	4	190.4 ± 14.7***
propranolol** + isoprenaline*	4	53.5 ± 4.4***
control	4	58.9 ± 7.0
PBA**	4	58.5 ± 6.5
isoprenaline*	4	224.9 ± 22.5
PBA** + isoprenaline*	4	237.3 ± 29.2

* concentration was 10^{-6} mol 1^{-1}, ** 3×10^{-6} mol 1^{-1} *** $P < 0.001$

pressed the effects of isoprenaline, but PBA failed to inhibit the isoprenaline effects.

The results of dose-response studies with isoprenaline are given in Table 3. The difference of the cyclic AMP level between the treated and

Table 3. The dose-response study on the isoprenaline effects.

	cyclic AMP (mean ± S.E.)		
isoprenaline (mol 1^{-1})	pmol / mg protein control	treated	percent increase
10^{-9}	67.0 ± 11.8	56.4 ± 9.8	96.9 ± 14.3
10^{-8}	40.3 ± 4.7	58.5 ± 6.6	145.7 ± 5.9*
10^{-7}	42.5 ± 6.8	114.1 ± 10.9	283.9 ± 32.3**
10^{-6}	48.3 ± 6.4	168.4 ± 15.5	358.3 ± 30.3**
10^{-5}	45.4 ± 9.5	165.4 ± 22.4	388.9 ± 56.0*
10^{-4}	57.5 ± 8.7	184.4 ± 27.5	323.0 ± 24.3*

Number of experiments was 5 for each concentration.
* $P < 0.005$ ** $P < 0.001$

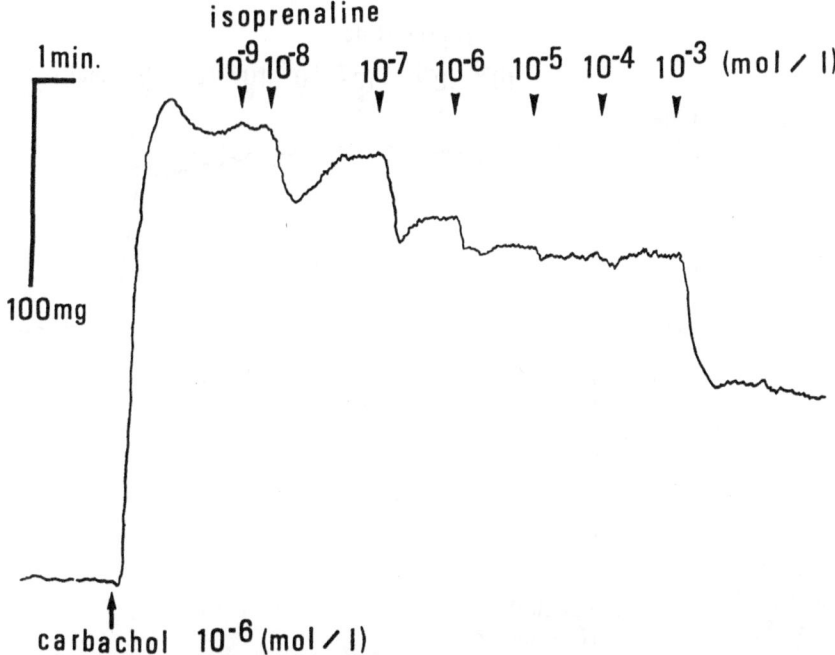

Fig. 1. Effects of cumulative doses of isoprenaline on contraction of the sphincter muscle induced with carbachol. An example from 5 experiments.

control strips was not significant in the isoprenaline concentration of 10^{-9} mol 1^{-1}, but it was significant with higher concentrations. The percent increase over the control level was dose-dependent in the concentration range between 10^{-8} and 10^{-4} mol 1^{-1}. The average percentage increases in various concentration groups were compared to that with 10^{-5} mol 1^{-1} of isoprenaline and the ED_{50} was calculated to be 4.47×10^{-8} mol 1^{-1}.

2. The drug effects on muscle tension

An example of the effects of cumulative doses of isoprenaline on the muscle tension in the presence of 10^{-6} mol 1^{-1} carbachol is shown in Fig. 1. A significant dose-dependent relaxation was observed in the range of the iso- prenaline concentrations from 10^{-8} to 10^{-4} mol 1^{-1}. A marked relaxation was observed with 10^{-3} mol 1^{-1}. An example of the similar experiments with pretreatment using propranolol, 3×10^{-6} mol 1^{-1}, is shown in Fig. 2. The muscle relaxation did not occur with isoprenaline concentrations from 10^{-9} to 10^{-4} mol 1^{-1} but a marked relaxation similar to that shown by Fig. 1 took place with 10^{-3} mol 1^{-1} of isoprenaline. Consequently, it was thought that the effects of 10^{-3} mol 1^{-1} of isoprenaline were not due to beta-adren- ergic stimulation, and this was excluded from the following analysis. The effects with 10^{-4} mol 1^{-1} were taken as the reference and the percentage

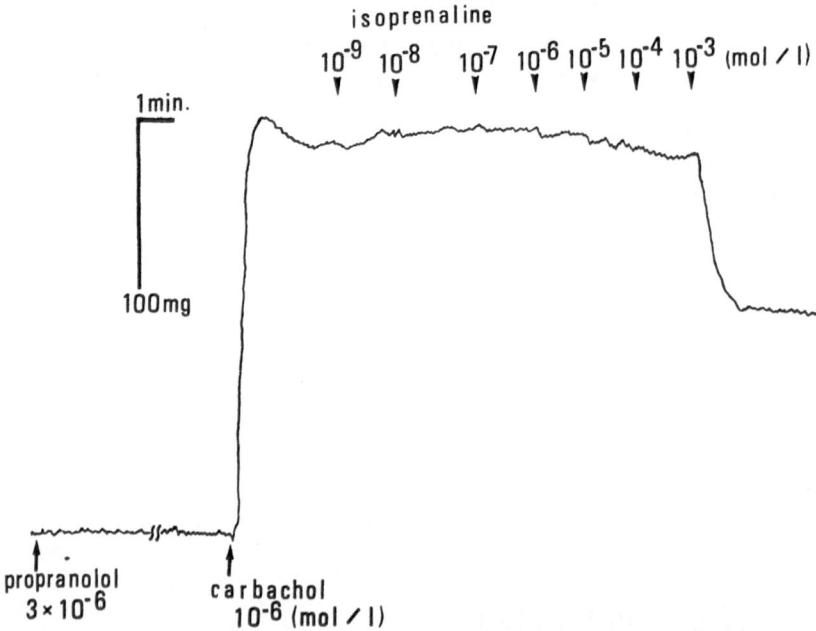

Fig. 2. Influence of propranolol on the isoprenaline effects. An example from 5 ex- periments.

relaxation was calculated for other concentrations. The dose-response relationship was thus obtained on the basis of 5 experiments and is illustrated in Fig. 3. The ED_{50} was calculated to be $4.78 \pm 0.56 \times 10^{-8}$ (mean ± S.E.) mol l^{-1}.

DISCUSSION

The anterior uvea of the rabbit produces prostaglandins (PGs) in response to trauma (Eakins, 1974). Furthermore, the PGs have been reported to increase the level of cyclic AMP in various cells (Harbon & Clauser, 1971; Waitzman & Woods, 1971; Neufeld & Sears, 1974). Consequently, it was thought that the present method of isolating the sphincter muscle strip is

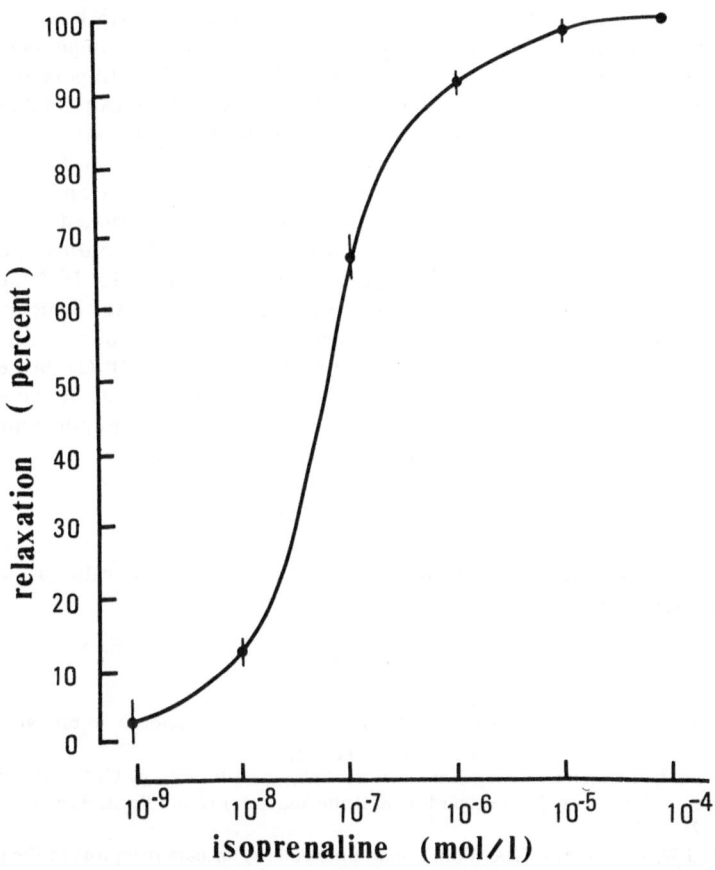

Fig. 3. The dose-response relationship in the isoprenaline effects on the tension of the sphincter muscle. Mean ± S.E. of 5 experiments is shown.

likely to initiate PGs synthesis thereby affecting the level of cyclic AMP in the muscles. For this reason, the indomethacin oil-drop was instilled before the sacrifice of the animals, according to the protocol which was shown to effectively inhibit PGs production in the eye following paracentesis (Masuda et al., 1977). The preliminary incubation studies revealed that the cyclic AMP level and its variation was the lowest with the incubation time of 30 minutes. This suggests that the influence of dissection was present in the early period and the condition of the tissue was stabilized in 30 minutes. The cyclic AMP level of the control muscles showed a considerable variation among animals, but the difference between the paired muscles from the same animal was small. Accordingly, the paired muscles were used for the drug studies.

The cyclic AMP of the sphincter muscle was significantly increased with isoprenaline and epinephrine but not with phenylephrine. The isoprenaline effects were completely suppressed with 3×10^{-6} mol 1^{-1} of propranolol but not with PBA, both of which did not affect the cyclic AMP level of the muscles. Furthermore, the effects of isoprenaline were dose-dependent and these results lead to a conclusion that the effects were due to beta-adrenergic stimulation. The dose-dependent muscle relaxation with isoprenaline and inhibition thereof with propranolol indicate that the effects are also due to beta-adrenergic stimulation. The maximum increase in the cyclic AMP of the sphincter muscles was obtained with 10^{-5} mol 1^{-1} of isoprenaline at which concentration the relaxation of the muscles also reached the maximum. Furthermore, the ED_{50} of this drug was similar for both responses, 4.47×10^{-8} mol 1^{-1} in increasing cyclic AMP level and 4.78×10^{-8} mol 1^{-1} in the relaxation. For several smooth muscles, experimental evidence has been accumulated to show that the muscle response to beta-adrenergic stimulation is mediated by intracellular increase of cyclic AMP (Dobbs et al., 1968; Andersson & Nilsson, 1972; Inatomi et al., 1974). Thus, it is possible that a similar mechanism is also operating in the sphincter pupillae muscles of rabbits. Further experiments are underway to confirm this.

ACKNOWLEDGEMENT

The authors are grateful to Professor I. Takayanagi for his valuable advices during this work.

REFERENCES

Andersson, R. & Nilsson, K. Cyclic AMP and calcium in relaxation in intestinal smooth muscle. *Nature New Biol.* 238: *119-120* (1972).

Bär, H.P. Cyclic nucleotid and smooth muscle, in Advances in Cyclic Nucleotides Research, Vol. 4, (ed. Greengard, P. & Robison, G.A.) Raven Press, New York 1974 pp. *195-237.*

Dobbs, J.W. & Robison, G.A. Functional biochemistry of beta receptors in the uterus. *Fedn. Prd. Fedn. Am. Socs. exp. Biol.* 27: *352* (1968).

Eakins, K.E. Prostaglandins and prostaglandin synthetase inhibitors: action in ocular disease, in Prostaglandin Synthetase Inhibitors (ed. Robinson, H.J. & Vane, J.R.) Raven Press, New York 1971 pp. *343-352*.

Harbon, S. & Clauser, H. Cyclic adenosine 3', 5' monophoshate level in rat myometrium under the influence of epinephrine, prostaglandins and oxytocin. Correlation with uterus motility. *Biochem. biophys. Res. Commun.* 44: *1496-1503* (1971).

Inatomi, N., Takayanagi, I., Uchida, M. & Takagi, K. Intracellular cyclic AMP level and intestinal smooth muscle relaxation. *Eur. J. Pharmacol.* 26: *73-76* (1974).

Kawasaki, A., Kashimoto, T. & Yoshida, H. Effects of 3', 5'-cyclic adenosine monophosphate and its dibutyryl derivative on the motility of isolated rat ileum. *Jap. J. Pharmac.* 19: *494-501* (1969).

Lowry, O.H., Rosebrough, N.J., Farr, A.L. & Randall, R.J. Protein measurement with the folin phenol reagent. *J. biol. Chem.* 193: *265-275* (1951).

Masuda, K., Izawa, Y. & Mishima, S. Breakdown of the blood: aqueous barrier and prostaglandins. *Bibl. Anat.* 16: *99-104* (1977).

Moore, P.E., Iorio, L.C. & McManus, J.M. Relaxation of the guinea-pig tracheal chain preparation by N^{-6}, 2'-0-dibutyryl 3', 5'-cyclic adenosine monophosphate. *J. Pharm. Pharmac.* 20: *368-372* (1967).

Neufeld, A.H. & Sears, M.L. Cyclic- AMP in ocular tissue of the rabbit, monkey and human. *Invest. Ophthalmol.* 13: *475-477* (1974).

Ohara, K. Effects of cholinergic agonists on isolated iris sphinter muscles: A pharmacodynamic study. *Jap. J. Ophthal.* 21: *516-527* (1977).

Robison, G.A., Butchner, R.W. & Sutherland, E.W. Cyclic AMP. *A. Rev. Biochem.* 39: *149-174* (1968).

Sachs, E. & Heath, P. The pharmacological behavior of the intraocular muscles. *Am. J. Ophthal.* 23: *1376-1387* (1940).

Sato, K., Miyachi, Y., Mizuchi, A., Ohsawa, N. & Kosaka, K. Enzymatic radioiodination of succinyl cyclic AMP tyrosine methyl ester by lactoperoxidase and radioimmunoassay for cyclic AMP. *Endocr. jap.* 23: *251-257* (1976).

Steiner, A.L., Kipnis, D.M., Utiger, R. & Parker, C. Radioimmunoassay for the measurement of adenosine 3', 5'-cyclic phosphate. *Proc. Natn. Acad. Sci.* 64: *367-373* (1969).

Takayanagi, I., Uchida, M., Inatomi, N., Tomiyama, A. & Takagi, K. Intracellular cyclic adenosine 3', 5'-monophosphate and relaxing effects of isoprenaline and papaverine on smooth muscle of intestine. *Jap. J. Pharmac.* 22: *869-871* (1972).

van Alphen, G.W.H.M., Holland, L., Kern, R. & Robinette, S.L. Adrenergic receptors of the intraocular muscles. *Arch. Ophthal.* N.Y. 74: *253-259* (1965).

Waitzman, M.B. & Woods, W.D. Some characteristics of an adenyl cyclase preparation from rabbit ciliary process tissue. *Expl. Eye Res.* 12: *99-111* (1971).

Authors' address:
Department of Ophthalmology
University of Tokyo
School of Medicine
Hongo, Bunkyo-ku
Tokyo, 113, Japan

Docum. Ophthal. Proc. Series, Vol. 18

EPITHELIAL CELL CYSTS OF THE ANTERIOR CHAMBER TREATED BY ACID INJECTIONS

By

KENNETH C. SWAN

(Portland, Oregon U.S.A.)

ABSTRACT

Seven large epithelial cysts of the anterior chamber were aspirated, injected with 20 percent trichloracetic acid and then collapsed by re-aspiration. Two patients had recurrences and required a second injection. Post-treatment follow-ups ranged from two to seven years. Serial photographs document the effectiveness of this treatment and the minimal postoperative inflammatory reaction. There were no significant complications or sequellae in this series. Accidental injections of the acid through the cyst wall into the aqueous or cornea presented a potential hazard which can be minimized by exacting microsurgical techniques.

John E. Harris is best known as an investigator and educator, but ability to apply scientific methodology to clinical problems, coupled with a warm personality and a concern for the welfare of patients also have brought him recognition as a clinical consultant. The subject of this report, chemical treatment of epithelial cysts of the anterior chamber, is an outgrowth of a consultation with Dr. Harris in 1952, when he still was at the University of Oregon Medical School. The subject is timely because extracapsular cataract extraction again has become a commonly used technique. It is resulting in an increased incidence of epithelial ingrowth into the anterior chamber because accidental incarcerations of lens capsule in limbal or corneal wound may occur and establish tracks for the ingrowth of epithelium. This is most likely to occur during the primary procedure but it may complicate discission of after-cataract. Epithelial ingrowth develops under other circumstances; for example, along sutures which penetrate the limbal or corneal stroma following traumatic perforations. Also, there are congenital epithelial cysts.

Epithelial invasion of the anterior chamber usually occurs either in a membranous form or as a cyst. The course of such cysts is variable. They may remain small and asymptomatic. However, repeated examinations always are indicated, because these cysts may enlarge dramatically after a dormant period. In most cases, a gradual enlargement of the cyst takes place so that a major part of the anterior chamber may be occupied and vision obstructed. Symptoms also result from corneal disturbances, uveitis and glaucoma. Relatively radical treatment then is justified to prevent loss of the eye.

363

Many techniques of treating cysts of the anterior chamber have been reported with varying degrees of success. In addition to surgical excision with and without corneal transplantation, cysts have been treated by x-ray radiation, diathermy, electrolysis, photocoagulation, cryotherapy and the injection of various sclerosing solutions. At the University of Oregon Health Sciences Center, it has been the policy to excise small epithelial inclusion cysts if they show evidence of growth. Since 1952 large cysts with extensive involvement of the iris and the posterior surface of the cornea have been treated by aspiration and injection of trichloroacetic acid. It is the purpose of this report to document the effectiveness of this relatively simple and reasonably safe therapy by summarizing the favorable course of seven eyes which developed epithelial cysts of such magnitude that surgical excision would have been extremely hazardous, if not impossible.

The first patient to be treated with chemical cauterization was an eight-year-old girl referred with a large epithelial inclusion cyst which was causing discomfort and reducing vision in her only eye. She had had multiple discissions of congenital cataracts. Complications had led to enucleation of referral, she had had a discission of an after-cataract in her remaining eye. The cyst became manifest about a year later and steadily enlarged. As shown in Figure 1 (top), it filled approximately one half of the lower anterior chamber and involved the iris. The corneal epithelium was bedewed inferiorly. There was extensive angle closure, and the ocular tension averaged 22-24 mm. Maximal visual acuity was 2/200 with the aphakic correction. Aspiration of the cyst, with injection of a sclerosing solution, offered the best hope with the least risk of the measures known to us at that time. The injection of one-half strength tincture of iodine had been recommended, but John Harris suggested that the injection of the cyst with dilute organic acid probably would be a more effective coagulant of the cells lining the cyst and that furthermore, the coagulation would tend to limit the solution to the interior of the cyst. We chose to use trichloroacetic acid, because its use as a 'chemical cautery' had been established, including injection into cysts of the anterior chamber. For this purpose, Lindner (1938) had recommended use of a 10% concentration but trials on anesthetized eyes of laboratory animals indicated that a concentration of 20% in aqueous solution would instantly and consistently produce a sharply delimited coagulum of the conjunctival epithelium. A 20% concentration, therefore, was selected for injection into the cyst in the child's eye where the cyst was in direct contact with the cornea.

The technique of injection of the cyst was similar to that detailed by Kirby (1950) for the injection of one-half strength tincture of iodine. Operating microscopes with para-axial illumination were not yet available, but we (Swan & Christensen, 1948) already had adapted a laboratory type of wide-field dissecting microscope for ophthalmic surgery. Mounted on an adjustable stand, this microscope could be swung over the operative field so that the position of the needle tip could be visualized clearly under magnification of 10 to 16 times.

Kirby (1950) recommended the introduction of a sharp needle directly

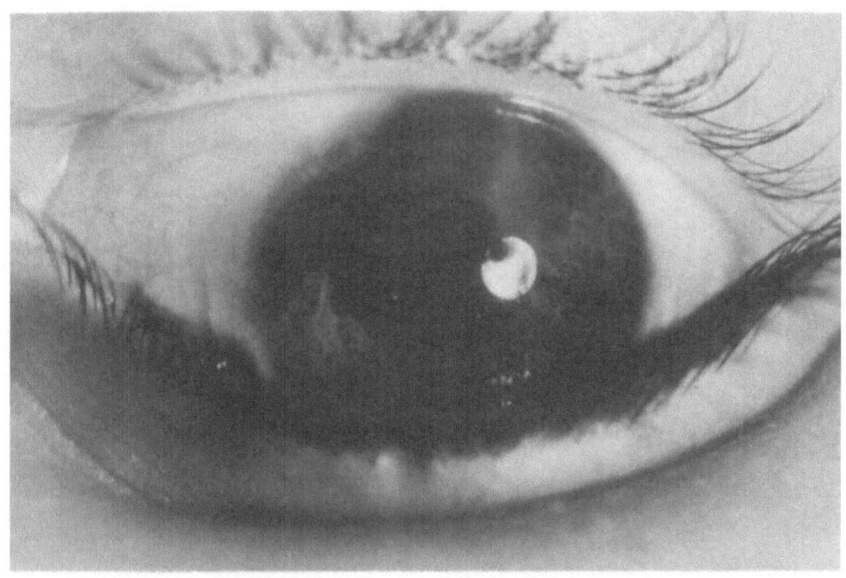

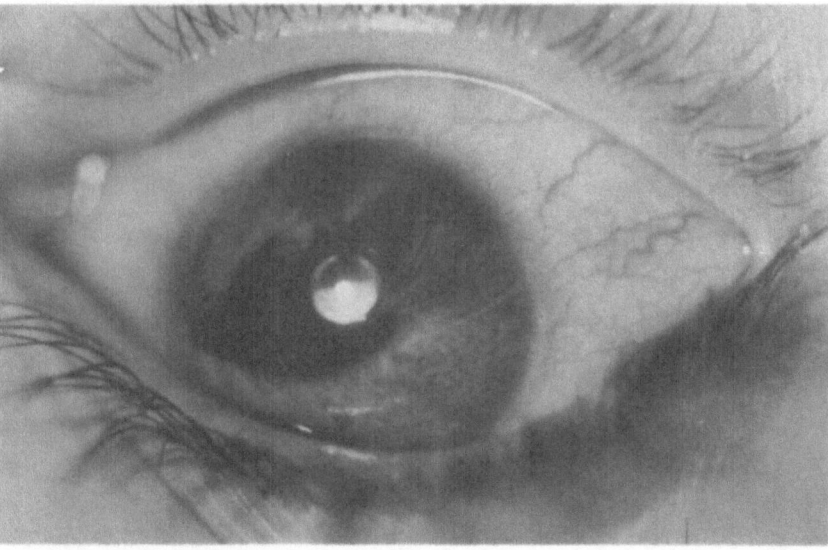

Fig. 1. Epithelial cyst (top) following discission of an after-cataract. The visual axis was blocked. Three years after injection of the cyst with trichloroacetic acid (bottom) the cyst had not reformed.

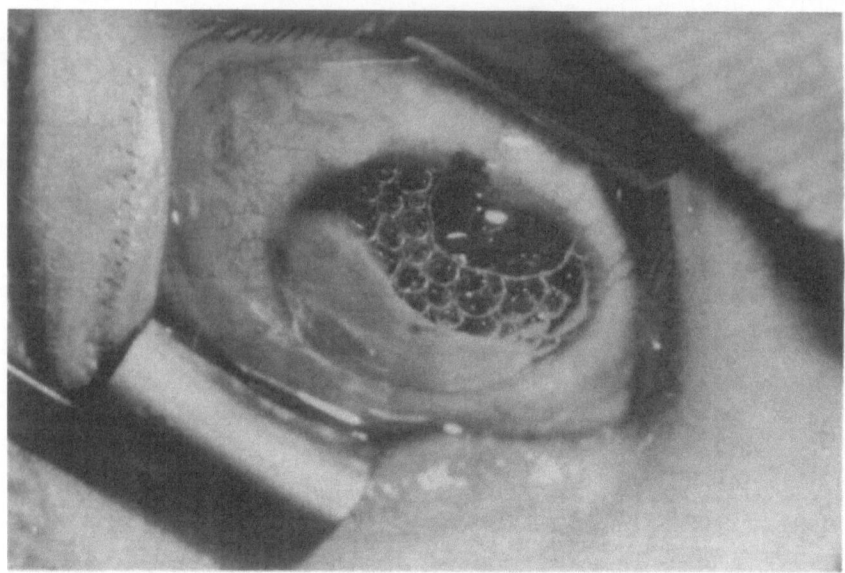

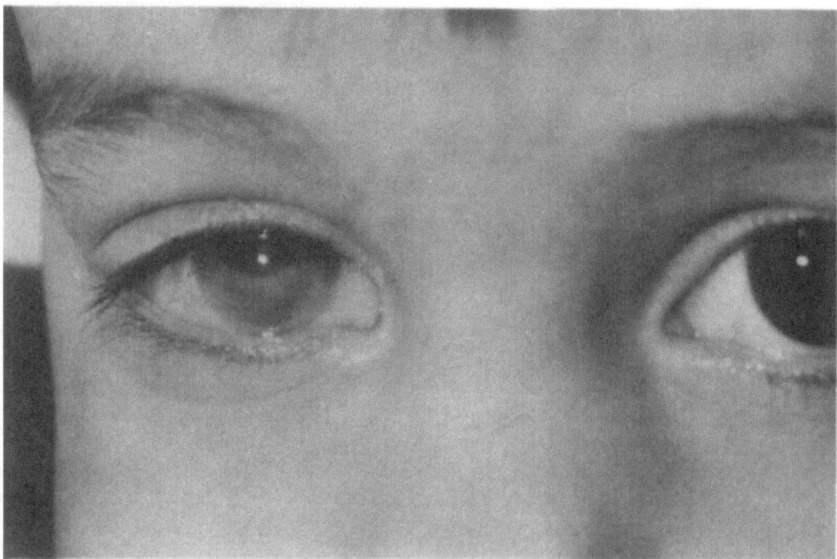

Fig. 2. Immediate postoperative appearance (top) of congenital cyst. The cyst walls are white due to coagulation. The cyst was so large that air was injected through a separate limbal puncture wound to restore the anterior chamber and to completely collapse the walls of the cyst. Three days later (bottom) there was minimal inflammatory reaction, the conjunctival and episcleral vessels were not congested and the child had little discomfort.

366

into the cyst but we were concerned that the thin cyst wall might be punctured when it was collapsed onto the sharp needle tip during the aspiration phase of the surgery. For this reason a discission knife was used to make a track into the cyst. The knife then was withdrawn and a short blunt-tipped 30-gauge needle attached to a 2 ml syringe containing .5 ml of the 20% trichloracetic acid was introduced. The cyst was aspirated, and then without withdrawal of the needle, the mixture of cyst fluid and trichloroacetic acid was carefully injected. The clear walls of the cyst and the protein in cyst fluid immediately turned white. The cyst contents then were aspirated to completely collapse the cyst before the needle was withdrawn. Suction was maintained as the needle was withdrawn to avoid spread of the acid into stroma. Only a minimal coagulation of the conjunctiva occurred at the puncture site.

Postoperative inflammatory reaction was minimal. The white coagulum in the collapsed cyst cleared in a few days. Ocular tension dropped to 15-16 mm. When the child was last examined three and one-half years later, she was comfortable and there had been no recurrence of the cyst or evidence of untoward cicatricial reaction either in the eye or at the puncture site (Fig. 1 bottom). Visual acuity was 20/100.

Following the successful treatment of the epithelial cyst in this child's eye, similar treatment was effectively used on another child who developed a large cyst following an accidental puncture wound of the cornea and also on a young child with a congenital cyst which filled the entire lower half of the anterior chamber. An attempt by the referring ophthalmologist to excise the congenital cyst surgically had been ineffective. Fig. 2 shows the minimal reaction which was present only three days after injection of the congenital cyst in the child's right eye which had filled more than one-half of the anterior chamber.

During the period 1954 through 1977, this injection-aspiration treatment also was used to treat four elderly adults who had developed large epithelial cysts of the anterior chamber and iris following extracapsular cataract extractions. These cysts filled at least one-fourth or more of the anterior chamber. Two of the four adult patients had had unsuccessful treatment prior to referral to the University of Oregon Medical School. One had been treated by transcorneal applications of cryotherapy, but the details of the treatment were not available. The other patient had been treated with diathermy by the technique described by Hogan & Goodner (1960). The referring physician reported that this cyst had returned within a month after treatment.

The typical appearance of an anterior cyst before and after trichloroacetic acid injection is shown in the stereograms in Fig. 3. Three of the four adults had no recurrence of the cyst over the period from three and one-half to seven years. After the initial reaction to the operation had subsided, which usually occurred within ten days, there were no undesirable sequellae which could be attributed to the treatment. Visual acuity was improved or unchanged.

Five of the seven eyes required only one treatment. The infant with the

367

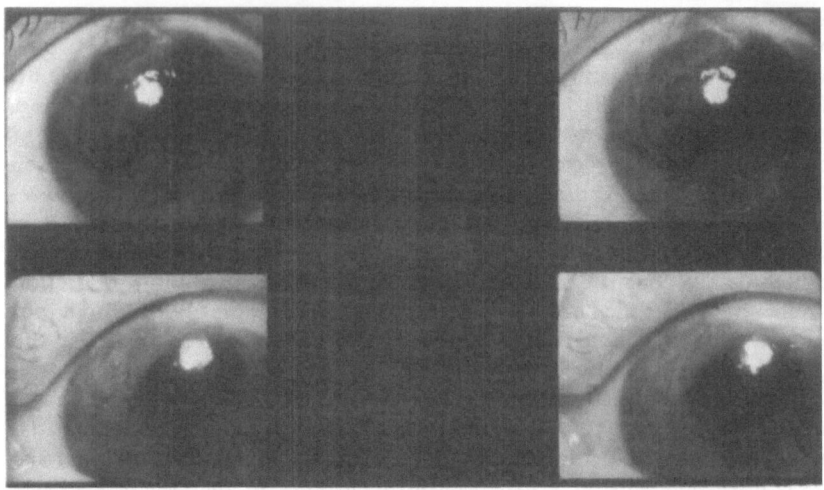

Fig. 3. Stereophotographs (top) of a cyst which developed after cataract extraction. It filled the superior part of the anterior chamber and split the iris down to the 7 o'clock position. Appearance (bottom) seven days after injection with 20 percent trichloroacetic acid. There had been no recurrence 7 years later.

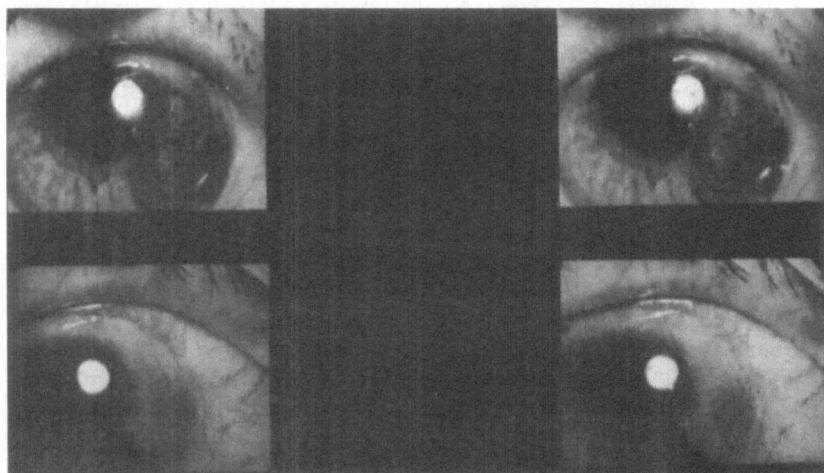

Fig. 4. Stereophotographs (top) of a large iris cyst which followed extracapsular cataract extraction. During the first injection the cyst wall was punctured accidentally and the trichloracetic acid solution had to be withdrawn before complete coagulation occurred. Despite the escape of some trichloroacetic acid into the aqueous, there was minimal postoperative reaction 6 days later (bottom). When the cyst partially recurred it was reinjected and completely coagulated. Thirty-four months later there had been no recurrence.

368

large congenital cyst required two injections five weeks apart. The only adult who required more than one injection and aspiration had had an extracapsular cataract extraction two years before referral to the University of Oregon Health Sciences Center. She did not return to the surgeon until she had developed pain and blurred vision in the eye due to a large cyst in the peripheral anterior chamber from 11 to 4 o'clock on the temporal side of her left eye. (Fig. 4 top). The cyst wall was accidentally perforated by the tip of the needle, as was evidenced by appearance of a tiny white cloud of coagulated protein in the aqueous at one edge of the cyst. The needle was withdrawn immediately rather than risk introducing additional acid into the anterior chamber. Minimal inflammatory followed this accident but the cyst was incompletely coagulated (Fig. 4 bottom). The cyst gradually reformed in the iris. Eleven months after the initial injection the procedure was repeated through the same injection site with complete collapse of the cyst. There has been no recurrence of the cyst.

DISCUSSION

It is beyond the scope of this paper to review the extensive literature on the subject of epithelial cysts in the anterior chamber, to discuss their prevention, or to make comparative evaluations of the many ingenious methods of their treatment; rather, it has been my purpose to document with serial photographs the effectiveness of treating these cysts by aspiration injection with trichloracetic acid and one re-aspiration to collapse the cyst.

It is a relatively simple procedure with surprisingly little postoperative inflammatory reaction if performed with great care to be certain that the injection is limited to the interior of the cyst. There were no complications in any of the seven eyes injected with the acid, but there is no doubt that the acid would be highly destructive if any significant amount were to escape from the cyst into the aqueous. Csapody (1962) reported that a permanent opacity followed unintentional intracorneal injection. All of the injections which I made were at sites where the cyst was in contact with the corneal or limbal stroma, so that the injected solution would be confined to the cyst. No attempts have been made by our staff to inject isolated cysts of the iris or cysts in eyes with a clear lens. Five of the seven treated eyes were aphakic. Both the child with congenital cyst and the child with the perforating injury already had partially cataractous lenses.

The optimal concentration of trichloroacetic acid for injection has not yet been established. Despite the wide spread use of trichloroacetic acid in many fields of medicine, especially in dermatology, there is a paucity of information about its tissue effects. Such studies have been initiated in our laboratories.

Finally, it should be noted that an epithelial cyst can be dormant for years and then begin to enlarge. It is, therefore, possible that recurrences of the cyst still may occur in some of the above described cases which have been observed from two to seven years.

REFERENCES

Csapody, J. Chemical obliteration of a large iris cyst. *Klin. Mbl. Augenheilk.* 139: *674-6*, (1962).

Hogan, M. & Goodner, E. Surgical treatment of epithelial cysts of the anterior chamber. *Archs. Ophthal.* 64: *286-291*, 1960.

Kirby, D. Surgery of Cataract, J.B. Lippincott. Philadelphia. p. *545* 1950.

Lindner, K. Treatment of iris cysts. *Z. Augenheilk. 93-96*, (1937).

Swan, K., Emmens, T. & Christensen, L. Tumors of the limbus. *Trans. Am. Acad. Ophthal. and oto-lar.* 52: *458*, 1948.

Author's address:
University of Oregon
Health Sciences Center
3181 S.W. Sam Jackson Park Road
Portland, Oregon 97201 U.S.A.